Type 1 Diabetes in 2023 - From Real Practice to Open Questions

Edited by Rudolf Chlup

Published in London, United Kingdom

Type 1 Diabetes in 2023 - From Real Practice to Open Questions
http://dx.doi.org/10.5772/intechopen.100991
Edited by Rudolf Chlup

Contributors
Nithyakalyani Mohan, Anusha Sunder, Sharad Purohit, Tiffanie Leeman, Katherine P. Richardson, Paul M.H. Tran, Om Prakash Sah, Anna Vladimirovna Lugovaya, Vladimir Phylippovich Mitreikin, Natalia Mikhailovna Kalinina, Rudolf Chlup, Josef Bartek, Ondřej Krystyník, Petr Mlčák, Jana Zapletalová, Edna S. Majaliwa, Emmanuel Ameyaw, Janet Bulemela, Asmahan T. Abdalla, Irina Buckle, Josephine M. Forbes, Gordon Ogweno, Edwin Murungi, Noemi Nováková, Martin Nezval, Marie Anna Robenková

First published in London, United Kingdom, 2023 by IntechOpen
IntechOpen is the global imprint of INTECHOPEN LIMITED, registered in England and Wales, registration number: 11086078, 5 Princes Gate Court, London, SW7 2QJ, United Kingdom

British Library Cataloguing-in-Publication Data
A catalogue record for this book is available from the British Library

Additional hard and PDF copies can be obtained from orders@intechopen.com

Type 1 Diabetes in 2023 - From Real Practice to Open Questions
Edited by Rudolf Chlup
p. cm.
Print ISBN 978-1-80356-395-4
Online ISBN 978-1-80356-396-1
eBook (PDF) ISBN 978-1-80356-397-8

For EU product safety concerns:
IN TECH d.o.o., Prolaz Marije Krucifikse Kozulić 3, 51000 Rijeka, Croatia,
info@intechopen.com or visit our website at intechopen.com.

Meet the editor

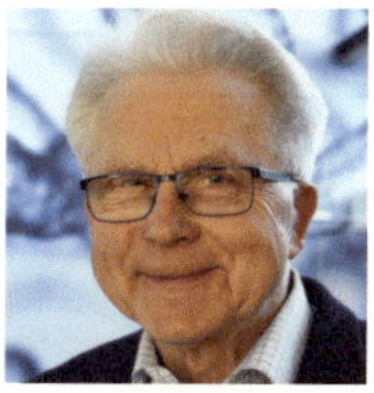

Rudolf Chlup graduated from Palacký University Olomouc, Czechia, and attended postgraduate courses in Prague, Karlsburg, Edinburgh, London, Bucharest, Moscow, Sophia, Düsseldorf, and San Francisco. He is a consultant for internal medicine and diabetology at the Teaching Hospital Olomouc. He became Dr. med. habil. at the University of Greifswald in 1993 and since 2020 he has been a Professor of Medicine at Palacký University Olomouc. His research interests include diabetes management comprising diet, exercise, education, and technology. He became a member of the Czech, German, European, and American Diabetes Associations and the executive committee of the Diabetes Education Study Group of the European Association for the Study of Diabetes (DESG/EASD). In 2015, Dr. Chlup received the "Rudolf Korec Award" from the Slovakian Diabetes Association.

Contents

Preface

This book provides a comprehensive overview of type 1 diabetes, ranging from its bleak history to contemporary practices and targets for the future. It includes nine chapters organized into two sections. The first section includes five chapters that address the management of type 1 diabetes. The second section includes four chapters that examine the etiopathogenesis of diabetes. Written by specialists in diabetes from around the world, including Africa, America, Asia, Australia, and Europe, chapters include figures and tables to illustrate important concepts. With its comprehensive coverage of the state of the art in diabetes, this volume is a useful resource for family physicians, diabetologists, educators, nurses, students, and other interested readers.

I would like to thank the staff at IntechOpen, especially Author Service Managers Ms. Silvia Sabo and Ms. Sara Debeuc, for their assistance throughout the publication process.

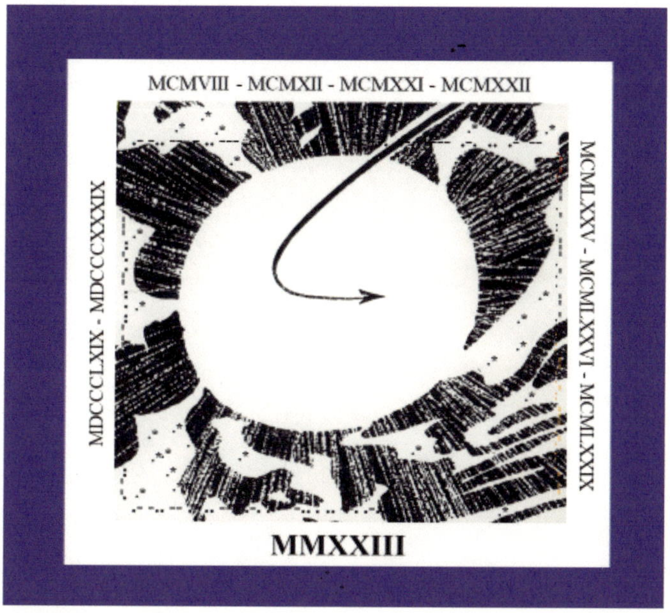

Mission: from recent history to dawning future (Years of milestones in diabetes management). Roman numerals at figure margins serve as reminders of important dates related to pancreas function [1, 2], insulin discovery [3–6], technology for insulin substitution [7], therapeutic exercise [8], and risk of atherosclerosis [9], which created a base for topics presented in chapters of this book [10].

Rudolf Chlup
2nd Department of Medicine,
Gastroenterology and Geriatrics,
Teaching Hospital Olomouc,
Olomouc, Czech Republic

Faculty of Medicine and Dentistry,
Department of Physiology,
Palacký University Olomouc,
Olomouc, Czech Republic

References

[1] Langerhans P. Beiträge zur mikroscopischen Anatomie der Bauchspeicheldrüse. (Contributions to microscopic anatomy of Pancreas. German.) Wilhelms-Friedrich Wilhelm Universität zu Berlin, printed by G. Lange; 1869

[2] Mering J, Minkowski O. Diabetes mellitus nach Pankreas extirpation. (Diabetes mellitus following the pancreatectomy. German.). Zbl Klin Med. 1889;**10**:393-394

[3] Zülzer G. Über Versuche einer spezifischen Ferment Therapie des Diabetes. (On experiments with a special enzymtherapy in diabetes. German.) Zeitschrift f exp Pathologie u Therapie. 1908;**5**:307-318

[4] Scott EL. On the influence of intravenous injections of an extract of the pancreas on experimental pancreatic diabetes. American Journal of Physics. 1912;**9**:306-310

[5] Paulescu NC. Action de l'éxtrait pancréatique injecté dans le sang chez un animal diabétique. (Effects of an injection of the pancreatic extract to blood stream in an animal with diabetes. French.) Comptes rendus des séances de la Société de biologie. 1921;**85**(27):556-559

[6] Banting FG, Best CH. Pancreatic extracts. Journal of Laboratory and Clinical Medicine. May 1922;7(8):3-11

[7] Pickup JC, Keen H, Parsons JS, et al. Continuous subcutaneous insulin infusion: an approach to achieving normoglycaemia. British Medical Journal. 1978;**282**:347-350

[8] Koivisto VA, Shervin RS. Exercise in diabetes. Therapeutic implications. Postgraduate Medicine 1979;66:87

[9] Stout RW. Diabetes and atherosclerosis – the role of insulin. Diabetologie 1979;16: 14110

[10] Type 1 Diabetes 2023 – From Real Practice to Open Questions. London, UK: IntechOpen; 2023

Section 1

Real Clinical Practice

Chapter 1

Intensive Management of Type 1 Diabetes in Adults: One Centre Experience 1970–2022

Rudolf Chlup, Ondřej Krystyník, Petr Mlčák, Jana Zapletalová and Josef Bartek

Abstract

This chapter deals with clinical trials and routine management of persons with type 1 diabetes (PWD1) carried out at the Teaching Hospital and Palacký University Olomouc since 1970 in cooperation with experts from other centres. The following outcomes are presented: (1) physical training resulted in (a) enhancement of physical working capacity; (b) increased insulin effectiveness (c) increased S-HDL cholesterol; (d) improvement of neuropathy, memory, attention and general condition of PWD1. (2) Intensive basal and prandial insulin substitution with only short-acting insulin given seven times a day and night appeared to be the most effective approach to the conventional insulin substitution; group education and pens motivated to the intensification of insulin therapy. (3) Continuous subcutaneous insulin infusion, conventional self-monitoring, continuous/flush glucose monitoring and prolongation of time in range opened new horizons. Intensive education, early application of hybrid insulin pumps and specialised prevention of late diabetes complications are deemed to improve the life expectancy and quality. Cooperation with insurance companies should be acknowledged.

Keywords: insulin, glucose monitoring, insulin pen, insulin pump, diabetes education, life style, food, muscular exercise

1. Introduction

Type 1 diabetes (T1D) is a chronic syndrome of disturbed metabolism of saccharides, proteins and fat. This syndrome is characterised by the destruction of insulin-producing B-cells of the pancreas which is mostly (in 80%) due to a lasting influence of autoantibodies of uncertain origin. Multiple factors could simultaneously explain the increasing T1D incidence [1]. Impact of HLA phenotype and previous contact with viral antigens should be mentioned [2, 3].

Clinical signs and symptoms of insulin deficiency comprise abundant passing of water, thirst, loss of body mass (up to several kilograms per week), hunger, overeating, weakness, loss of appetite and finally nausea, vomiting, dehydration, breathlessness, abdominal pain, disturbed consciousness, coma and death. These signs are accompanied by fasting hyperglycaemia ≥ 7 mmol/l and high or low plasma concentrations of minerals and lactate; acidosis, uraemia and infections may also be present [4, 5]. The only possibility how to interrupt this deleterious chain is to recover the homeostasis with adequate amounts of fluids, the substitution of missing insulin combatting the acidosis.

The exciting milestones of the insulin era have already been described [6–12]. In the year 1922, the pharma industry started production of short-acting bovine/porcine insulin (Iletin, Eli Lilly, Indianapolis, USA). Long-acting Protamin Insulin was discovered by Hagedorn in 1934 [13]. In the year 1940, NPH (Neutral Protamin Hagedorn, Nordisk, Denmark) was discovered by Rosenberg and Krayenbühl in Hagedorn´s laboratories and published after the war in 1946 [11]. Human insulins have been produced since 1980. Short-acting insulin analogues lispro, aspart and glulisine have been used since 2000 [14], followed by long-acting analogues (glargine, detemir), ultralong analogue degludec and biosimilars. The pharmacokinetics of individual insulin preparations were studied [15]. Insulin concentrations were unified from 20 IU/ml or 40 IU/ml or 80 IU/ml to the mandatory concentration of 100 IU/ml. However, in disposable pens, there are some exceptions: glargine (Toujeo) 300 IU/ml, degludec (Tresiba) 200 IU/ml. Faster-acting insulin (FIASP) has been used since 2017 [16].

The evolution of technologies for insulin application enhanced the flexibility of insulin substitution which became more physiologic [17]. In the seventies, glass syringes were replaced by plastic disposable syringes. Continuous subcutaneous insulin substitution (CSII) using Mill Hill Infuser as a personal insulin pump was described in Guy´s Hospital London in 1978 [18]. Convenient pocket insulin syringes appeared in England before 1980. According to personal communication, Dr. Ireland in Glasgow, following an idea of Dr. Reith, invented an insulin pen injector produced then by Hypoguard ([17, 19], personal communication). Development of insulin pens (later they have received the name MADI) was supported by Palacký University Olomouc, Czech Republic. Their production started in 1983 (Meta Ostrava, Czech Republic) [20–22] . The NOVO Laboratories, Copenhagen, Denmark, started the production of Novopen [23, 24]. Their technical evolution continued up to the smart pens of today [25]. Haemoglobin A1c [26], Dextrostix and Glucometer-strips systems followed by continuous glucose monitoring (CGM) [27–31], flash glucose monitoring (FGM) [32] and by the assessment of time in range (TIR) [33] became prerequisites for effective metabolic control.

Primary insulin regimens were based on insulin boluses prescribed by a physician. These "mandatory" insulin doses resulted in diabetic diets with fixed amounts of nutrients. Then, limitations of muscular exercise were a measure for the prevention of hypoglycaemias [34]. In contradiction, a few specialists emphasised a liberalised approach to food consumption which was based on adaptations of frequent prandial boluses of regular insulin [35, 36]. The vital mission of insulin and the harmful angiopathic consequences of hyperinsulinaemia and hyperglycaemia [37–41] should be considered. Potential risks of hypoglycaemia are always worthy of attention [42].

In healthy people, the insulin production was found to be mostly 30–40 IU per 24 h [43]. So, the daily amount of injected insulin needs to be "as high as necessary and simultaneously as low as possible" [44]. This paradigm became the leading idea of our therapeutic strategy.

Active individual and/or group therapeutic education was suggested in Genf and Düsseldorf [45, 46]. A series of teaching letters was issued by the Diabetes Education Study Group of the European Association for the Study of Diabetes (DESG/EASD). Scheduled educational programmes of various structures were applied in diabetes centres all over the world [47–54].

This chapter is focused on selected clinical trials and routine management of people with type 1 diabetes (PWD1) carried out since the year 1970 at the Teaching Hospital and Palacký University Olomouc [55, 56], mostly in cooperation with experts from diabetes centres in the Czech and Slovak Republics [57], Institute of Diabetes G. Katsch Karlsburg [58–76], Heinrich Heine Universität Düsseldorf [77], Royal Infirmary Edinburgh [62] and St. Thomas Hospital London [62, 78].

The targets of the presented topics and single-centre "real world trials" have been to encourage physicians and health care professionals to implement flexible insulin substitution along with adequate exercise into routine management of PWD1. Sensor-augmented CSII and/or recent insulin analogues are going to be the core of this intention.

2. Influence of dynamic physical training on metabolic, hormonal and clinical parameters in adolescents and men with Type 1 diabetes mellitus (1978 to 1982)

A prospective single-centre study with 19 PWD1 males (age 15–35 years, diabetes duration from 2 months to 20 years (mean 6,8 years) improved insights on the effects of physical training [62]. The study protocol was based on several previous studies [79–88] At the beginning of the training period, proband was admitted to the hospital for one week. His Physical Working Capacity (PWC 170) was investigated using the bicycle ergometer Zimmermann [89]. At the end of the following outdoor training period (duration 157 ± 43 days), the second and third tests were performed whereas a one-week quiet break between them without any exercise was included into the study schedule (**Figure 1**). Each test was performed one hour after breakfast in the morning. PWC 170 and other parameters at the first, second and third tests were compared (**Figures 2** and **3**).

Here are the effects of the 5–6-month dynamic training (athletics, cycling and swimming) in PWD1:

1. Increase of PWC 170. PWC 170 is the submaximal ergometer load resulting in a heart rate of 170 beats/min which is reached at the 4th step. This load was calculated using linear extrapolation of heart rates at previous steps. Each step lasted 10 min (In future studies maximum oxygen capacity VO2 max. has been used instead of PWC 170).

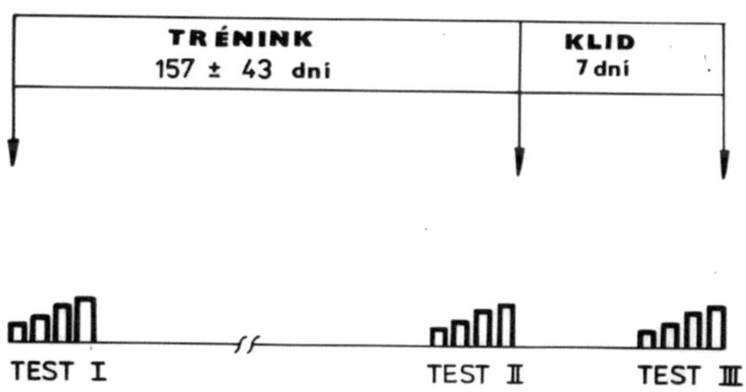

Figure 1.
Design of the training and quiet (klid) period with three ergometer tests.

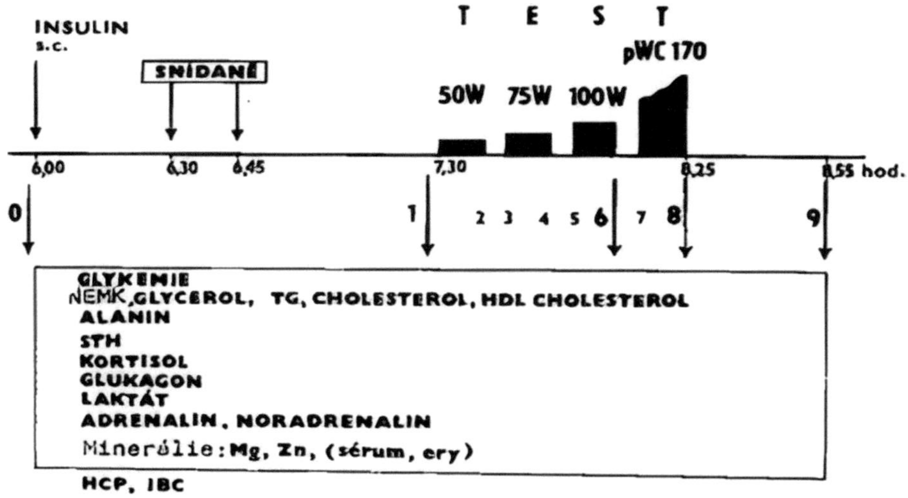

Figure 2.
Schedule of PWC 170 ergometer step test [89] and respective investigations.

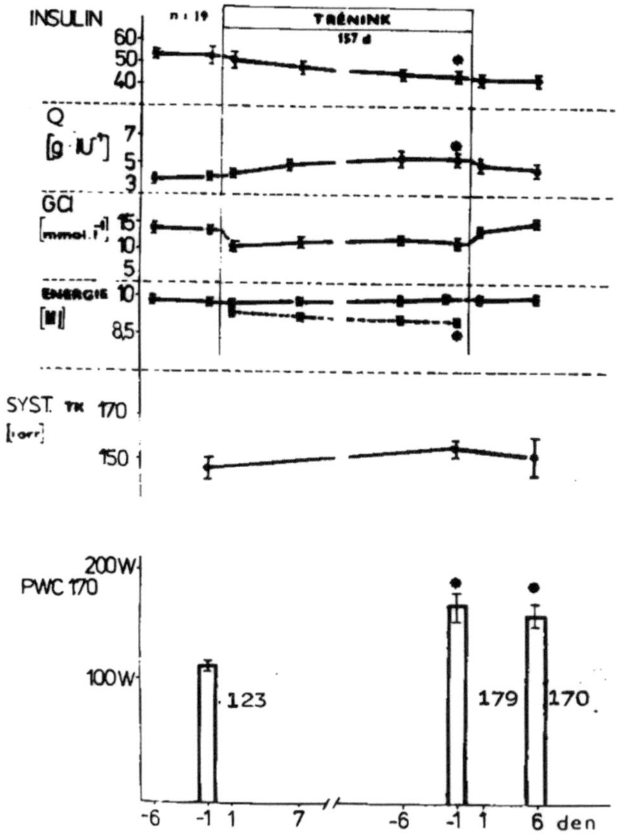

Figure 3.
Amount of injected insulin [IU/d], quotient Q [g Carb/IU] (saccharide relation), Michaelis glycaemic control index GCI [90] estimated energy expenditure [MJ/d], systolic blood pressure (syst TK) at the 3rd step (100 W) of ergometer test and PWC 170 [W] over the study n = 19.

DOI: http://dx.doi.org/10.5772/intechopen.108032

2. An improvement of saccharide (carbohydrate) metabolism was demonstrated by increased insulin effectiveness (quotient Q) without any change in blood glucose control. Quotient Q describes how many grams of consumed carbohydrates are metabolised due to 1 IU of injected insulin. An approximate relation between insulin effectiveness Q and physical working capacity PWC 170 can be calculated using a new formula derived from our observations:

$$Q\ [\text{g Carb./IU}] = 0{,}03\ \text{PWC 170}\ [\text{W}] - 0{,}5, \tag{1}$$

(where PWC 170 reached values 90 W <PWC 170 <295 W).

The increase of PWC 170 depends on the amount of estimated energy expended for the submaximal training. Following training interruption (as it may happen e.g. after admission to the hospital) the insulin effectiveness drops in relation to the decrease of PWC 170 due to reduced physical exercise (**Figure 3**).

The insulin effectiveness Q in this study reached values ranging from 2.5 to 22.4 g Carb./IU. Its evolution appears to be related to the value of the physical working capacity PWC 170 (**Figure 4**).

No influence of training either on venous blood glucose concentration (vBG) at the beginning of ergometer test or on the speed of vBG reduction in the course of tests I, II and III was shown. The reduction of vBG became significant ($p < 0{,}05$) as soon as at the end of step 2 (75 W) (**Figure 5**).

An improvement of lipoprotein metabolism was recognised by an increase in HDL cholesterol concentration (1.19 ± 0.08 vs 1.86 ± 0.22 mmol/l, $p < 0.05$) (**Figure 6**) and by a decrease in the index of total cholesterol/HDL cholesterol. These significant changes could also be found 7 days after the end of the training [58].

A beneficial influence on some signs of neuropathy [59], on memory, attention and on the general condition of diabetic patients could also be demonstrated [60].

The important results of our study are comprised in the Abstract book (**Figure 7**).

Hence, based on this study, a submaximal dynamic physical training may be recommended as an additive treatment of type 1 diabetic patients with no signs of

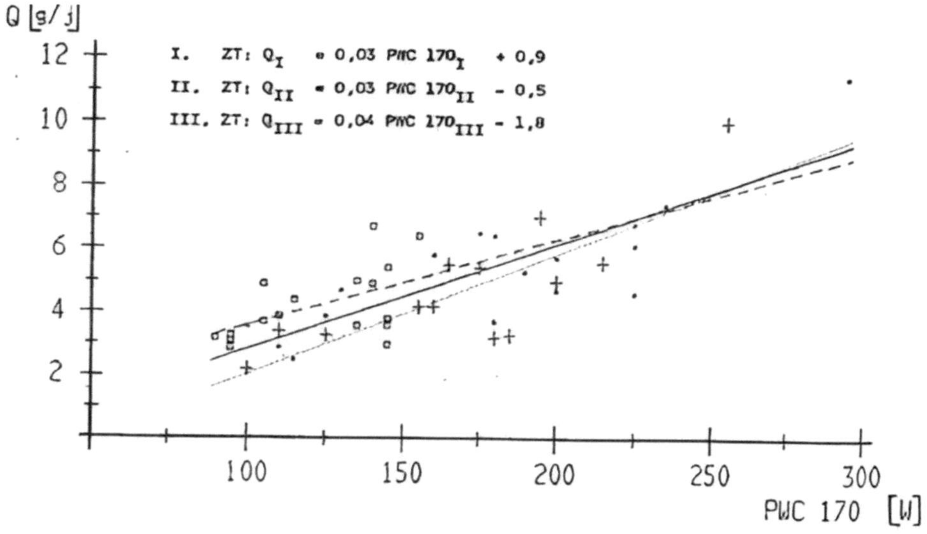

Figure 4.
Relation of insulin effectiveness Q_I, Q_{II}, Q_{III} and respective PWC 170.

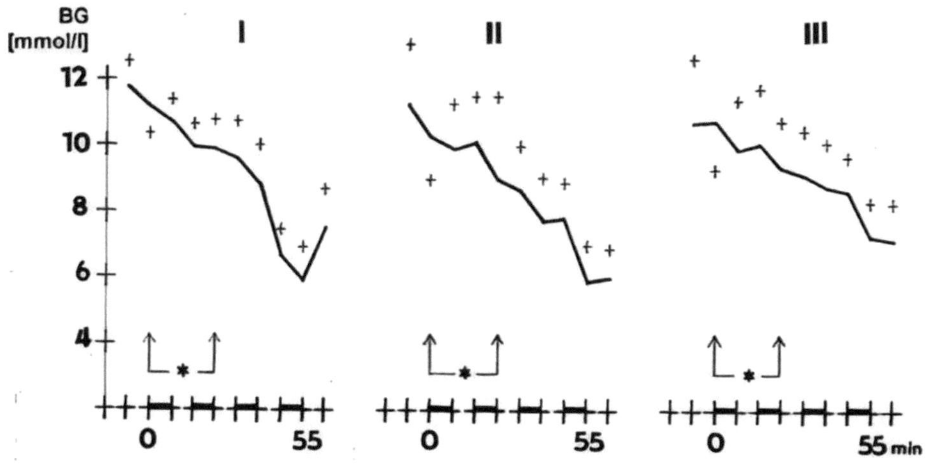

Figure 5.
Development of vBG in the course of the bicycle ergometer test I (before training), II (end of training) and III (after 6 days of quiet) n = 19.

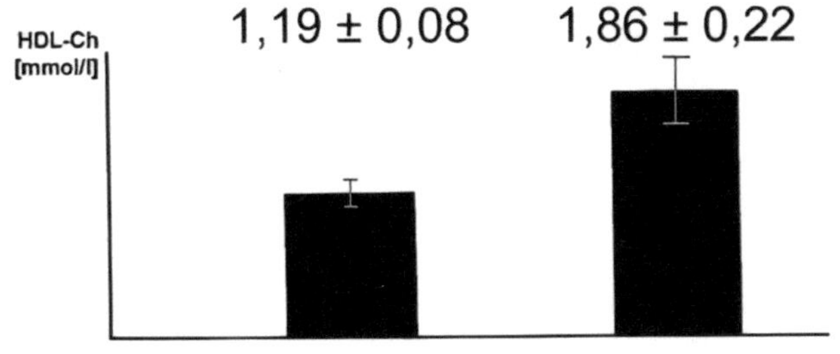

Figure 6.
Increase of serum HDL cholesterol concentration between the start and end of the 6-month training (n = 19).

catabolism. At the beginning, the insulin should be reduced or the amount of carbohydrates in food increased along with the change of insulin effectiveness. Even in patients with high physical working capacity, it is not possible to replace insulin by physical exercise. Following the training cessation, the amount of injected insulin should be increased or the amount of carbohydrates in food reduced along with the decrease of insulin effectiveness.

3. Randomised cross-over clinical trial on metabolic effectiveness and feasibility of three intensive insulin regimens with particular consideration of night period in PWD 1 (Institute of Diabetes Karlsburg, Germany, 1989–1990)

Subjects: A group of 36 T1D (males, age 18 to 50 years, duration of diabetes at least 3 years, C-peptide 0,037 ± 0,013 nmol/l, BMI 23,6 ± 0,5 kg/m^2, PWC 170 172,5 ± 6,8 W, retinopathy 1st grade in 7 and 2nd grade in 7 of them, traces of proteinuria in 11 of them, proteinuria > 2 g/d in one of them) completed the study.

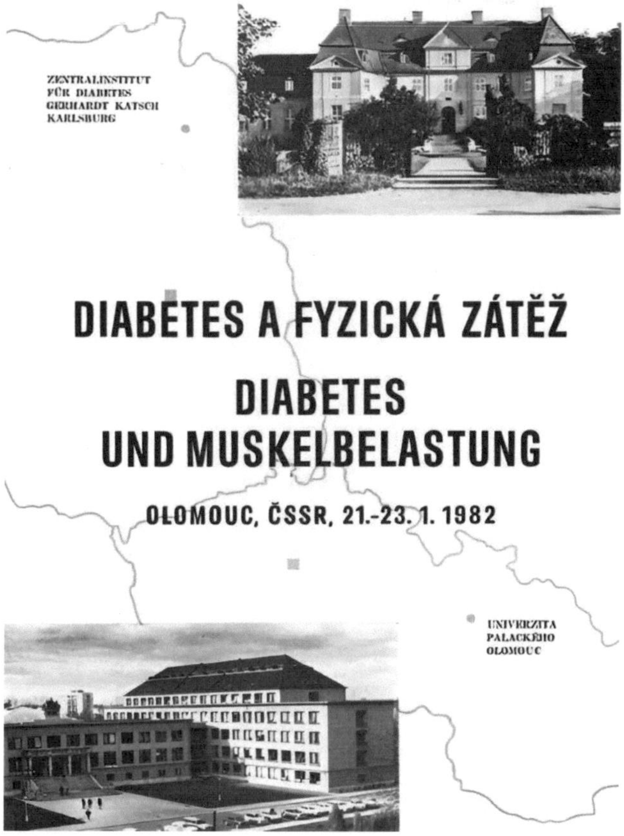

Figure 7.
Abstract book Symposium on Diabetes and exercise, 21.-23.1.1982, Olomouc, Czechoslovakia, organised by Palacký University Olomouc and Central Institute of Diabetes G. Katsch Karlsburg; Olomouc, 1982 p 102 [63, 91–96].

Study design: The suggested protocol considered our previous experience and outcomes of other studies on dawn phenomena and pharmacokinetics of various insulin preparations [97–105]. After admission, each of the three insulin regimens A, B, and C (**Tables 1** and **2**) was randomly tested over two weeks and then replaced by another one. At discharge (6 weeks after admission) the tested person could choose the preferred regimen for the 8-week treatment period at home/at work. Final in-patient examination targeted to the complex assessment of respective clinical and laboratory parameters.

Results: The basal and prandial insulin substitution with only purified porcine shortacting insulin (SNC, Berlin Chemie) given seven times a day (regimen A) was the most effective kind of the conventional insulin therapy as assessed by the mean cBG (MBG 16) of 16-point BG profiles at the end of the respective test period (**Figure 8**).

The regimen A led to the best metabolic control in 21/36 (58%) of patients (**Figures 9** and **10**).

The insulin regimen B with one animal intermediate insulin preparation (BS, Berlin Chemie) at 10 p.m. or the regimen C with a long-acting insulin (Ultratard HM, NovoNordisk) at 5.30 p.m. led to the best control in 6/36 (17 %) or in 9/36 (25%) of all patients, respectively.

Randomisation	**Hospital**			**At home**	**Hospital**
Each PWD was randomized to 1 of 6 subgroups	12 d	14 d	14 d	8 weeks	3 days
	A	B	C	Individually selected insulin regimen A or B or C	
	A	C	B		
	B	A	C		
	B	C	A		
	C	A	B		
	C	B	A		
Diet				Free adopted diet	
BG-profiles					
FIRI-profil					
Fruktosamin					
Lipoproteins					
C-peptid, IBC					
STH					
Psychology					
PWC 170					
HbA_1					
U-glucose, U-aceton					
Selfmonitoring			Strips for capillary blood measurements		

Table 1
Schedule of PWD randomisation into six groups with different sequences of insulin regimens; hospital and home study periods; clinical and laboratory check-ups.

Time	**6,30**	**9,00**	**11,30**	**15,00**	**17,30**	**22,00**	**2,30**
Regimen A	R	R	R	R	R	R	R
Regimen B	R	R	R	R	R	B intermediate	
Regimen C	R	R	R	R	R + Ultratard		

Table 2.
Tested insulin regimens: A (regular insulin R only), B (R in the course of day plus intermediate insulin at 10 p.m.), C (R in the course of day combined with Ultratard insulin at 5.30 p.m.).

Even though the capillary FIRI concentrations (which were investigated parallel with cBG) were significantly higher than in healthy men (**Figure 11**), the cBG values in the best PWD when compared to a group of 9 healthy men remain significantly higher.

In addition, in the last two regimens (B and C), the total daily insulin dose was higher than in regimen A. On the other hand, the fasting BG concentrations were in regimen A 60 of 72 BG measurements below 10 mmol/l. In regimen B, it was only in

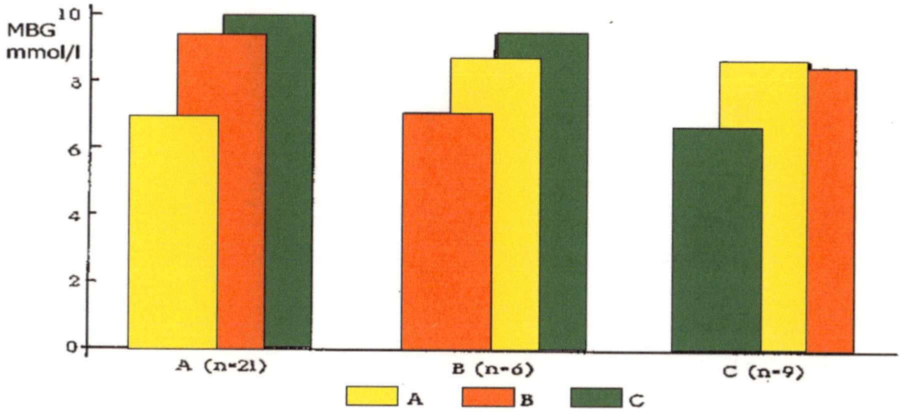

Figure 8.
MBG 16 in the group with the best regimen A (n=21)—left, in the group with the best regimen B (n = 6) —middle, and in the group with the best regimen C (n = 9)—right, in comparison with MBG 16 of other two regimens in the respective group.

14 of 72 measurements and in regimen C in 19 of 70 measurements (2 values were missing) (**Figure 12**).

The group education and an insulin pen motivated the diabetic patients to an intensification of insulin therapy including injections of insulin at 2.30 a.m. [73]. The feasibility (acceptance) of night injections (insulin regimen A) increased from 2/36 (6 %) at the beginning to 15/36 (42 %) at the end of the study. On the contrary, the optimistic patients´ hopes expecting the best effects from the long-acting insulin preparation Ultratard declined from 26/36 (72 %) on recruitment to 12/36 (33 %) on the final assessment at the end (**Figure 13**).

Neither the intensive insulin treatment enabled a long-lasting normalisation of B-glucose and B-FIRI concentrations.

A significant impact of regimen A on MBG 16 was only seen in a subgroup of 19 PWD who on discharge preferred regimen A for their future treatment.

No metabolic differences were seen when using the MADI 7/2ml needle pen (**Figure 14**) or catheter pen [78, 106]. The needle pen was preferred in 54 % of all patient days.

4. Continuous subcutaneous insulin infusion (CSII)

Since the year 1978 CSII by means of an external insulin pump became the best near-physiological way of insulin substitution [18, 107–115].

CSII supported by intensive self-monitoring mostly resulted in improved metabolic control as well as in increased satisfaction and quality of life in thousands of PWD1.

In our diabetes centre the first pump (Promedos E 1, Siemens, Germany) was introduced in December 1981 (**Figure 15**) [115]. From 2003 to 2012, DAHEDI Elektronics (**Figure 16**), H tron (**Figure 17**), Minimed (**Figure 18**) and Animas IR 1000, 1200 and 2020 (**Figure 19**) were inserted and regularly upgraded beyond the date of their 4-year expiry period. There were two pumps produced in Czechoslovakia: Insulin Injektor Kovo Brno developed by Hirš, Institute of Physiology, Academy

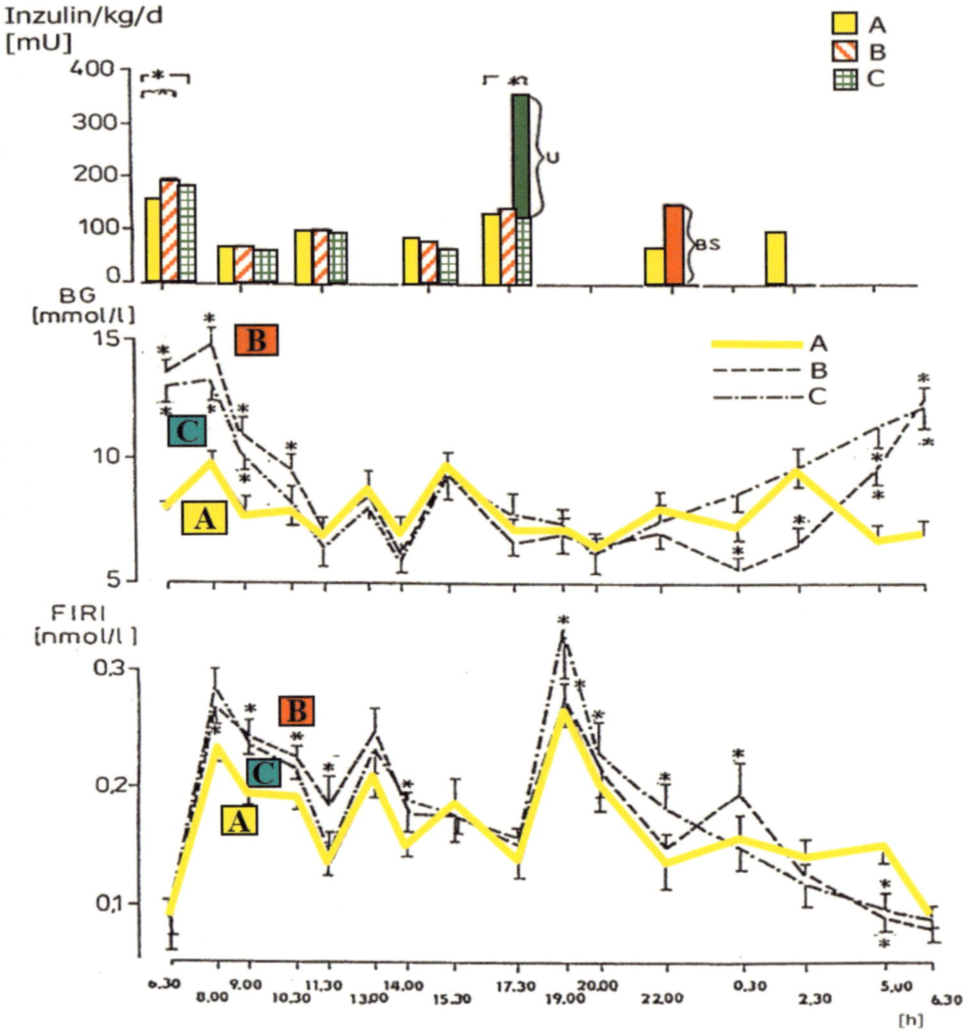

Figure 9.
*Comparison of insulin doses, 16-point cBG profiles and 16-point free immunoreactive insulin (FIRI) profiles at the end of respective insulin regimen period. See **Figures 9** and **10** for further details.*

of Sciences, Prague (**Figure 20**) [108–112] and programmable pump DI2 PC, developed by Vojtek, MEDIPO Brno. Thirty prototypes of this pump were produced, seven of them successfully tested in 1991–1993 in Olomouc (**Figure 21**) [53].

Paradigm 712, 722, 522, VEO 754 and 554 enabled the "low glucose suspend" if connected to CGM (**Figure 22**).

4.1 Single centre pilot study on metabolic effectiveness of CSII in PWD1 (1993–1998)

Subjects: Thirteen PWD1 males and females were put on an insulin pump (Dahedi, H-Tron, Minimed) in the period of years 1993–1998 demonstrated that the continuous subcutaneous insulin infusion resulted as soon as in 72 days in a decrease of concentrations of HbA1c in blood (NGSP scale 9.3 ± 0.46 vs 7.6 ± 0.28 %, $p < 0.05$)

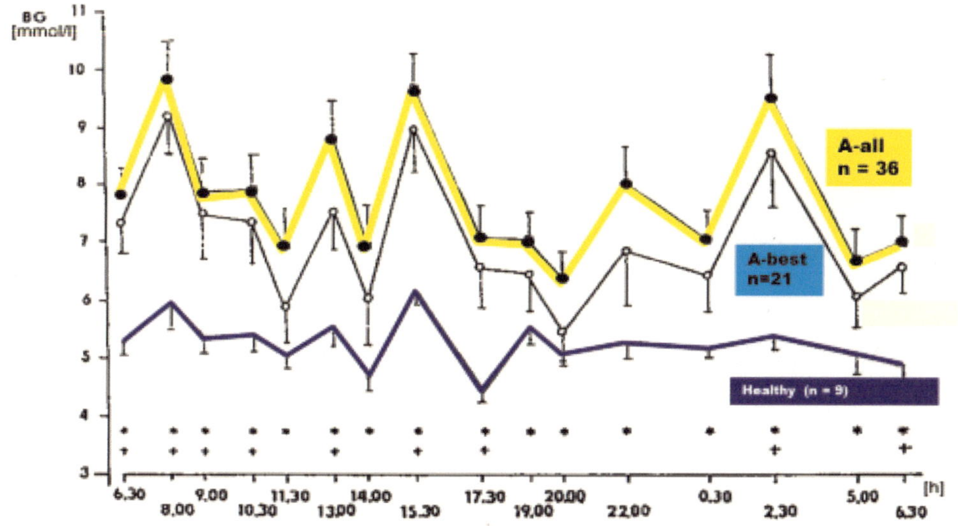

Figure 10.
*The 16-point cBG profiles at the end of insulin regimen A in 36 PWD (A) and in 21 of them who reached the best BG values with regimen A (A-best). cBG values in the group A-best remain significantly higher than in a control group of 9 healthy men. See also **Figure 11**.*

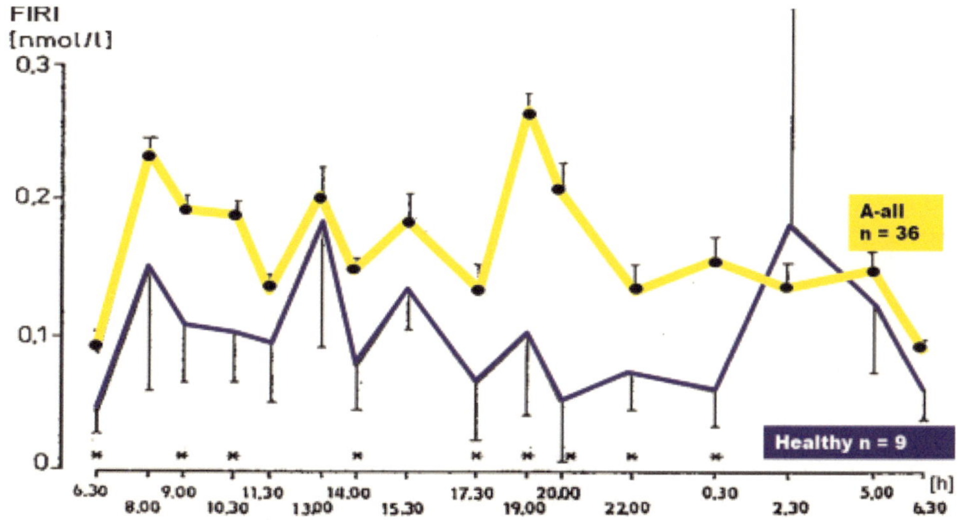

Figure 11.
*The 16-point FIRI profiles at the end of insulin regimen A in 36 men (A-all) and in a control group of 9 healthy men. * $p < 0.05$.*

(**Figure 23**), of total serum cholesterol (5.47 ± 0.29 vs 4.85 ± 0.19 mmol/l, $p < 0.05$) (**Figure 24**) and triacylglycerols (1.58 ± 0.24 vs 1.13 ± 0.15 mmol/l, $p < 0.05$). The total daily dose of insulin was reduced (47.8 ± 2.75 vs 41.3 ± 2.3 IU/d, $p < 0.05$) and the body mass did not change. An improved metabolic control was also found in a check-up 554 days later. There were no serious complications resulting from the usage of a pump.

In the third milenium, insulin pumps enable adaptation of basal rate up to 48 times per 24 h. Based on the biorhythm of insulin sensitivity and

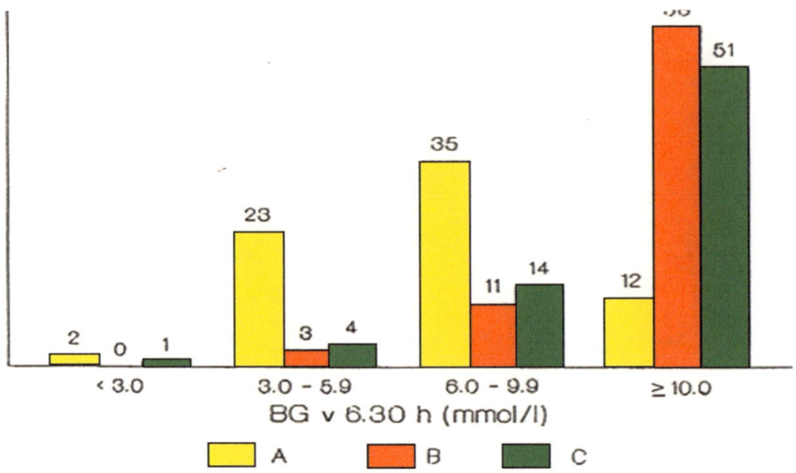

Figure 12.
Frequency of fasting cBG concentrations at BG profiles in the course of respective regimen.

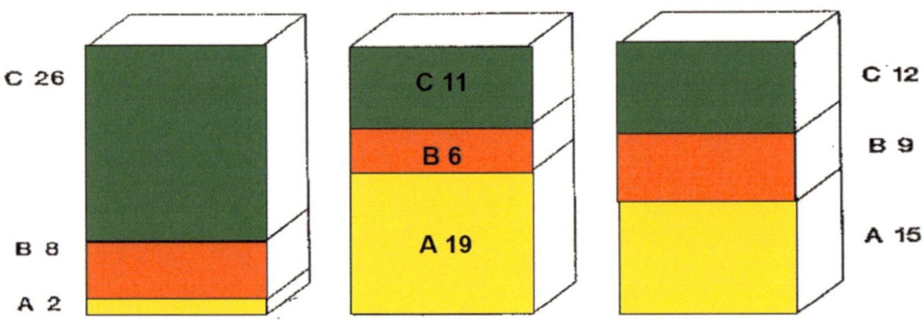

Figure 13.
Preference of regimens A, B, C at the beginning, at the end of the in-patient period and after 8-week home therapy with self-selected regimen.

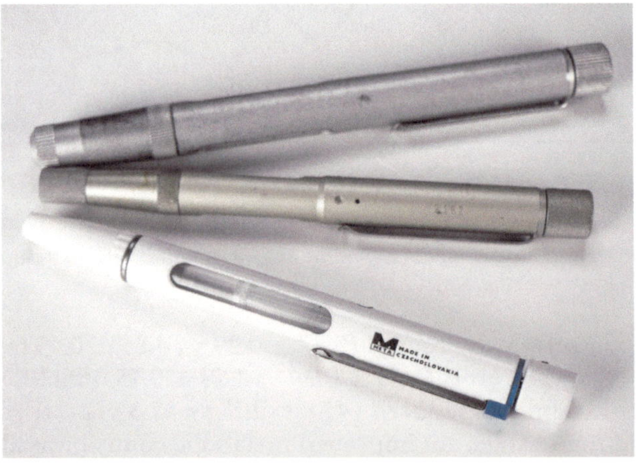

Figure 14.
First insulin pens MADI (MAnual Device for Insulin) developed at Palacký University Olomouc in 1983–1990 [20, 21, 78] MADI 5/5 ml (above), MADI 7/2 ml—used in this study (middle), MADI 8/3 ml (below). Photo V. Kupčík, www.diabetesmuseum.cz.

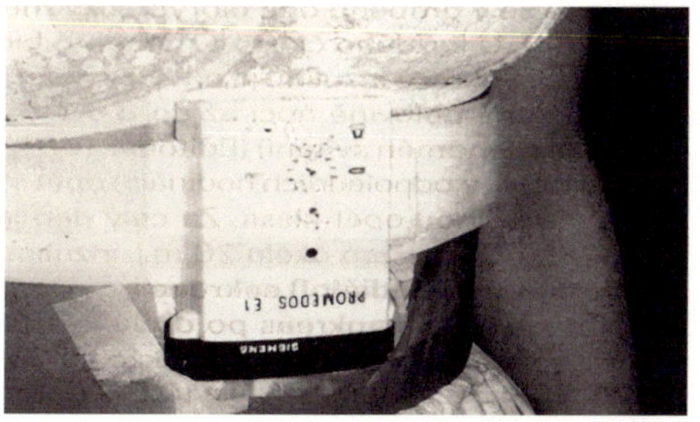

Figure 15.
Promedos E 1, Siemens, Germany [115].

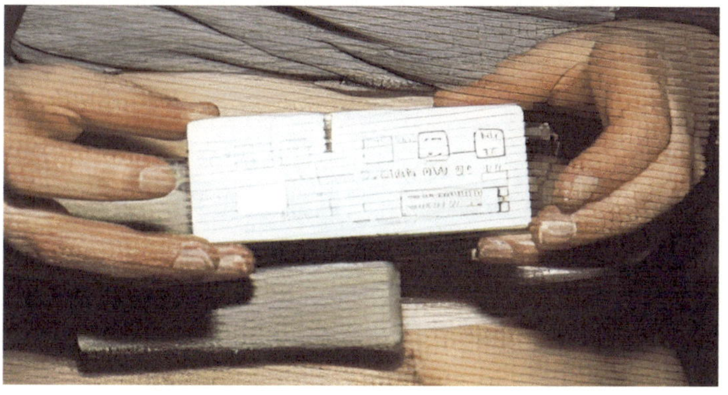

Figure 16.
Dahedi Elektroniks, Netherlands.

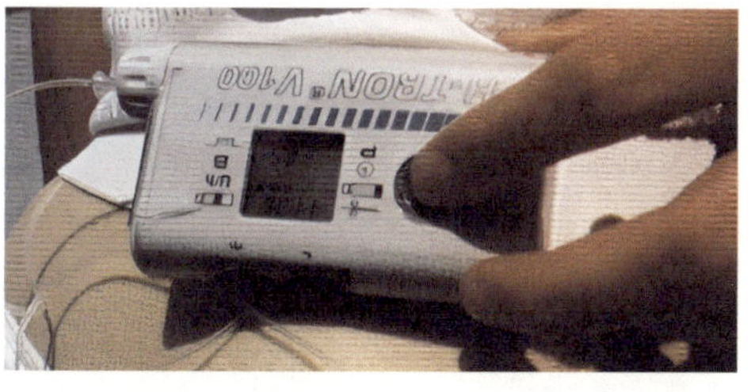

Figure 17.
H tron, Disetronic, Switzerland.

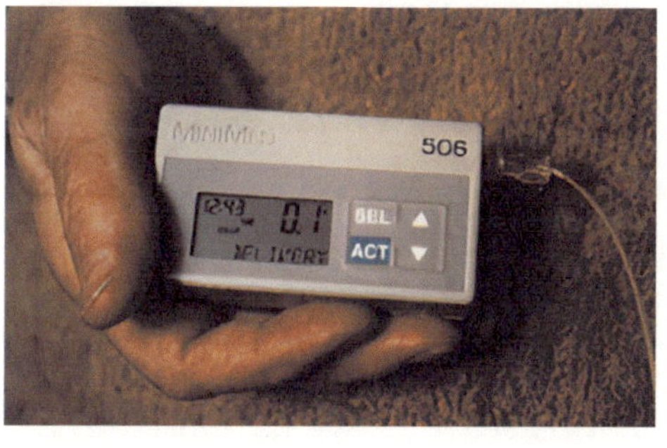

Figure 18.
Medtronic-Minimed 506, CA, USA.

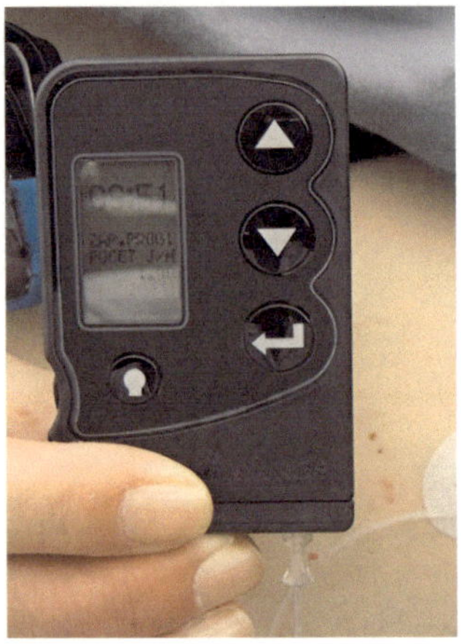

Figure 19.
Animas IR.

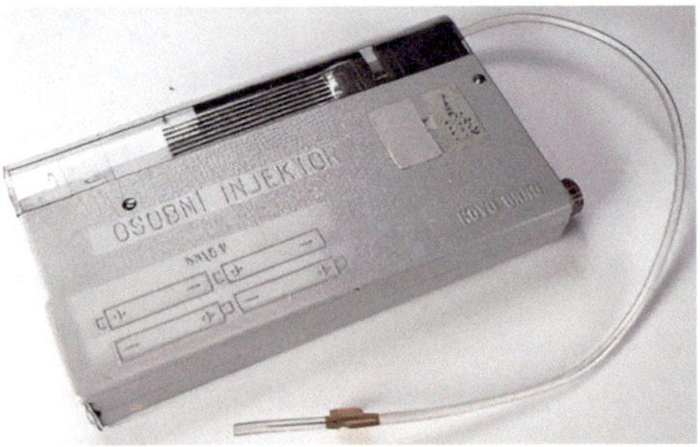

Figure 20.
Osobní Injektor, Institute of Physiology Prague, Kovo Brno, CR. Hundreds of pumps were widely used in Prague, Brno and Hradec Králové in the period of years 1984–1991 [108–112]. Photo V. Kupčík, www.diabetesmuseum.cz

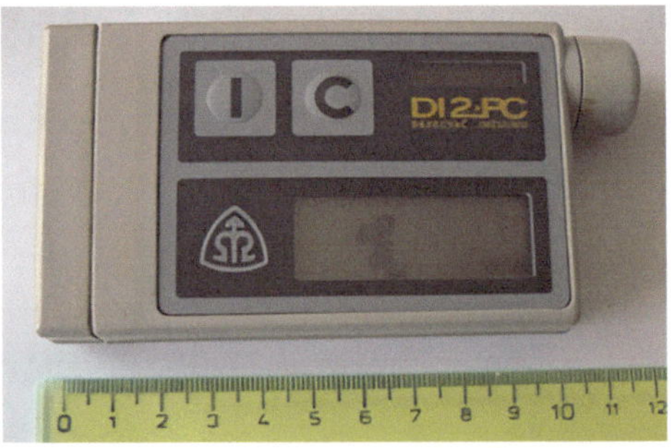

Figure 21.
DI2 PC, MEDIPO Brno, CR.

carbohydrate ratio and on our clinical experience with CGM-augmented CSII (**Figure 25**) [65, 98, 100, 103, 116], we have introduced a dynamic schedule of basal rates (**Figure 26**). This schedule we have used in PWD1 at the beginning of CSII therapy, to be adopted individually. Intensive conventional self-monitoring or CGM or FGM are prerequisites for an effective CSII.

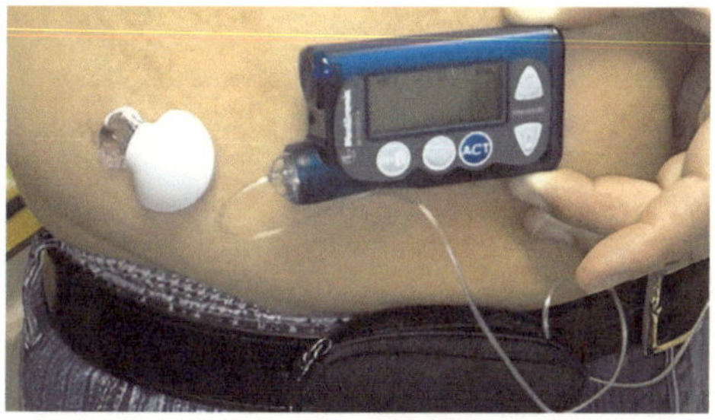

Figure 22.
Paradigm 722, Sensor and transmitter, Minimed-Medtronic, CA, USA. These sensor-augmented pumps [116] opened the door for the effective application of CGM or FGM in metabolic control and prevention of late complications in PWD1.

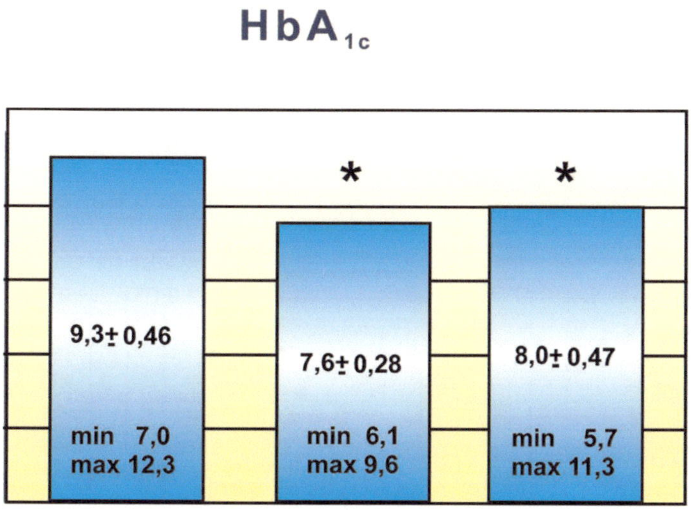

Figure 23.
HbA1c (NGSP %) at baseline, after 72 d and 554 d on CSII n = 13.

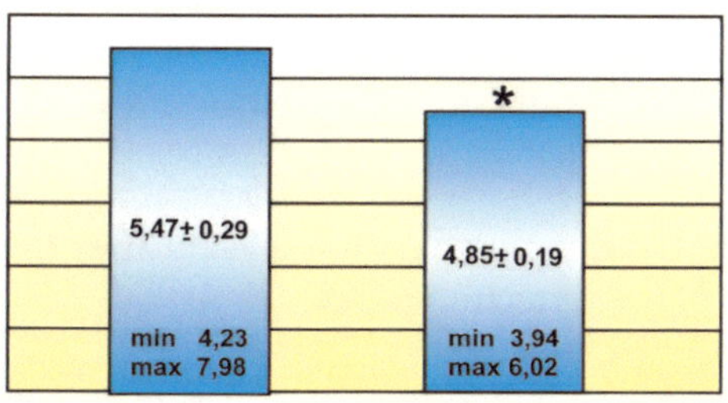

Figure 24.
Total cholesterol (mmol/l) at baseline and after 72 d on CSII n = 13.

4.2 Retrospective single centre study on feasibility of CSII in PWD1 and PWD2 (1981–2013)

In a period of 31 years we summarised our observations (**Figures 27** and **28**) [117]:

- a total of 185 PWDs (113 type 1, 72 type 2), aged 18–78 years, duration of diabetes from 0 to 56 years, were put on insulin pumps;

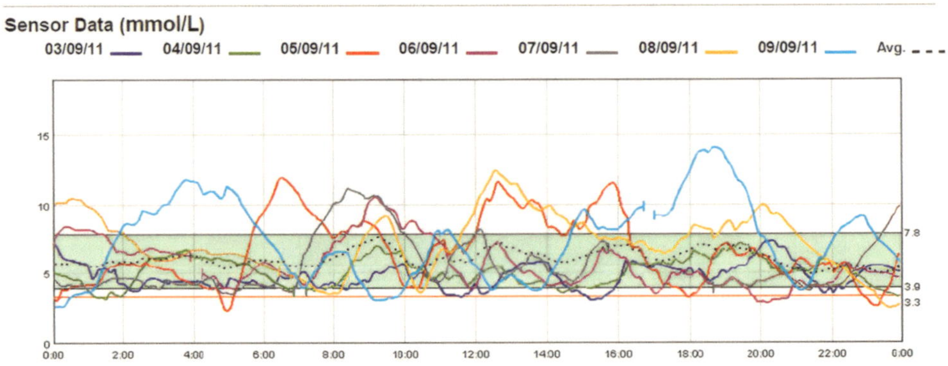

	Sat 3 Sep	Sun 4 Sep	Mon 5 Sep	Tue 6 Sep	Wed 7 Sep	Thu 8 Sep	Fri 9 Sep	Average / Total
# Sensor Values	288	284	288	285	254	285	285	1,969
High SG (mmol/L)	7.3	7.2	11.9	10.6	11.2	12.3	14.1	14.1
Low SG (mmol/L)	3.1	3.1	2.3	2.8	3.5	2.4	2.6	2.3
Average SG (mmol/L)	4.8	5.1	6.6	5.7	5.6	7.2	7.3	6.0
Standard Dev.	0.9	1.0	2.4	1.7	2.0	2.2	2.9	2.2
MAD %	19.5	8.9	25.1	3.6	1.5	9.8	5.5	13.4
# Valid Calibrations	4	3	3	3	2	2	3	20

Figure 25.
Continuous glucose monitoring (CGM) using a transcutaneous sensor in the course of 7 days. Each day has a different colour. Up to 288 sensor values per day.

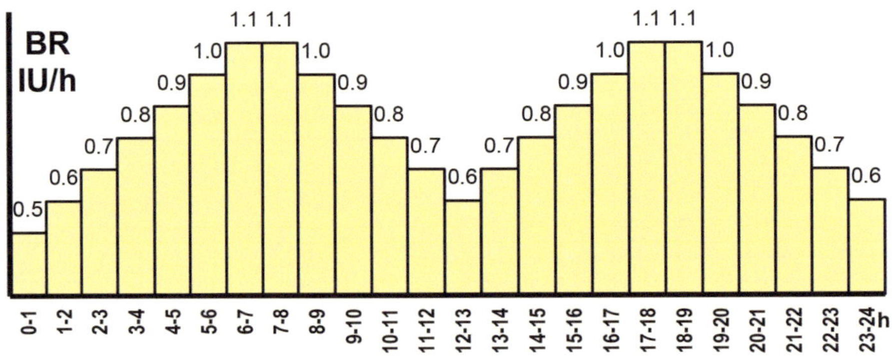

Figure 26.
CSII start: suggested distribution of basal rates over 24 h; to be individually adopted according to glycaemic profiles and clinical experience.

- six PWDs (3%) rejected the pump within 6 years after the commencement of use due to stress related to new technologies.
- seven PWDs (4%) were switched to other treatments (pancreas transplantation 2, liraglutide 2, multiple daily insulin 3).
- twenty pump-treated PWDs (11 %) died (heart failure 12, stroke 2, renal failure 2, pneumonia 2, M. Alzheimer 2).
- in the year 2013, 152 of 185 (82 %) CSII-treated PWDs registered in our working group PARASEN (since 1981) have been profiting from insulin pumps.

Insulin pumps are the optimum available and safe means for insulin substitution in PWD1 [117, 118]. From insulin pumps may also profit some PWD 2 [106, 119].

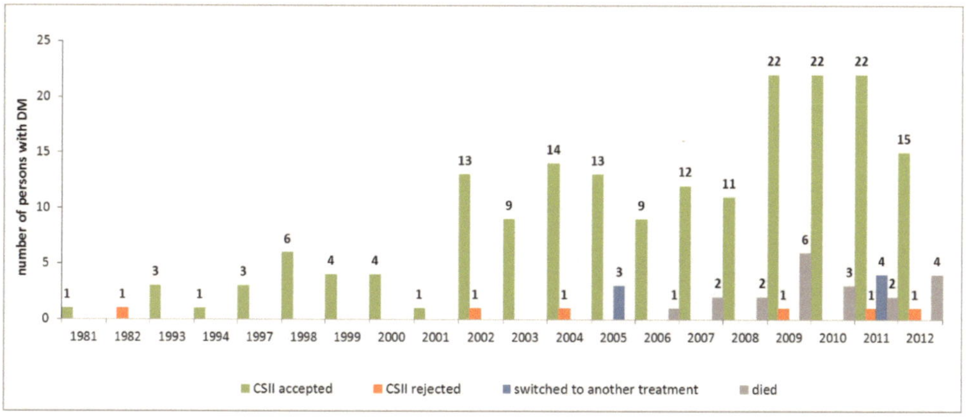

Figure 27.
Distribution of PWD (PARASEN Group) with accepted or rejected insulin pump or switched to other treatments or decreased over the period of 31 y.

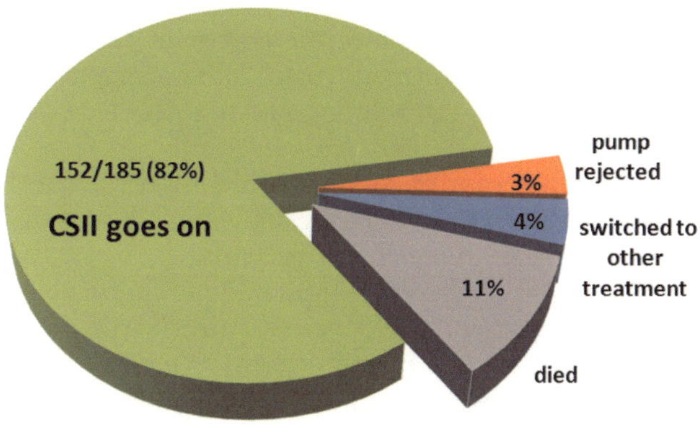

Figure 28.
Summary of outcomes from insulin pump treatment of PWD (PARASEN Group) over the 31-year period 1981–2012.

However, in PWD2 incretins and gliflozins recently appear to offer better cardioprotective and nephroprotective perspectives.

4.3 Retrospective single centre study on the safety and microbial hazards of prolonged transcutaneous sensor insertion (2004–2007)

Inflammation is a potential adverse event at the site of sensor insertion. In eight studies, there were 364 transcutaneous sensors used in 169 men and women with diabetes and in 40 healthy persons. The skin was sprayed with an antiseptic before sensor insertion. In the course of 2117 sensor days, there was only one serious complication: an abscess in the gluteal region. We demonstrate this case report [120].

History: A man born in 1972 with T1D from 1981, on insulin pump since 2002, from 2003 he used 15 sensors without any complication except occasional slight redness and increased sensitivity at the site of insertion. On 14.3.07, the patient inserted a sensor in the middle of the right gluteal area 14 cm below spina illiaca posterior superior. Before insertion, the site was sprayed by antiseptic. The third day

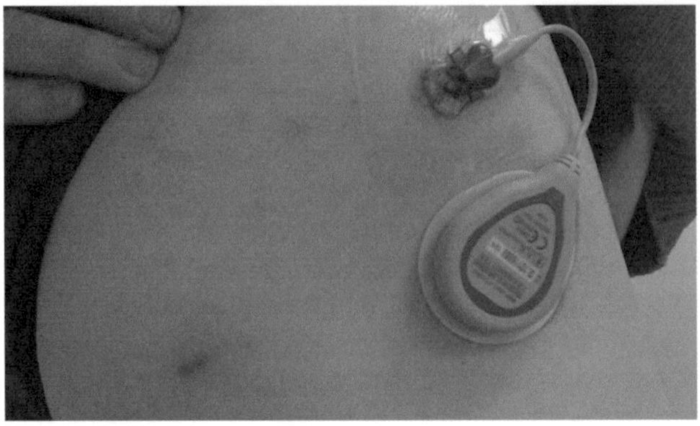

Figure 29.
Healing serious adverse events after sensor insertion. Scar after the abscess drain (left lower corner). New sensor and transmitter (right upper corner).

after insertion pain and aedema appeared, the fourth day the sensor was removed, the pain became more severe so 5 days later (23.3.07) he contacted the diabetes centre.

On examination: Redness and infiltration 5 cm of diameter. Small incision in local anaesthesia (Mesocain 1%) was performed, 10–20 ml of purulent fluid was evacuated. The wound rinsed using physiological solution and drained. New sensor was inserted (**Figure 29**).

Microbial culture: Streptococcus pyogenes. No antibiotics were given. Within 14 days after surgical intervention, the local redness and pain disappeared and no signs of secretion or retention were seen. A small scar remains.

Conclusions: In the course of the FDA-approved period for sensor insertion only one serious adverse event occurred. There were no other serious adverse events in sensors used for up to 9 days. Hence, from the point of view of potential microbial hazards prolonged insertion of sensors appears to be safe. These conclusions are supported by other studies [72].

4.4 Interests in long-term continuous glucose monitoring in persons on insulin pumps-one centre experience (2006–2012)

The purpose of this prospective study [57] was to assess the real patient´s interest in routine use of transcutaneous sensors related to hypothetic optimum state of "always on CGM".

Methods and results: In the course of 7 years (from 2006 to 2012), the sensor augmentation of Continuous Subcutaneous Insulin Infusion (CSII) was repeatedly offered free of charge to all PWD on pumps (n=123) attending the regular check-ups supported by Carelink Personal software. The CGM was accepted for a variable number of days by 63 (51%) of them. The real percentage of time spent on CGM shows the present study (**Table 3**).

SPSS v 15.0, SPSS Inc., Chicago, IL, was used for statistical analysis. $P < 0.05$ was considered significant. Fisher´s exact test and Mann–Whitney U test revealed no significant differences in number of PWD, duration of diabetes, duration of CSII, duration of offer of CGM, total number of days with real use of CGM and rates of real use of CGM compared between PWD1 vs. PWD2 and men vs. women, except the age of PWD1 vs. PWD2 at start of CSII ($P = 0.0001$). The interests of PWD on CGM augmented CSII and their real-life conditions resulted in median of up to 14.1 % time

Parameter	Unit	PWD1 Men	PWD1 Women	PWD1 M+W	PWD2 M+W
N	#	26	27	53	10
Age at the start of CSII	y	30.5 (23.2, 52.2)	31.7 (23.8, 45.2)	31.0 (24, 48)	57.7 (52, 66)
Duration of DM at CSII start	y	18.5 (5.8, 29.0)	9.0 (3.0, 20.0)	12.0 (3.5, 25.0)	7.0 (3.8, 21.5)
Duration of CSII	y	4.1 (2.4, 10.3)	6.3 (2.4, 12.1)	5,8 (2.4, 10.9)	3.2 (2.5, 4.5)
Unlimited offer of CGM	d	1491 (868, 2147)	1491 (883, 2252)	1491 (883, 2221)	1123 (746, 1499)
Real use of CGM	d	154 (72, 339)	189 (27, 337)	175 (56, 333)	66 (6, 137)
Days on CGM/ Days of offer	%	10.9 (5,1, 26.9)	14.1 (4.1, 28.0)	12.1 (5, 26.1)	7.7 (0.4, 12.2)

Table 3.
Characteristics of PWD on insulin pumps and their interest in sensor-augmented CSII (median, percentile 25 and 75).

of CGM use. So, having made available sensors and CGM education for unlimited time for all 123 PWD on insulin pumps in our centre, their attitudes and motivation remained to be adopted.

5. Prevention, early diagnosis and treatment of gestational diabetes, T1D and late complications in PWD1 at Teaching Hospital Olomouc (2014–2022)

5.1 Gestational diabetes mellitus (GDM)

GDM is transient glucose intolerance first detected during pregnancy. Manifestation usually occurs in the second and third trimesters. After delivery, the impaired glucose metabolism is corrected, and the glucose level moves within the normal range.

At the beginning of pregnancy, the main goal of the mother's metabolism is to build up sufficient reserves of energy to be used for foetal growth [121]. With the end of the first trimester, insulin resistance of muscle and adipose tissue gradually begins to develop, reaching its peak during the third trimester. The volume of adipose tissue decreases and the supply of free fatty acids increases, which newly become the main source of energy for the maternal organism. Glucose is redirected by the placenta to the foetus. Despite significant insulin resistance development of diabetes in pregnancy usually does not occur.

The HAPO study in 2008 demonstrated a strong association between glycaemia values and the perinatal complications which was almost linear and already evident at the level of glycaemia, which until then was considered completely physiological [122]. This study led to the development of a new guideline for screening and diagnosis of gestational diabetes [123]. Our centre, like others in the Czech Republic, adopted these criteria in 2015 (**Table 4**).

The primary treatment of GDM consists of dietary control, adequate physical activity and weight management remain the cornerstones of GDM treatment.

First antenatal visit	24– 28 week of gestation (75g oGTT)
FPG ≥5,1mmol/l[1]	PG ≥ 5,1mmol/l (fasting) PG ≥ 10,0mmol/l (1h) PG ≥ 8,5 mmol/l (2h)

FPG=fasting plasma glucose; PG=plasma glucose; 75g oGTT=oral glucose tolerance test with 75g of glucose. [1] *At least 2 measurements on separate days.*

Table 4.
Diagnostic criteria for GDM (adopted from IADPSG).

FPG	<5,3 mmol/l
PPG (1h)	<7,8 mmol/l
PPG (2h)	<6,7 mmol/l

FPG=fasting plasma glucose; PPG=postprandial plasma glucose.

Table 5.
Glucose targets recommended for GDM treatment [124].

Pharmacological (mainly insulin) treatment of GDM is considered in cases where we are unable to achieve the treatment goals through dietary modification and lifestyle management. Insulin is indicated when glycaemia exceeds the recommended range (**Table 5**).

In GDM, the reason for insulin preference dominance is good efficacy in glycaemic control and the low risk of foetal harm with the negligible transplacental transfer. Metformin has the most experience worldwide. However, in our centre, metformin is not currently recommended in the management of GDM. It is known to cross placenta and a long-term safety for offspring is still of some concern [124].

The relationship between hyperglycaemia at 24–28 weeks of pregnancy and the incidence of perinatal complications is well established. This is not entirely true for the detection of hyperglycaemia in early pregnancy. We have insufficient data to establish target glycaemic values for the diagnosis and treatment of early onset gestational diabetes. However, increased fasting glycaemia in early pregnancy has shown to be closely associated with higher body mass and BMI in the initial weeks of pregnancy [125]. Women with GDM had more pronounced features of metabolic syndrome than pregnant women without GDM in terms of lipid profiles (triglycerides) and increased insulin production (C-peptide) [126]. Women with early onset GDM also showed altered adipokine production. Increased A-FABP and decreased adiponectin levels are correlating with visceral adiposity and glucose control and may be affected by treatment later in pregnancy [127].

It turns out that gestational diabetes is a heterogeneous condition. Further research is now focusing on finding potential different screening strategies and diagnostic criteria in early and late pregnancy. At the same time, it is necessary to look for appropriate treatment approaches for women with hyperglycaemia at different stages of pregnancy in terms of efficacy and safety [128].

5.2 Sensor-augmented insulin pumps

Continuous subcutaneous insulin infusion (CSII) represents the most physiological substitution of insulin in PWD1. However, without frequent glycaemic control

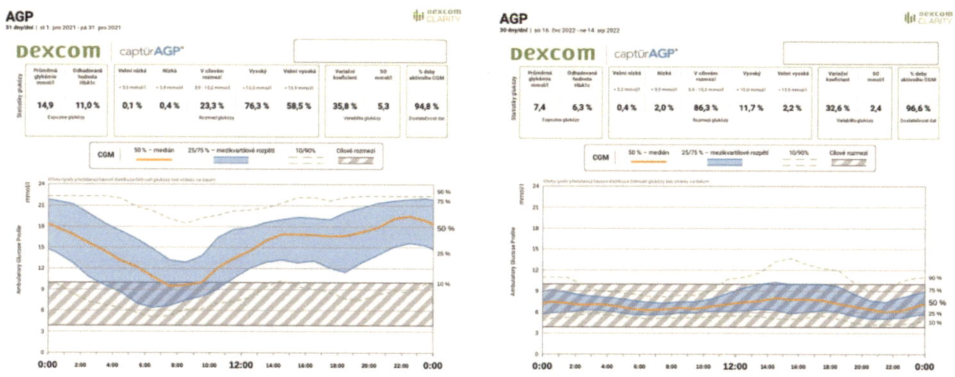

A) TIR (3.9-10.0mmol/l) 23,3%   B) TIR (3.9-10.0mmol/l) 86,3%

Figure 30.
A—Ambulatory glucose profile (AGP) on multiple-dose injection regiment (MDI) with real-time glucose monitoring. B—Ambulatory glucose profile (AGP) after 6 months of sensor-augmented pump therapy with a hybrid close loop system (Control-IQ ™; t:slim X2™).

and insulin dose correction, it fails to keep glycaemia within the recommended range. Real-time continuous glycaemic monitoring system (rtCGM) on the other hand improves the metabolic outcomes regardless of insulin delivery method [31]. Sensor-augmented pump therapy (SAP) integrates these two technologies into one functional system. In the course of the last few years, it has been further improved by a mathematical algorithm that allows semi-autonomous adjustments of subcutaneous insulin infusion according to the current glycaemia (hybrid close loop system—HCL). For the last 2 years, we have been using the Minimed™ 780G system (Medtronic) with the SmartGuard™ and also t:slim X2™ (Tandem) with the Control-IQ™. Those systems have been certified and fully approved for the treatment of T1DM in the Czech Republic. Our experience with the HCL system shows that it is possible to achieve very good results, surprisingly not only in well-cooperating and trained PWD1. **Figure 30** shows the increase of the TIR (Time In Range) and the enormous improvement of daily glucose pattern in a woman, who has been using Control-IQ hybrid close loop function of t:slim X2 inuslin pump for 6 months.

5.3 Prospective uncontrolled single-centre study ROXINEGLYD (Contribution of Retinal OXimetry to the assessment of impact of INternal Environment, GLYcaemia and Diabetes control on retinal vessel oxygen saturation in PWD) (2016–2020)

Retinal oximetry is a method for measuring retinal oxygen saturation ($SatO_2$). Changes of retinal oxygen saturation were described in various clinical conditions such as retinal vein occlusion, retinitis pigmentosa, glaucoma, cataract, after pars plana vitrectomy, Alzheimer's disease and also in diabetic retinopathy [129, 130]. An increase in venous oxygen saturation was shown to be related to the severity of retinopathy [131–133]. Lower arteriovenous difference of oxygen saturation reflects reduced oxygen delivery to tissues [134]. The question is whether early regular investigations of retinal oxygen saturation might help to assess the risk and progress of diabetic retinopathy.

Purpose of the pilot study [135] was to find an association of retinal oxygen saturation with acid-base balance, carboxyhaemoglobin concentration, current plasma glucose concentration (PG), mean PG and PG variability over the last 72 hrs, HbA_{1c}. and other conditions.

Methods: Forty-one adults (17 men) with T1D (n=14) or T2D (n=27), age 48.6±13.5 years, diabetes duration 9 (0.1–36) years, BMI 29.4±6.3 kg/m^2, HbA_{1c} 52±12.7 mmol/mol completed the study. The 4-day study comprised two visits (Day l, Day 4) including 72 hrs of CGM by iPro®2 Professional CGM (Medtronic, MiniMed, Inc., Northridge, CA, USA). Retinal oximeter Oxymap T1 (Oxymap ehf., Reykjavik, Iceland) was used to assess retinal oxygen saturation.

Results: Wilcoxon signed-rank test showed no $SatO_2$ difference between eyes and visits. A significant correlation between arterial $SatO_2$ and PG variability in T2D, a positive correlation of venous $SatO_2$ with HbA_{1c} and with finger pulse oximetry was found. No correlation of retinal oxygen saturation with acid-base balance, carboxyhaemoglobin, current PG, mean PG over the 72 hrs, age, diabetes duration, BMI, lipoproteinaemia, body temperature, systolic and diastolic blood pressure, heart rate, central retinal thickness and retinal nerve fibre layer thickness was shown.

Conclusion: This study confirmed the association of venous retinal oxygen saturation with long-term but not with short-term diabetes control and not with acid-base balance or other conditions. The increased oxygen saturation and questionable impact of PG variability should be clarified further on.

6. Conclusions

This chapter summarises the authors′experience along with outcomes of respected trials and inventions from the insulin era. It became clear that the intensive management of T1D comprising insulin, diet, exercise and control of therapeutic effectiveness may recover the balance between energy intake and expenditure. Active approach to the diagnosis of diabetes and to prevention of retinopathy, nephropathy, diabetic foot and other cardiovascular complications may reduce their potential risks. Adequate education focused on knowledge, skills, attitudes and communication has created a

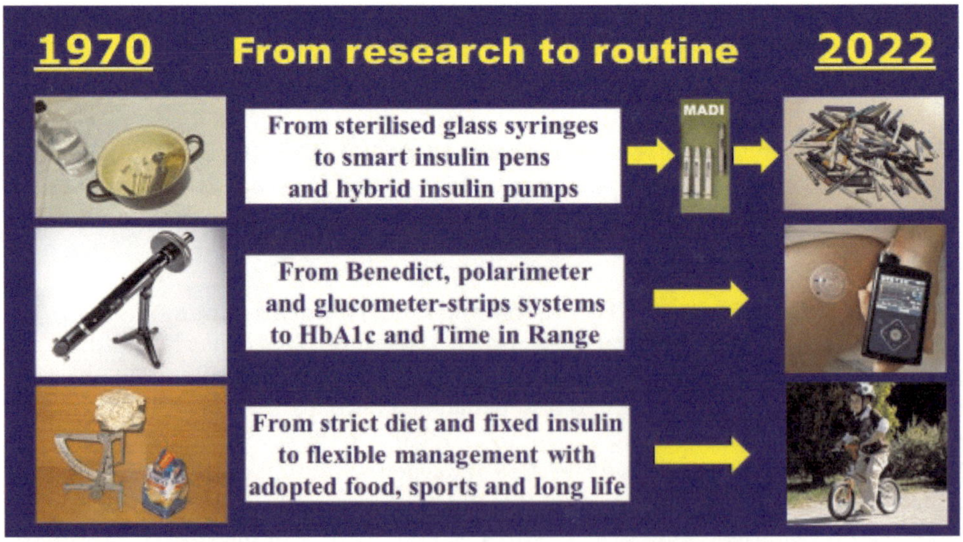

Figure 31.
Journey from the known past to perspectives of unknown future.

reliable base for effective approach. Recent technologies including smart insulin pens, hybrid insulin pumps, CGM, FGM and glucometer-strips systems as well as new insulin analogues, and transplantation of Langerhans islets and stem cells are offerring great perspectives (**Figure 31**).

Shall we always be strong enough to transfer the practice-related research outcomes to our daily routine?

7. Dedication

This chapter is dedicated to the memory of *Leslie James Park Dun*can (*Sumatra, 1922 – + Scotland 2005), unforgetable diabetologist who created a centre of excellence at the Royal Infirmary of Edinburgh [42, 136–140], for his empathy with patients, students and colleagues, as it was recognized by one of the authors of this Chapter in the course of his postgraduate training in Edinburgh in 1980.

Acknowledgements

Those who found this chapter worthy of reading surely appreciate the long-lasting support provided by Palacký University Olomouc, Teaching Hospital Olomouc and Institute of Specialized Treatments Paseka, all of them represented by experienced specialists, nursing and other staff, students etc., and, last but not least by insurance companies and other important institutions … .

Author details

Rudolf Chlup[1,2,3*], Ondřej Krystyník[4], Petr Mlčák[1,5], Jana Zapletalová[6] and Josef Bartek[7]

1 Faculty of Medicine and Dentistry, Department of Physiology, Palacký University Olomouc, Czech Republic

2 2nd Department of Medicine, Teaching Hospital Olomouc, Czech Republic

3 Department of Diabetes Moravský Beroun, Institute of Specialized Treatments, Paseka, Czech Republic

4 3rd Department of Medicine, Teaching Hospital Olomouc and Faculty of Medicine and Dentistry, Palacký University Olomouc, Czech Republic

5 Department of Ophthalmology, Teaching Hospital Olomouc and Faculty of Medicine and Dentistry, Palacký University Olomouc, Czech Republic

6 Faculty of Medicine and Dentistry, Department of Medical Biophysics, Palacký University Olomouc, Czech Republic

7 Faculty of Medicine and Dentistry, Department of Medical Chemistry and Biochemistry, Palacký University Olomouc, Czech Republic

*Address all correspondence to: rudolf.chlup@fnol.cz

References

[1] Atkinson MA, Eisenbarth GS, Michels AW. Type 1 diabetes. Lancet. 2014;**383**: 69-82

[2] Irvine WJ, Dimario U, Feek CM, Ting A, Morris PJ, Gray RS, et al. Insulin-antibodies in relation to islet cell antibodies and HLA antigens in insulin-dependent (type-I) diabetes. Journal of Clinical & Laboratory Immunology. 1978;**1**(2):111-114

[3] Lenhart K, Bartova A, Lenhartova E. Frequency of HLA DR genes in the district of Olomouc (first report). Acta Universitasis Palackianae Olomoucensis (Olomouc) Facultatis Medicae. 1981;**99**:95

[4] Zander E, Strese J, Schulz B. Coma diabeticum. Zeitschrift für klinische Medizin-ZKM. 1990;**45**(24):2137-2141

[5] Rosival V. Interesting Development in the Pathophysiology of Diabetic Ketoacidotic Coma. Journal of Diabetes Metabolism. 2014;**5**:455. DOI: 10.4172/2155-6156.100045

[6] Engelhardt D. Diabetes – Its Medical and Cultural History: Outlines, Texts, Bibliography. New York: Springer-Verlag; 1989

[7] Korec R. 75th anniversary of insulin discovery: NC Paulescu´s and FG.

[8] Ionescu-Tirgoviste C. The re-discovery of Insulin. Romania: Editura Geneze; 1996

[9] Jörgens V. They got very near the goal: Zülzer, Scott, and Paulescu. In: Jörgens V, Porta M, editors. Unveiling Diabetes – Historical Milestones in Diabetology. Basel: Karger; 2020. pp. 58-72

[10] Porta M. One hundred years ago: The dawning of the insulin era. Acta Diabetologica. 2021;**58**(1):1-4

[11] Jörgens V. Die Geschichte der Diabetes-forschung vom Opium zum Insulin. 1st ed. Mainz: Verlag Kirchheim +Co GmBH; 2022. p. 303

[12] Bolli GB, Cheng AYY, Owens DR. Insulin: Evolution of insulin formulations and their application in clinical practice over 100 years. Acta Diabetologica. 2022;**59**:1129-1144

[13] Hagedorn H. Protamine insulinate. Proceedings of the Royal Society of Medicine. 1937;**30**(6):805-814

[14] Standl E. Insulin analogues – state of the art. Hormone Research. 2002;**57**: 40-45

[15] Skyler JS. Lessons from studies of insulin pharmacokinetics. Diabetes Care. 1986;**9**:666-668

[16] Chlup R, Zapletalová J, Zálešáková H, Kochtová J, Kaňa R. Vliv léčby inzulinem Fiasp na glykemii, HbA1c a tělesnou hmotnost u osob s diabetem 1. a 2. typu: studie z reálné praxe. Diab Obez. 2019;**19**(38):90-97

[17] Sharp P, Ives E. Insulin delivery devices 100 years on. Practical Diabetes. 2021;**38**(4):21-26

[18] Pickup JC, Keen H, Parsons JS, et al. Continuous subcutaneous insulin infusion: An approach to achieving normoglycaemia. British Medical Journal. 1978;**282**:347-350

[19] Paton JS, Wilson M, Ireland JT, Reith SB. Convenient pocket insulin syringe. The Lancet. 1981;**317**(8213):189-190

[20] Janů K, Chlup R, Chleboun J. Ruční mechanický dávkovač kapaliny (Manual mechanical device for fluid dosing).

Patent and Inventions Office Prague (Úřad pro patenty a objevy v Praze): Application number PV 6160 submitted on (podaná dne) 24. 8. 1983, Patent number (číslo patentu) 237521, was granted by the patent office on (datum udělení patentu) 24. 4. 1985.

[21] Chlup R, Menzel R, Kolesár P, Rybka J, Svoboda Z, Škarpová O, Venháčová J, Zander E, Abel P, Rosenfeld R, Hildebrandt R, Janů K, Jutzi E. Erste Erfahrungen mit dem MADI-multizentrische technische und klinische Studie. VIII. internationales Donau-Symposium über Diabetes mellitus, Bratislava, 18-21. Juni 1985. Wien: Robidruck 1985, Abstrakt 79. 1985

[22] Janů K, Chlup R. Konstrukční řešení ručního dávkovače inzulínu MADI. Jemná mechanika a optika (Fine mechanics and optics). 1992;**37**(1):14-15

[23] Rex J, Vogeley OA. Dispenser. U.S. patent number 4,592,745 [Application Number 06/584,876], submitted on 1984-02-29, was granted by the patent office on 1986-06-03.

[24] Jefferson IG, Marteau TM, Smith MA, Baum JD. A multiple injection regimen using an insulin injection pen and pre-filled cartridged soluble human insulin in adolescents with diabetes. Diabetic Medicine. 1985;**2**(6):493-495

[25] Heinemann L, Schnell O, Gehr B, Schloot NC, Görgens SW, Görgen C. Digital diabetes management: A literature review of smart insulin pens. Journal of Diabetes Science and Technology. 2022;**16**(3):587-595

[26] Hanas R, John G, On behalf of the International HbA1c Consensus Committee. 2010 Consensus statement on the worldwide standardization of the hemoglobin A1C measurement. Diabetes Care. 2010;**33**:1903-1904

[27] Bode BW, Hirsch IB. Using the continuous glucose monitoring system to improve the management of type 1 diabetes. Diabetes Technology & Therapeutics. 2000;**2**(Suppl 1):43-48

[28] Mlčák P, Fialová J, Trnková K, Chlup R. A continuous glucose monitoring system (CGMS) – a promising aproach for improving metabolic control in persons with type 1 diabetes mellitus treated by insulin pumps. Biomedical Papers. 2004;**148**(1):33-38

[29] Chlup R, Jelenová D, Chlupová K, Zapletalová J, Chlupová L, Bartek J. Function and accuracy of glucose sensors beyond their stated expiry date. Diabetes Technology & Therapeutics. 2005;**8**(4): 495-504

[30] Peterson K, Zapletalová J, Kudlová P, Matušková V, Bartek J, Novotný D, et al. Benefits of three-month continuous glucose monitoring for persons with diabetes using insulin pumps and sensors. Biomed Papers. 2009;**153**(1): 47-52

[31] Šoupal J, Petruželková L, Grunberger G, Hásková A, Flekač M, Matoulek M, et al. Glycemic outcomes in adults with T1D are impacted more by continuous glucose monitoring than by insulin delivery method: 3 years of follow-up from the COMISAIR Study. Diabetes Care. 2020;**43**(1):37-43

[32] Edelman SV, Argento NB, Pettus J, Hirsch IB. Clinical implications of real-time and intermittently scanned continuous glucose monitoring. Diabetes Care. 2018;**41**(11):2265-2274

[33] Battelino T, Danne T, Bergenstal RM, et al. Clinical targets for continuous glucose monitoring data interpretation: Recommendations from the international consensus on time-in-range. Diabetes Care. 2019;**42**:1593-1603

[34] Frier BM. Hypoglycaemia and diabetes. Diabetic Medicine. 1986;**3**: 513-525

[35] Stolte K, Wolff J. Die Behandlung der kindlichen Zuckerkrankheit bei freigewählter Kost. In: Czerny A, Müller F, Pfaundler M, Schittenhelm A, editors. Ergebnisse der inneren Medizin und Kinderheilkunde. Berlin: Verlag von Julius Springer; 1936. pp. 154-193

[36] Mores A. Probleme des Kinderdiabetes. Bratislavské lekárske listy. 1939;**19**(9):1-19

[37] Stout RW. Diabetes and atherosclerosis – The role of insulin. Diabetologia. 1979;**16**:141

[38] Jarett RJ. Is insulin atherogenic? Diabetologia. 1988;**31**:71-75

[39] Keen H, Jarret RJ, Fuller JH, McCartney P. Hyperglycaemia and arterial disease. Diabetes. 1981;**30**:49

[40] Alvarsson ML, Grill VE. Effect of long term glycemic control on the onset of retinopathy in IDDM subjects. A longitudinal and retrospective study. Diabetes Research. 1989;**10**:75-80

[41] Reichard P, Nilsson BY, Resenquist U. Retardation of the development of the microvascular complications after long-term intensified insulin treatment: The Stockholm Diabetes Intervention. The New England Journal of Medicine. 1993; **329**:304-309

[42] Frier BM, Matthews DM, Steel JM, Duncan LJ. Driving and insulin-dependent diabetes. Lancet (London, England). 1980;**1**(8180):1232-1234

[43] Waldhäusl WK, Bratusch-Marrain RP, Francesconi M, Nowotny P, Kiss A. Insulin production rate in normal man as an estimate for calibration of continuous intravenous insulin infusion in insulin-dependent diabetic patients. Diabetes Care. 1982;**5**:18-24

[44] Katsch G. Regulationskrankheit Diabetes. Wissenschaftliche Zeitschrift der Universität Greifswald. 1951;**I**:1-9

[45] Assal JP, Mühlhauser I, Pernet A, Gfeller R, Jörgens V, Berger M. Patient education as the basis for diabetes care in clinical practice and research. Diabetologia. 1985;**28**:602-613

[46] Berger M, Jörgens V, Mühlhauser I, Zimmermann H. Die Bedeutung der Diabetikerschulung in der Therapie des Typ-I-Diabetes. Dtsch med Wschr. 1983; **108**:424-430

[47] Joslin EP. The treatment of diabetes. In: Joslin EP, editor. TheTreatment of Diabetes Mellitus. 6th ed. London: Henry Kimpton; 1937. pp. 263-313

[48] Mühlhauser I, Bruckner I, Berger M, Cheta D, Jörgens V, Ionescu-Tirgoviste C, et al. Evaluation of an intensified insulin treatment and teaching programme as routine management of type I (insulin-pendent) diabetes. Diabetologia. 1987;**30**:681-690

[49] Howorka K. Insulinabhängig? Funktioneller Insulingebrauch: Der Weg zur Freiheit mit nahezu normalem Blutzucker. 2nd ed. Mainz: Verlag Kirchheim; 1987

[50] Anděl M, Slabochová Z, Dryaková M, et al. Všeobecné základy intenzifikované konvenční terapie cukrovky 1. typu inzulínem. (Basics of intensified conventional insulin therapy. Czech.). Vnitř Lék (Intgernal Medicine). 1987;**33**:475-484

[51] Chantelau EA, Frenzen A, Gösseringer G, Hansen I, Berger M. Intensive insulin therapy justifies

simplification of the diabetes diet: A prospective study in insulin-dependent diabetic patients. The American Journal of Clinical Nutrition. 1987;**45**:958-962

[52] Menzel R, Brunstein U, Wilke W, Rosenbaum F, Knigge E, Staritz B, Gengelbach E. Kleiner Ratgeber für Anwender von Insulinpumpen. Zentralinstitut für Diabetes Gerhardt Katsch Karlsburg. 1989

[53] Chlup R, Navrátilová L, Řehořová J, Vaverková H, Venháčová J, Bartek J, Ficker L, Slezáková L. Programová léčba diabetu. (Czech. Programmed diabetes therapy) Galén, Praha (pp. 196). 1996

[54] Kudlova P, Chlup R, Zapletalova J. The benefits of postgraduate therapeutic education in diabetology in the Czech Republic. In: Bekirogullari Z, Minas MY, Thambusamy RX, editors. 3rd icH& Hpsy International Conference on Health and Health Psychology, July 5–7, 2017. Viseu, Portugal: The European Proceedings of Social & Behavioural Sciences EpSBS; 2017. pp. 217-227

[55] Chlup R. The Diabetes Centre at Olomouc University in the Czech Republic. Practical Diabetes International. 1997;**14**(2):51

[56] Chlup R. Outcomes of clinical diabetes research at the Teaching hospital and Faculty of Medicine, Palacký University Olomouc (1971–2014). Bulletin of the Karaganda University Biology, Medicine, Geography. 2015;**19**:34-50

[57] Milata V. Využívání kontinuální monitorace glykémie u osob léčených inzulínovou pumpou [The use of continuous glucose monitoring in patients treated with insulin pump. Czech.] [thesis] St. Elizabeth University College of Health and Social Work Bratislava, External Teaching Dept. of blessed Metod D. Trčka Michalovce; 2013.

[58] Bartek J, Chlup R. HDL-Cholesterin und Gesamtcholesterin während der Muskelbelastung bei untrainierten Typ-1-Diabetikern. In: Wiedermann B, Bibergeil H, editors. Symposium Diabetes a fyzická zátěž – Diabetes und Muskelbelastung, Olomouc, ČSSR, 21.-23.1. Olomouc; 1982

[59] Steidl L, Chlup R. Einfluß eines Trainingsprogrammes auf Neuropathie bei Diabetikern vom Typ-1. In: Wiedermann B, Bibergeil H, editors. Symposium Diabetes a fyzická zátěž-Diabetes und Muskelbelastung, Olomouc, ČSSR, 21.-23.1. Olomouc: Univerzita Palackého v Olomouci; 1982

[60] Bartošová S, Vybíralová J, Chlup R. Einfluß eines Trainingsprogrammes auf psychologische Parameter bei Diabetikern vom Typ-1. In: Wiedermann B, Bibergeil H, editors. Symposium Diabetes a fyzická zátěž – Diabetes und Muskelbelastung, Olomouc, ČSSR, 21.-23.1. Olomouc; 1982

[61] Bartek J, Chlup R. Ambulante Tagesprofile mittels Selbstblutentnahmen. In: Wiedermann B, Bibergeil H, editors. Symposium Diabetes a fyzická zátěž Diabetes und Muskelbelastung, Olomouc, ČSSR, 21.-23.1. Olomouc; 1982

[62] Chlup R. Vliv trénnku na metabolické, hormonální a klinické ukazatele u diabetu 1. typu (Impact of training on metabolic, hormonal and clinical parameters in T1D. Czech.) [thesis]. Palacký University Olomouc; 1983.

[63] Chlup R. Klinisch-experimentelle Studie zur metabolischen Wirksamkeit und Akzeptanz von verschiedenen Regimen der intensiven konventionellen

Insulintherapie unter besonderer Berücksichtigung der Nachtphase bei insulinpflichtigen (Typ-1)-Diabetikern [thesis]. Greifswald University; 1993

[64] Zander E, Schulz B, Chlup R, Woltansky P, Lubs D. Muscular exercise in Type-1-Diabetics: II. Hormonal and metabolic responses to moderate exercise. Experimental and Clinical Endocrinology. 1985;**85**(1):95-104

[65] Zander E, Schulz B, Woltansky P, Wulfert P, Chlup R. Hormonal and metabolic effects of moderate exercise in Type-1-Diabetics with hypo-and hyperinsulinemia. Acta Universitatis Palackianae Olomucensis – Tomm III facultatis medicae pp. 1985:281-286

[66] Chlup R, Zander E, Hildmann W, Bartek J, Jutzi E. Vliv tělesného tréninku na metabolismus sacharidů a tuků u diabetiků I. typu. In: Horniak E, editor. Sport ve zdraví a nemoci: Práce IV. Evropského kongresu sportovního lékařství. Praha; 1985. pp. 245-251

[67] Zander E, Chlup R, Schulz B. Über den Einfluß des Muskeltrainings auf die Insulinsensitivität bei adipösen Personen mit gestörter Kohlenhydrattoleranz und auf Parameter im Kohlenhydratstoffwechsel bei Typ-1-Diabetikern. Medizin und Sport. 1986;**26**(5):153-154

[68] Zander E, Schulz CR. Die Bedeutung des sportlichen Trainings beim Diabetes mellitus. Z ärztl Fortbild (Jena). 1987;**81**: 1265-1267

[69] Chlup R, Menzel R, Keilacker H, Heinke P, Jutzi E. Ist die Einführung der nächtlichen Injektion von Normalinsulin bei Typ-1-Diabetikern gerechtfertigt? Akt Endokr Stoffw. 1990;**11**:81

[70] Chlup R, Janů K, Mořkovský J, Venháčová J. Six models of insulin pen MADI: Description and first controlled trial. In: Electronic Book (Bayer) 15th International Diabetes Federation Congress Abstracts. Kobe, Japan; 1994

[71] Menzel R, Chlup R, Jutzi E, Hildmann W. Catheter Pens an alternative to insulin pump treatment? Experimental and Clinical Endocrinology. 1990;**95**:64

[72] Chlup R, Maršálek E, Bruns W. Prospective study of the hazards of multiple use of disposable syringes and needles in intensified insulin therapy. Diabetic Medicine. 1990;**7**: 624-627

[73] Chlup R, Menzel R, Keilacker H, Heinke P, Jutzi E. Night injections of regular insulin improve diabetes control in C-peptide negative patients. Diabetologia. 1997;**40**(Suppl 1):328

[74] Kohnert KD, Augstein P, Heinke P, Zander E, Peterson K, Freyse EJ, et al. Chronic hyperglycemia but not glucose variability determines HbA1c levels in well-controlled patients with type 2 diabetes. Diabetes Research and Clinical Practice. 2007;**77**:420-426

[75] Peterson K, Chlup R, Zapletalová J, Kohnert K, Kudlová P, Bartek J, et al. Influence of oral antidiabetic drugs on hyperglycemic response to foods in persons with type 2 diabetes mellitus as assessed by continuous glucose monitoring system: A pilot study. Journal of Diabetes Science and Technology. 2010;**4**(4):983-992

[76] Chlup R, Janů K, Menzel R, et al. Léčba diabetu pomocí ručního dávkovače inzulinu MADI. (Diabetes management by means of a MAnual Device for Insulin application MADI. Czech.). 1st. ed. Olomouc: Univerzita Palackého v Olomouci; 1985. p. 64

[77] Berger M, Jörgens V, Chlup R. Léčba inzulínem v každodenním životě. Praha: Victoria Publishing; 1995

[78] Chlup R, Janů K, Venháčová J, Bartek J. Six models of a new insulin pen (MADI): Description and first clinical trial. Practical Diabetes International. 1995;**12**(1):32-35

[79] Lawrence RO. The effect of exercise on insulin action in diabetes. Brit Med J. 1926;**1**:648

[80] Seliger V, Bartunek Z. Mean values of various indices of physical fitness in the investigation of czechoslovak population aged 12-55 years. In: International Programme Results of Investigations 1968–1974. Prague; 1976

[81] Jahnke K, Mehnert H, Reis HD. Muskelstoffwechsel, körperliche Leistungsfähigkeit und Diabetes mellitus. New York, Schattauer: Stuttgart; 1977

[82] Koivisto VA, Felig P. Effects of leg exerice on insulin absorption in diabetic patients. New England Journal of Medicine. 1978;**298**:79

[83] McMillan DC. Exercise and diabetic microangiopathy. Diabetes. 1979;**280** (Suppl 1):103

[84] Soman VR, DeFronzo RA. Direct evidence for downregulation of insulin receptore by physiologic hyperinsulinemia in man. Diabetes. 1980;**29**:159

[85] Vranic M, Berger M. Exercise and diabetes mellitus. Diabetes. 1979;**28**:147

[86] Wahren J, Felig P, Hagenfeldt L. Physical exercise and fuel homeostasis in diabetes mellitus. Diabetologia. 1979; **14**:213

[87] DeFronzo RA, Ferrannini E, Sato Y, Felig P. Synergistic interaction between exercise and insulin on peripheral glucose uptake. The Journal of Clinical Investigation. 1981;**68**:1468

[88] LeBlanc J, Nadeau A, Richard D, Tremblay A. Studies on the sparing effect of exercise on insulin requirements in human subjects. Metabolism. 1981;**30**:1119

[89] Markusas F. Die Bestimmung der PWC 170 durch einen submaximalen Belasstunstest mit Hilfe des nomograms von Astrand-Ryhming. Medicina dello Sport. 1997;**27**:362

[90] Michaelis D, Rjasanowski I, Bombor H, Haubenreiser H, Semmler H, Gottschling D, et al. Die Beurteilung des Stoffwechselkompensationsgrades beim Diabetes mellitus mittels des Glykämiwertes (GW). Dt Gesundh-Wesen. 1982;**37**:634-637

[91] Kemmer FW. Muskelarbeit u nd Diabetes. In: Wiedermann B, Bibergeil H, editors. Symposium Diabetes a fyzická zátěž Diabetes und Muskelbelastung, Olomouc, ČSSR, 21.-23.1. Olomouc; 1982

[92] Zander E, Schulz B, Bruns W, Wulfert P, Lubs D, Besch W, et al. Hormonelle und metabolische Veränderungen während akuter Muskelarbeit bei Typ-1-Diabetikern – in Abhängigkeit von der Insulinverfügbarkeit und Arbeitsintensität. In: Wiedermann B, Bibergeil H (eds), Symposium Diabetes a fyzická zátěž Diabetes und Muskelbelastung, Olomouc, ČSSR, 21.-23.1. Olomouc; 1982

[93] Chlup R, Bartek J, Hildmann W, Lubs D, Wodrig W, Jutzi E, et al. Vliv Tréninku na potřebu inzulínu a na látkovou výměnuu diabetu 1. typu. In:

Wiedermann B, Bibergeil H, editors. Symposium Diabetes a fyzická zátěž Diabetes und Muskelbelastung, Olomouc, ČSSR, 21.-23.1. Olomouc; 1982

[94] Michalková D, Černay J, Birčák J, Kolář J, Zmeková E. Skusenosti z prázdninových rekondičných táborov pre deti s diabetes mellitus. (Experience from vacation recondition camps for children with diabetes mellitus. Slovak.). In: Wiedermann B, Bibergeil H, editors. Symposium Diabetes a fyzická zátěž-Diabetes und Muskelbelastung, Olomouc, ČSSR, 21.-23.1. Olomouc; 1982

[95] Piroch V, Šuchmanová V. Vliv kondičního tréninku na metabolické ukazavele při diabetu. (Influence of recondition-training on metabolic parameters in diabetes mellitus. Czech.). In: Wiedermann B, Bibergeil H, editors. Symposium Diabetes a fyzická zátěž Diabetes und Muskelbelastung, Olomouc, ČSSR, 21.-23.1. Olomouc; 1982

[96] Besch W, Keilacker H, Ziegler M, Woltanski KP, Kohnert KD. Zur radiologischen Bestimmungdes Glukagons, Huuman C-Peptids, Wachstumshormons und der Insulinantikörper. In: Wiedermann B, Bibergeil H, editors. Symposium Diabetes a fyzická zátěž Diabetes und Muskelbelastung, Olomouc, ČSSR, 21.-23.1. Olomouc; 1982

[97] Bruns W. Is good control possible with several insulin injections per day? Can late complications be prevented or reduced? In: Irsigler K, Kunz K, Owens DR, Regal H, editors. New Approaches to Insulin Therapy. Lancaster: International Medical Publishers; 1980

[98] Bruns W, Jutzi E, Fischer U, Bombor H, Woltanski KP, Jahr D, et al. Über tagesrhythmische Veränderungen der Insulinkonzentrationen und der Plasmaglukose bei Nichtdiabetikern sowie des Insulinbedarfs bei insulinpflichtigen Diabetikern. Ber Ges Inn Med. 1980;**12**:258-260

[99] Schiffrin A, Belmonte M. Multiple daily self-glucose monitoring: Its essential role in long term glucose control in insulin-dependent diabetic patients treated with pump and multiple subcutaneous injections. Diabetes Care. 1981;**4**:595-600

[100] Bruns W, Bombor H, Jutzi E, Ratzmann KP, Schulz B, Abel P, et al. Reproducibility of insulin dosage on consecutive days of blood glucose control by an artificial beta-cell in brittle diabetic patients. Diabetes Care. 1983;**6**: 112-117

[101] Schade DS, Santiago JV, Skyler JS, Rizza RA. Intenzive Insulin Therapy. Amsterdam Geneva Hong Kong Princeton Tokyo: Medical Examination Public; 1983

[102] Dimitriadis GD, Gerich JE. Importance of timing of preprandial subcutaneous insulin administration in the management of diabetes mellitus. Diabetes Care. 1983;**6**:374-377

[103] Schmidt MI, Lin QX, Gwynne JT, Jacobs S. Fasting early morning rise in peripheral insulin: Evidence of the dawn phenomenon in nondiabetics. Diabetes Care. 1984;**7**:32-35

[104] Campbell PJ, Bolli GB, Cryer PE, Gerich JE. Pathogenesis of the dawn phenomenon in patients with insulin-dependent diabetes mellitus. The New England Journal of Medicine. 1985;**312**: 1473-1479

[105] Hirsch IB, Farkas-Hirsch R, Skyler JS. Intensive insulin therapy for treatment of type I diabetes mellitus. Diabetes Care. 1990;**13**:1265-1283

[106] Chlup R, Kaňa R, Hanáčková L, Zálešáková H, Doubravová B. Pathophysiologic approach to Type 2 diabetes management: One Centre Experience 1980–2020. In: Stoian AP, editor. Type 2 Diabetes - From Pathophysiology to Cyber Systems. London: IntechOpen; 2021

[107] Home PD, Capaldo B, Burrin JM, Worth R, Alberti KGMM. A crossover comparison of continuous subcutaneous insulin infusion (CSII) against multiple insulin injections in insulin-dependent diabetic subjects: Improved control with CSII. Diabetes Care. 1982;**5**:466-471

[108] Hirš P, Bureš J, Zahálka A. Programovatelná osobní infusní pumpa pro parenterální aplikaci. (Programmable insulin pump for parenteral application. Czech.). Prakt Lék. 1984;**64**:548-550

[109] Svoboda Z. Přenosné infúzní inzulínové pumpy v léčení cukrovky. (Transportable insulin pumps for the treatment of diabetes. Czech.). Prakt Lék. 1984;**64**(14):545-546

[110] Dvořáková L, Svoboda Z, Hájková E. Dlouhodobá léčba insulinovými pumpami (Longlasting therapy by means insulin pumps. Czech.). Prakt Lék. 1984;**64**(14):551-554

[111] Vavřinec J, Kopecký A, Žižkovský J, et al. Léčba diabetu přenosnými inzulínovými pumpami. (Therapy of diabetes by means of transportable insulin pumps Czech.). Čs Pediat. 1985; **40**(12):700-704

[112] Dryáková M, Vondra K, Hirš P, Štolba P. New ways in treatment on insulin-dependent diabetes. Czechoslovak Medicine. 1987;**2**:175-184

[113] Marshall SM, Home PD, Taylor R, Alberti KGMM. Continuous subcutaneous insulin infusion versus injection therapy: A randomized cross-over trial under usual diabetic clinic conditions. Diabetic Medicine. 1987;**4**: 521-525

[114] Jeitler K, Horvath K, Berghold A, Gratzer TW, Neeser K, Pieber TR, et al. Continuous subcutaneous insulin infusion versus multiple daily insulin injections in patients with diabetes mellitus: Systematic review and meta-analysis. Diabetologia. 2008;**51**(6): 941-951

[115] Chlup R, Možíšová L. Léčba diabetiků pomocí inzulínové pumpy – teorie a praxe. Diabet Metabol Endokrin Výž. 2000;**3**(1):3-17

[116] Cohen O, Körner A, Chlup R, Zoupas C, Ragozin A, Wudi K, et al. Improved glycemic control through continuous glucose sensor – augmented insulin pump therapy: Prospective results from a community and academic practice patient registry. Journal of Diabetes Science and Technology. 2009; **3**(4):804-811

[117] Chlup R, Tomčalová J, Kudlová P, Zapletalová J. Pump away: Patient´s rejection of continuous subsutaneous insulin infucion, physician´s decision to switching to other treatments and death rates. Diabetes Technology Therapy. 2013;**15**(1):37

[118] Ĺoyková K, Krystyník O, Loyková V, Chlup R, Gajdová J, Číhalíková D, et al. Léčba kontinuální podkožní infuzí inzulínu z pohledu diabetologického centra. (Therapy using CSII from the point of view of a diabetic centre. Czech.). Diabetes Metabololic Endokr Výž. 2018;**17**:51

[119] Chlup R, Runzis S, Castaneda J, Lee S, Nguyen X, Cohen O. Complex assessment of metabolic effectiveness of

insulin pump therapy in patients with type 2 diabetes beyond HbA1c reduction. Diabetes Technology & Therapeutics. 2018;**20**(2):153-159

[120] Matušková V, Fajkusová Z, Přibylová H, Jadviščoková T, Langová K, Chlup R. Abscess at the site of CGMS sensor insertion in a man with type 1 diabetes. In: 27th Workshop of the AIDPIT Study Group. 2008. p. 106. Available from: www.aidpit.org

[121] Catalano PM, Roman-Drago NM, Amini SB, et al. Longitudinal changes in body composition and energy balance in lean women with normal and abnormal glucose tolerance during pregnancy. American Journal of Obstetrics and Gynecology. 1998;**179**(1):156-165

[122] Group HSCR, Metzger BE, Lowe LP, Dyer AR, Trimble ER, Chaovarindr U, et al. Hyperglycemia and Adverse Pregnancy Outcomes. New England Journal of Medicine. 2008;**358**(19): 1991-2002

[123] Panel IA of D and PSGC, Metzger BE, Gabbe SG, Persson B, Buchanan TA, Catalano PA, et al. International association of diabetes and pregnancy study groups recommendations on the diagnosis and classification of hyperglycemia in pregnancy. Diabetes Care. 2010;**33**(3):676-682

[124] Draznin B et al. Management of diabetes in pregnancy: Standards of medical care in diabetes-2022. Diabetes Care. 2022;**45**:S232-S243

[125] Harreiter J, Simmons D, Desoye G, Corcoy R, Adelantado JM, Devlieger R, et al. IADPSG and WHO 2013 gestational diabetes mellitus criteria identify obese women with marked insulin resistance in early pregnancy. Diabetes Care. 2016;**39** (7):e90-e92

[126] Cibickova L, Schovanek J, Karasek D. Changes in serum lipid levels during pregnancy in women with gestational diabetes. A narrative review. Biomed Pap Med Fac Univ Palacký Olomouc Czech Repub. 2021;**165**(1):8-12

[127] Karasek D, Krystynik O, Kucerova V, Macakova D, Cibickova L, Schovanek J, et al. Adiponectin, A-FABP and FGF-19 levels in women with early diagnosed gestational diabetes. Journal of Clinical Medicine. 2022;**11**(9):2417

[128] Simmons D. Paradigm shifts in the management of diabetes in pregnancy: The importance of type 2 diabetes and early hyperglycemia in pregnancy: The 2020 Norbert Freinkel award lecture. Diabetes Care. 2021;**44**(5):1075-1081

[129] Stefánsson E, Olafsdottir OB, Eliasdottir TS, et al. Retinal oximetry: Metabolic imaging for diseases of the retina and brain. Progress in Retinal and Eye Research. 2019;**70**:1-22

[130] Hübnerová P, Mlčák P, Šínová I, Karhanová M, Šín M. Current use of the automatic retinal oximetry. Cesk Slov Oftalmol. 2020;**76**:3-11

[131] Hammer M, Vilser W, Riemer T, Mandecka A, Schweitzer D, Kühn U, et al. Diabetic patients with retinopathy show increased retinal venous oxygen saturation. Graefe's Archive for Clinical and Experimental Ophthalmology. 2009; **247**:1025-1030

[132] Hardarson SH, Stefánsson E. Retinal oxygen saturation is altered in diabetic retinopathy. The British Journal of Ophthalmology. 2012;**96**:560-563

[133] Šínová I, Chrapek O, Mlčák P, Řehák J, Karhanová M, Šín M. Automatic retinal oxymetry in patients with diabetic retinopathy. Ceská a Slovenská Oftalmologie. 2016;**72**:182-186

[134] Jørgensen CM, Bek T. Lack of differences in the regional variation of oxygen saturation in larger retinal vessels in diabetic maculopathy and proliferative diabetic retinopathy. The British Journal of Ophthalmology. 2017;**101**:752-757

[135] Mlčák P, Chlup R, Kudlová P, Krystyník O, Král M, Kučerová V, et al. Retinal oxygen saturation is associated with HbA1c but not with short-term diabetes control, glycaemic variability and internal environment - ROXINEGLYD Study. Acta Ophthalmologica. 2018;**100** (1):E142-E149

[136] Gray RS, Duncan LJP, Clarke BF. Seasonal onset of insulin dependent diabetes in relation to sex and age at onset. Diabetologia. 1979;**17**:29-32. DOI: 10.1007/BF01222974

[137] Fraser DM, Smith AF, Gray RS, Borsey DQ, Sinclair ME, Clarke BF, et al. Glycosylated haemoglobin concentrations in newly diagnosed diabetics before and during treatment. The British Medical Journal. 1979;**1**. DOI: 10.1136/bmj.1.6169.979Duncan

[138] Steel JM, Parboosingh J, Cole RA, Duncan LJP. Prepregnancy counceling: a logical preludeto the managementof the pregnant diabetic woman. Diabetes Care. 1980;**3**(2):371-373. DOI: 10.2337/diacare.3.2.371

[139] Steel JM, LJP D. Contraception for the insulin-dependent diabetic woman: The view from one clinic. Diabetes Care. 1980;**3**(4):557-560. DOI: 10.2337/diacare.3.4.557

[140] Young RJ, Duncan LJ, Paton L, Yap PL. Development of insulin-dependent diabetes in adult-onset hypogammaglobulinaemia. British Medical Journal (Clinical Research Ed.). 1981;**282**:1668. DOI: 10.1136/bmj.282.6277.1668

Chapter 2

The African Face of Childhood Diabetes

Edna S. Majaliwa, Emmanuel Ameyawak, Janet Bulemela and Asmahan T. Abdalla

Abstract

This chapter will talk about diabetes in African children living in Africa. It will cover diabetes, the classification in general, and the gray areas of diabetes in Africa. It will also cover part of the genetics of diabetes around Africa and its shortfall. The chapter will also look at the management of diabetes in an African setting, where insulin is stored in pots, and the challenges that a child with diabetes goes through in Africa. This chapter will be useful for pediatric endocrinologists, pediatricians, adult diabetologists, doctors, nurses, and everyone in the health sector dealing with children with diabetes.

Keywords: diabetes mellitus, sub-Saharan Africa, malnutrition, health care systems, type 1 diabetes mellitus

1. Introduction

Diabetes mellitus is a biochemical disorder caused by the defect in insulin secretion, action, or both, resulting in hyperglycemia [1]. Reduced insulin leads to abnormal metabolism of carbohydrates, fats, and proteins. There are different types of diabetes known globally, namely, type 1 diabetes mellitus (T1DM), type 2 diabetes mellitus (T2DM), gestation diabetes mellitus, and other forms of specific diabetes (e.g., maturity-onset diabetes of the young (MODY), neonatal diabetes, etc.) [2]. However, this classification may be difficult to locate in Africa due to challenges of diagnosis as well as other forms of diabetes that do not follow the global trend like malnutrition-related diabetes, [3] ketosis prone diabetes [4], and fibrocalculus pancreatic diabetes [5]. T1DM is an immune-mediated condition; however, in African people living in Africa, the picture might look different. Apart from the immune-mediated T1DM, which is attributed to most of the patients with type 1 diabetes in sub-Saharan Africa, other patients have diverse forms of type 1 diabetes, which are non-immune-mediated. Few studies done on autoimmunity in T1DM in sub-Saharan Africa showed less than 50% immunogenicity ranging from 30 to 40%. Most of them have a single autoantibody, mainly GAD65. Other forms also fall in the category of T1DM but are not immune mediated.

1.1 Sub-Saharan Africa and diabetes

Sub-Saharan is the term used to describe the area in the continent of Africa that is below the southern border of the Sahara Desert. It is a savanna grassland with some trees. Sub-Saharan Africa has about 42 countries and 5 islands, which are different geographically and culturally. It has a landmass of 23,890,896.1 sqm as o 2020 with 1.17 billion people. The annual population growth is 2.6%, and the GDP per capita is 1.92 (World Bank 2020). The number of prevalent (existing) cases of type 1 diabetes is 1,211,900. The number of incident (new) cases of type 1 diabetes per year is 149,500.

Diabetes mellitus used to be a disease of the developed countries, more so in children. However, the recent global data shows that about 536.6 million adult people with diabetes live in Africa, with the projection of 783.2 million people in 2045. In children up to 19 years, the number is at 1.2 million, with 184,100 new diagnoses each year (IDF Atlas). Among these, 1,211,900 are children aged 0–19 years with type 1 diabetes and 149,500 are those diagnosed yearly with type 1 diabetes. All of these are affected by missed diagnosis, which reaches to about 53.6% of the population in Africa, which is 72 million people (IDF). Few studies have been done on the prevalence and incidences of diabetes in children in Africa, and most of the prevalence studies are hospital based. The few incidence studies that have been carried out range from 1.9 to 11.2/100,000 population (**Table 1**) [6, 7].

There is variation in the incidence of diabetes in children in sub-Saharan Africa by region, with the population in the horn of Africa (e.g., Eritrea 11.2/100,000 population and Sudan 10.3/100,000) [6, 8] more affected compared to western regions (e.g., Nigeria 3.1% and Cote devoir 0.4%) [10, 11]. Probably, these are the regions that have more of missed diagnosis and early deaths, or it is true that there is less incidence of diabetes in those areas.

1.2 The healthcare systems in sub-Saharan Africa

Most of the sub-Saharan African health systems are designed in such a way that they are able to tackle the infectious diseases and their acute patterns. HIV has been a challenging situation, because of its chronicity nature, hence forcing the system to deal with chronic diseases and meeting the global sustainable development goals. The system has not been planned to tackle the NCD (diabetes in sub-Saharan Africa, from clinical care to policy). There is a move by the UN to reduce premature deaths from NCDs by 2030, in which case it requires a lot of co-ordinations that are difficult to achieve right now. As it has been studied, to

Country	Incidence /100,000 population
Sudan	10.3
Eritrea	11.2
Rwanda	2.7
Tanzania	1.8–1.9

Table 1.
Incidence studies of diabetes in children in sub-Saharan Africa [6–9].

manage diabetes, a broad-based health system is needed, which more often than not is not present there. Because of the way sub-Saharan Africa health systems are, most patients with diabetes will likely drop off the system, because the system cannot cater to their needs, including facilities to manage micro- and macrovascular complications; adding it to the present infectious disease program like HIV has not been successful yet.

1.3 Care of children and adults with diabetes

Diabetes care in Africa has been a subject of many challenges especially after being hit by triple burden of HIV, diabetes, and tuberculosis, among other infectious diseases [12]. To add to the fire, the COVID-19 pandemic brought in more challenges to the governments and the healthcare system that was already fragile. The system has been used to cater to acute and infectious conditions rather than chronic infections, which has a different model and high costs.

1.3.1 Types of diabetes in Africa

For the most part, the types of diabetes in sub-Sahara Africa are no more different from the global types. However, very few studies have investigated in detail on diabetes occurring in Africa. Apart from the classical global forms of diabetes, that is, type 1 diabetes, type 2 diabetes, gestational diabetes, and specific genetic types, there have been studies indicating other forms of diabetes that occur in Africa, such as atypical African diabetes, ketosis prone atypical diabetes mellitus, and malnutrition-related diabetes of tropical diabetes [13, 14]. This is a significant challenge in which intervention needs to be set and prevalence of complications observed.

1.3.2 Type 1 diabetes mellitus

T1DM is characterized by deficiency in insulin secretion. Its cause is unknown; however, genetic susceptibility, environmental factors, immune system, and β-cells are implicated. The interaction of these causes immune-mediated beta cell destruction and hence partial/absolute insulin deficiency. There are four stages toward the development of T1DM symptoms: 1. multiple islet antibodies and normal glucose; 2. multiple islet antibodies, raised blood glucose, but no symptoms; 3. islet autoimmunity, raised blood glucose, and symptoms (when the islet cells have diminished to about 90% lost); and 4. long-standing T1DM. However, in sub-Saharan Africa, some patients do not have auto-antibodies, and so it can be confused with other types of diabetes. Management of T1DM can be challenging in Africa because of lack of laboratory support and access to insulin.

1.3.3 Genetics of T1DM

Despite the great leap in technologies and advances in genetic studies in T1DM, numerous gaps in knowledge remain, especially in sub-Saharan Africa. More data and genetic studies from non-European ancestry population are needed to identify novel risk genes and novel variants in known genes. It has to be noted that environmental factors play a major role as the triggering stimulus to develop diabetes even in people with low genetic risk to develop T1DM.

1.3.4 Evidence of the role of genetics in diabetes

The overall risk of T1DM in the general population is 0.4%, but it is higher in relatives of patients. For example, siblings of patients have on average a 6–7% lifetime risk; the risk of T1DM is 1.3–4% in children of a female patient and 6–9% in children of a male patient. While the risk in identical twins with one positive autoantibody reaches up to 60% in some populations and is prone to development of diabetes within three years from detection, accumulated data showed that those with more than two positive autoantibodies will eventually develop diabetes. T1DM in non-identical twins is similar to that in siblings, which is about 6%.

Over the past 40 years, histocompatibility leukocyte antigen (HLA) regions, on chromosome 6p21, have been the first and largest loci that are linked to T1DM susceptibility, namely, class II HLA DR (especially DR3 and DR4) and DQ (mainly DQ2 and DQ8). These genes are felt to alter type 1 diabetes risk by affecting the ability of these class II molecules to bind to and present β-cell protein peptide fragments to T-cells and therefore to activate an autoimmune reaction. Up to 90% of individuals with type 1 diabetes carry either the DR3/DQ2 halotype, which is associated with glutamic acid decarboxylase autoantibody (GADA), or the DR4/DQ8 haplotype, which is associated with insulin autoantibodies (IAA) (both DQ2 and DQ8 are non-Asp alleles). In contrast, while 20% of the population carries the DQ6.2 alleles (with aspartate at position 57), this allele is rare in individuals with type 1 diabetes, marking this as a dominantly protective allele.

1.3.5 Genetics of T1 diabetes mellitus from sub-Saharan Africa

Data from certain areas in the world are very limited including sub-Saharan Africa. A recent study from Sudan by Tamador et al. has concluded that young Sudanese individuals with T1DM generally have similar characteristics as reported from European-origin T1DM populations. However, they have higher rates of DKA and slightly lower autoantibody rates than those reported from European-origin populations and a particularly strong association with *HLA-DRB1*03:01*. Another study from Ethiopia by Shitaye et al., which has studied specifically the Amhara genomes, has concluded that Amhara genomes were distinct from modern European and other African genomes. *HLA-DRB1*03:01 (p = 0.0014) and HLA-DRB1*04 (p = 0.0001)* were positively associated with this form of diabetes, while HLA-DRB1*15 was protective ($p < 0.0001$). This means type 1 diabetes genetic risk score (derived from European data) was higher in patients than in control participants ($p = 1.60 \times 10{-}7$). Interestingly, despite the modest sample size, autoantibody-positive patients revealed evidence of association with SNPs in the well-characterized MHC region, already known to explain half of type 1 diabetes heritability in Europeans.

1.3.6 Pathogenesis of type 1 diabetes

Type 1 diabetes is an insulin-dependent type of diabetes with an onset in childhood extending to early adulthood (≤ 30 years old); however, any age group can be affected.

Its pathogenesis involves three interlinked mechanisms:

Genetic susceptibility, immune system regulation abnormalities, and environmental factors; however, for type 1 b, the pathogenesis is idiopathic. The HLA locus on chromosome P21 contributes about 50% of susceptible genes. The HLA molecules are located close to peptide-binding pockets that are related to disease code alleles (HLA-DR3 or HLA-DR4) with features of antigen display. Then, there are environmental factors that have been associated with triggering the islet cell destructions; this includes some viral infections, for example, cytomegalovirus, which will either induce the destruction of islet cells releasing β-cells antigen that will cause activation of T-cell-mediated reactivation of antibodies, or virus release proteins that resemble β-cell antigen and the immune system cross-reacts with the self-tissue.

Therefore, the autoantibody produced against the islet cell antigens as a result of environmental exposure cause injury to the pancreases of people with genetic susceptibility.

1.3.7 Non-Type 1 diabetes mellitus

Because of lack of fancy laboratory support in sub-Saharan Africa like islet cell autoantibodies and molecular testing, it is sensible to know when to suspect a monogenic form of diabetes or non-type 1 diabetes. Symptoms of diabetes in the first six months of life are defined as neonatal diabetes, which is a rare type of monogenic diabetes due to single gene mutation. Symptoms are usually vague but physicians should be aware of the problem with high suspicion rate. A neonate with unexplained growth failure, dehydration, and irritability with frequent nappy changes (polyuria) although good appetite and frequent breast feeding should be subjected to a simple blood sugar measurement and urine ketones. Blood sugars levels more than 35 mmol/L are not usually a presentation of stress hyperglycemia. Communities with high consanguinity rate are prone to have this kind of gene mutations since most of

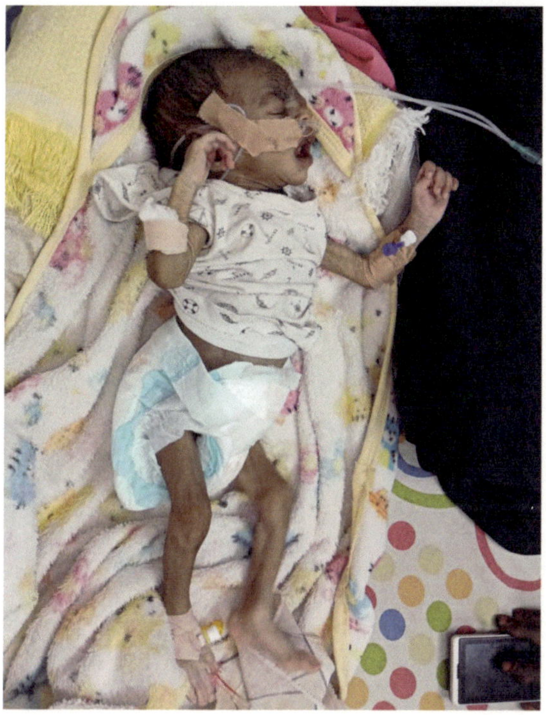

Figure 1.
Neonatal diabetes in sub-Saharan Africa.

the cases are recessive. For example, in Sudan, a country with 45% consanguinity rate, 56% of neonatal diabetes were found to be caused by EIF2AK3 recessive variants causing the Wolcott–Rallison syndrome, which usually presents with skeletal abnormalities and liver dysfunction, while only 8.1% and 5.4% were caused by mutations in KCNJ11 and ABCC8 genes, respectively (*local unpublished data*). This is completely different from what has been reported from Western and Asian populations, where ABCC8 was the commonest cause of neonatal diabetes (**Figure 1**).

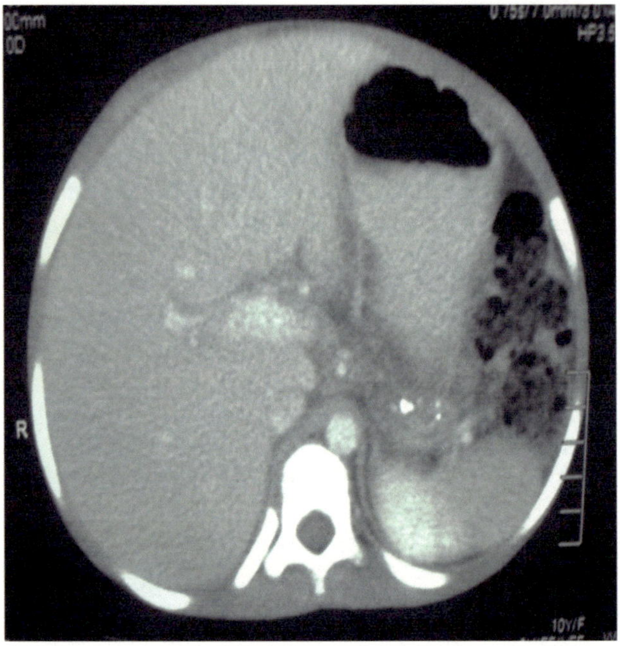

Figure 2.
Fibrocalcular pancreatitis causing diabetes and malnutrition.

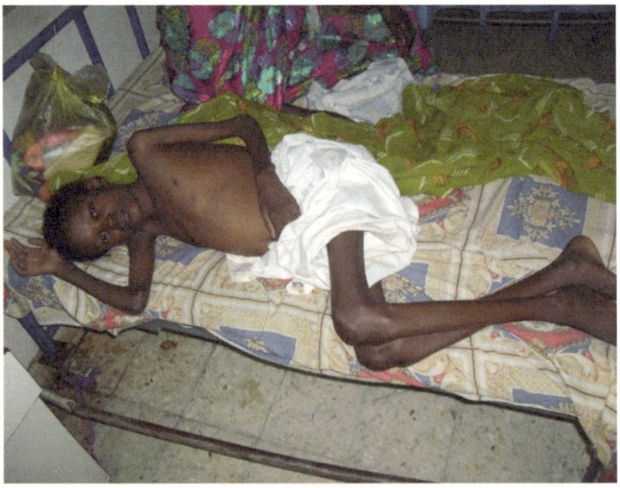

Figure 3.
Diabetes and malnutrition.

Other monogenic diabetes forms like MODY should be suspected clinically even when there is lack of laboratory facilities. A family history of diabetes in three subsequent generations, minimum or no requirements to insulin to maintain euglycemia, and bouts of unexplained hypoglycemia outside the honeymoon period should raise the suspicion of monogenic diabetes. Other clinical supportive findings of monogenic diabetes are presence of megaloblastic anemia that is responsive to thiamin (TRMA), deafness with diabetes insipidus and optic atrophy (DIDMOAD), deafness with renal anomalies in Roger's syndrome, and liver dysfunction and skeletal malformation (WRS). Early detection and correct diagnosis are crucial for a better outcome. Molecular testing is very helpful in such cases whenever feasible.

In a recent study from South Africa, 1643 diabetic adults who were diagnosed to have either type 1 or type 2 diabetes were subjected to molecular testing. A total of 6.6% were found to have monogenic diabetes caused by two genes mutations: HNF41A and GCK polymorphism [15]. This indicates that monogenic diabetes is underdiagnosed in our community, which might result in inappropriate treatment and exacerbation of related illnesses. Awareness should be increased among healthcare professional about when to suspect a non-type 1 diabetes mellitus.

1.3.8 Ketosis prone diabetes

Ketosis prone diabetes is a form of diabetes that is characterized by severe beta cell dysfunction presenting with DKA or unjustified diabetes.

It is a syndrome classified by four systems that are based on: immunological criteria; immunological criteria and insulin requirements; BMI and immunological criteria, or beta cell function. They are all non-autoimmune diabetes with severe insulin deficiency [4]. The classes are non-autoimmune diabetes with DKA, [16] the ketosis-prone insulin-dependent (clinical features of type 1 diabetes) and ketosis-prone non-insulin-dependent clinical characteristics of type 2 diabetes, [17] lean ketosis-prone features of Type 1. and obese Ketosis-prone features with features of type 2 diabetes [18, 19].

However, in Africa, these conditions were present in the past 4–5 decades [20–22]; with the usual characteristics of absence of autoimmunity and beta-cell function reduction in this category, there are those who may need insulin for a short time and those that may need insulin permanently. These patients present with DKA (**Figures 2** and **3**).

2. Presentation and diagnosis

Suspicion of the diagnosis of diabetes mellitus begins with the presence of clinical features, then doing random capillary blood glucose to confirm the diagnosis. Glycated hemoglobin supports the diagnosis. Urine glucose is important for diagnosis, especially in settings where laboratory support and glucometers are a challenge. However, the criteria involve having the symptoms of hyperglycemia and high levels of blood glucose.

The commonest symptoms are tiredness, polyuria, polydipsia, and weight loss despite polyphagia; however, there are other subtle symptoms that may indicate diabetes mellitus, including skin infections such as boils and recurrent fungal infections. Most of the occasions for diagnosis within the context of an acute illness.

It is common to measure random blood glucose either by using capillary blood (using glucometers) or venous blood where laboratory facilities are available. In settings where there are in the diagnosis, the most common form is the severe form of diabetes, where a patient presents with diabetes ketoacidosis (hyperglycemia, acidosis, and ketonemia/ketonuria). At this point, the diagnosis will involve random blood glucose for hyperglycemia greater than 11.1 mmol/L and urine dipstick to look for ketonuria of 2+ or more, weakness, unclear poor growth for children, neglects, and anger of youth.

The finger prick at any time should be the same or exceed 11.1 mmol/L along with clinical symptoms of short duration of loss of weight, polyuria, and polydipsia. This can be done in sick patients or outpatients. Thus, the diagnosis of diabetes is confirmed when:

1. Classical symptoms and signs of diabetes or hyperglycemia crisis and a plasma glucose of ≥11.1 mmol/L or

2. Fasting plasma glucose of ≥7 mmol/L on more than one occasion or

3. Two hours post-glucose load/standard ≥11.1 mmol/L (OGTT)

4. HbA1c > 6.5% two hours post-glucose load ≥11.1 mmol/L (OGTT)

Note: If there are no symptoms, there should be two blood glucose readings tested at different times.

At initial diagnosis, glycated hemoglobin (HbA1c) is an important parameter, but a normal value does not rule out the diagnosis of diabetes. HbA1c is used for monitoring hyperglycemia in 3 monthly checks because of its variation in availability.

Since type 1 diabetes is an autoimmune condition, the likelihood of other autoimmune conditions is high; hence, screening for other autoimmune conditions is important. These include: thyroid profile (TSH, FT4, and FT3) ± coeliac disease. Most of the times, patients in sub-Saharan Africa delay the diagnosis, resulting in a lot of loss in follow-up; therefore, there is need for screening for complications of diabetes, that is, urine examination for micro-albumin, lipid profile—triglycerides and lipoproteins, and renal function tests (serum creatinine, blood urea nitrogen) as well as the assessment for neuropathy using filament touch for sensation.

3. Management

Management of diabetes involves diagnosis of diabetes, which consists of taking history, conducting a physical examination and testing blood to confirm the high level of blood glucose.

Clinical features suggestive of diabetes with random blood glucose (RBG) of 11.1 mmol/L or more confirm diabetes. If there are suggestive clinical features but RBG is less than 11.1 mmol/L, fasting blood glucose test or oral glucose tolerance test (OGTT) and HbA1C are done. Fasting blood glucose of 7 mmol/L or more confirms diabetes. OGTT of 11.1 mmol/L or more after 2 hours confirms diabetes. It is important to do urine routine examination to look for ketone because in Africa many children with diabetes may present for the first time to hospital in diabetic ketoacidosis.

For first-time diagnosis, admit the patient to the ward and stabilize blood glucose with 0.1 units/kg of short-acting insulin until blood glucose level falls to 10 mmol/L or less. Then, put the patient on a multiple dose injection regimen; the total dose is divided over long-acting and short-acting insulin in a ratio of 1:1, that is, 50% each. The short-acting portion is divided into three portions and given at breakfast, lunch, and supper, 30 minutes before meals. The long-acting portion is usually given once a day usually at bedtime. Where an intermediate-acting insulin is given as long acting, the dose is divided into two, and each portion is given in the morning and evening. If there is no food, the patient should skip the short-acting insulin at that specific time. Patients and families are usually taught how to draw the dose, give injection, and adjust the insulin dosage. They are also taught about injection sites and how to rotate the injection sites to prevent ulcers and lipodystrophy.

3.1 Different regimens that are feasible in sub-Saharan Africa

3.1.1 Insulin access and storage

Due to the cost and availability of food, the insulin injection most of the times is not constant; there are different regimen being used, the commonest being multiple dosing regimen and twice daily dose regimen (**Figure 4**). With all these, the storage of insulin is a challenge with many families who store in a pot (**Figure 5**).

3.1.2 Multiple dosing regimen (MDI)

The multiple dose injection regimen is more physiological and usually gives better glycemic control. It involves giving 1–2 injections of basal insulin (long acting) and three or more times of prandial blood glucose. The total dose is divided over long acting and short acting in a ratio of 1:1. It is the recommended dose globally and

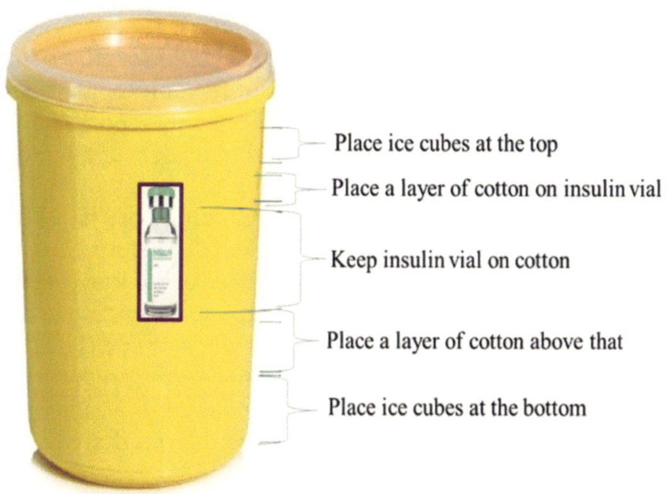

Figure 4.
Improvised container for transportation (courtesy of EADSG-guidelines).

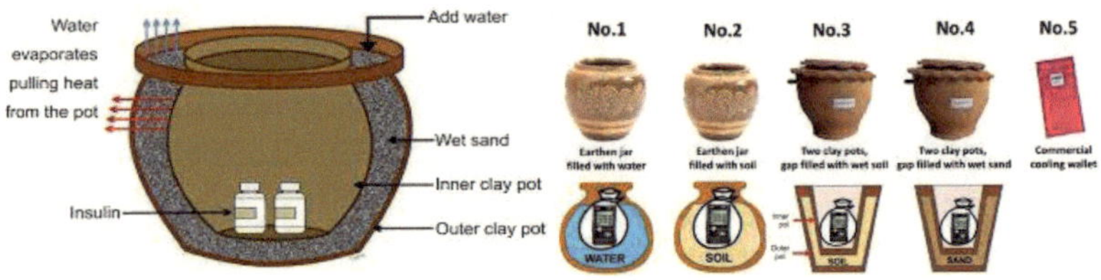

Figure 5.
Local pot for insulin storage.

gives better control; however, in sub-Saharan Africa, it has different challenges from no food to the time of getting food, the insulin access itself, etc.

3.1.3 Twice dosing regimen

This uses pre-mixed insulin, which is a combination of short-acting and NPH insulin insulin in a fixed proportion or a free mixture of regular insulin and intermediate-acting insulin. It is given two times a day. Two-thirds (2/3) of the total dose is given in the morning and 1/3 is given in the evening.

Patients should be educated on insulin use, storage dosage, and Side effects in simple terms and in a dialect they understand; this includes knowledge about insulin injections, injection sites and how to rotate, doses and dose adjustment, how to take care of injection sites, signs of hypoglycemia and its management, and short-term and long-term complications. And in both the regimen, the gadget for delivering insulin is mostly syringes; a few times there are pens, and rarely do they use pumps.

In Africa, a very sensible regimen of insulin use is the premixed Twice-daily dose. It is Cost-effective and available, and patients and their families love it because of the infrequent injections. With the progress of diabetes services in the continent, healthcare professionals (HCPs) started to modify this regimen by adding a fixed pre-lunch dose of short-acting insulin (since it is the biggest meal in most countries). In addition to that, the concept of the basal bolus regimen started to emerge especially among patients coming from the developed side of the world. Endocrinologists in the recent years have seen the benefits of the basal bolus regimen of delivering insulin in the form of a better glycemic control and fewer hypoglycemic bouts. What is currently observed from the developed world is the impact of continuous glucose monitoring on the time one spends in target blood glucose when using pumps and flash glucose monitoring [23–25].

As sweet as it sounds, continuous glucose monitoring goes hand in hand with carb counting, which has many challenges in Africa. Carb counting is a bit difficult in Africa since families eat in one plate, and it is difficult to know the exact amount of food the child is going to eat. To overcome that, a scale system is used based on the blood glucose readings (pre/post meals over a week or so). The daily pattern of the patient is figured out, and a fixed short- or rapid-acting insulin is given before each meal. The second challenge of using a basal bolus regimen is the resistance to regularly and frequently check blood glucose at home even if strips are given for free.

Regarding the insulin pumps, the number of patients who use them started to escalate, specifically among prosperous and highly educated people. The decision to shift a patient to use an insulin pump is not easy. It is highly recommended in

Africa that one should have experienced the use of insulin syringes and a basal bolus or premixed regimen prior to using a pump so as to adapt to the whole concept and learn how to use a syringe in case of any pump breakdown. The cost is still high, although it is subsidized and supported by the Governments of some sub-Saharan countries like Sudan. In spite of that, it still needs a high-class category of people who are dedicated and educated and can afford the pump expenses.

In a mini-survey done at the last African Society of Pediatric and Adolescent Endocrinology's (ASPAE) virtual conference in February 2022, 74% of the endocrinologists from sub-Saharan Africa have never used a pump for their patients. More than 50% of the endocrinologists have never educated their patients about carb-counting because they either do not know how to do it, or they think patients would not understand it, or because of the lack of local food exchange tables. From that survey, 44% of the patients could check their blood glucose twice daily, while about 20% would do it about 4–5 times a day, and these are the patients on the basal-bolus regime. In that survey, it was clear that training should be intensified among doctors about the benefits of basal bolus regimen and insulin pumps whenever feasible. Even for basal bolus regimen, NPH insulin can be used with short-acting insulin since these are much cheaper than insulin analogues.

Premixed insulin regimen, which has been widely used in sub-Saharan Africa, is associated with early diabetes complications like nephropathy and neuropathy in addition to Mauriac syndrome, which is rarely seen nowadays in Western countries. In a recent study from Sudan by Hana Ahmed et al., frequency of nephropathy and retinopathy has been found in 36% and 33% of the patients in the age category 10–18 years, respectively [26]. In another study from Sudan, 88% of the studied population had evidence of peripheral neuropathy [27]. All patients from the two studies were on premixed or modified premixed insulin regimen. Although the sample size was small in the two studies, it still rings a bell that early complications are common among premixed insulin users.

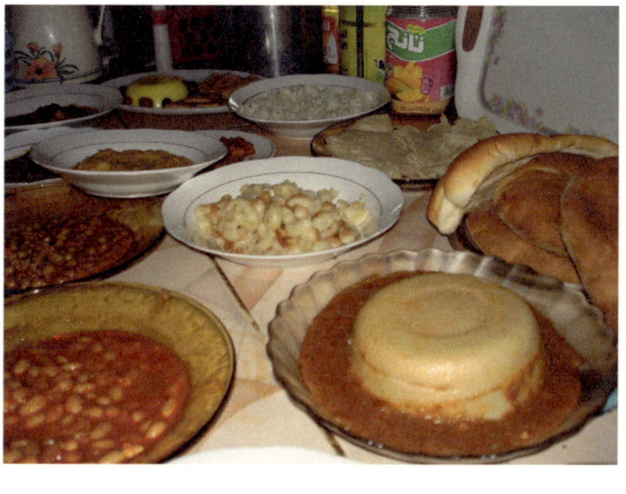

Figure 6.
Readily available foods (Mostly starch).

3.1.4 Diet

Diabetes diet is a balanced diet. It involves a dietician. Highly concentrated sugar drinks such as fizzy soft drinks should be avoided except in periods of hypoglycemia. In the hospital setting, food rich in starch are staple food and readily available; thus, education on portions and limiting consumption of these food types is insisted. Various food types are recommended in all Type 1 diabetes clinics in this setting; this includes proteins such as diaries along with vegetables and fruits.

Difficulties in carb counting are faced because in most of the foods, the carbohydrate content is not estimated (**Figure 6**).

3.1.5 Exercise

Exercise is important for all children with diabetes. Exercise improves insulin sensitivity, cardiac strength, and glucose absorption. Children may not comply with exercise. Involve the whole family because it is good for everyone, and it gives motivation to the patient.

3.1.6 Monitoring and appointments

Diabetic children are asked to monitor and document their blood glucose levels, two to three times a day, at home. Blood glucose logbook is reviewed each visit to the clinic. Based on blood glucose values, the insulin dose can be adjusted to make sure they attain the blood glucose target values.

HbA1C is checked every three months. The HbA1C is used to monitor blood glucose control in patients with diabetes. With good glycemic control, most blood glucose values will be within target ranges and HbA1C will come down to the normal range or closer. For children and adolescents, the desired value is less than 7.5%. In order to achieve better control, target values should be in place. Before meals: 4–7 mmol/L, after meals: 5–10 mmol/L, bed time: 5–10 mmol/L, 3 am: 5–8 mmol/L. The insulin dose is adjusted until most of the blood glucose levels are within the target range.

3.1.7 Screening for complications

It has been shown by different studies that complications start either after a duration of 5 years if a child is pre-pubertal or after 2 years if the patient is diagnosed within/after puberty. This is different from studies done in Africa, where achieving a good control is challenging, screening must be done much earlier after the initial diagnosis and then 1-2 yearly. Hence, every year, the following screening tests should be done:

1. Microalbuminuria. This screens for early kidney damage

2. Eye examination. Fundoscopy should be done by an ophthalmologist to rule out eye diseases

3. Lipid profile

4. Microfilament examination of the limbs to rule out neuropathy

5. ECG, Echoccardiography, etc

In the current century, a very rare diabetes complication is still seen in sub-Saharan Africa, which is Mauriac syndrome. It is a constellation of hepatomegaly, delayed growth, and puberty with cushingoid features in a poorly controlled diabetic. In addition to that, contracted small joints creating what is known as "a prayer sign" is a common clinical sign that junior staff are trained to look for when taking care of patients in the outpatient setting. No recent publication from the region has estimated its prevalence.

Other complications that are seen in the transitional clinics are problems related to final adult height, puberty delay, and infertility. At the same time, adolescents, commonly females, refuse to take frequent insulin injections so as not to gain weight. Learning difficulties like dyslexia and memory disturbances as well as psychological instabilities of poorly controlled diabetic children and adolescents are other serious complications that are not always discovered.

To prevent such complications in the coming future, more epidemiological studies are needed from the region to identify the burden of the disease. Continuous training to the HCP and Enhancing the awareness among the community about diabetes could play a role in improving the delivery and efficiency of diabetes services through better glycemic control, early complications detection, and timely intervention whenever needed. Intensive insulin therapy should always be the practice, targeting better glycemic control and less complications.

4. Challenges: in management of diabetes in Sub-Saharan Africa

Despite the improvement that is taking place, Africa still has a long way to go before realizing the standard of care. There are different challenges affecting the management of diabetes in Africa, including the following:

4.1 Education/awareness

Diabetes mellitus has been termed as a disease of the affluent, so there is a gap of knowledge on diabetes in the society as well as with the healthcare providers. Food security is poor, since majority of the rural clients are dependent and either work in

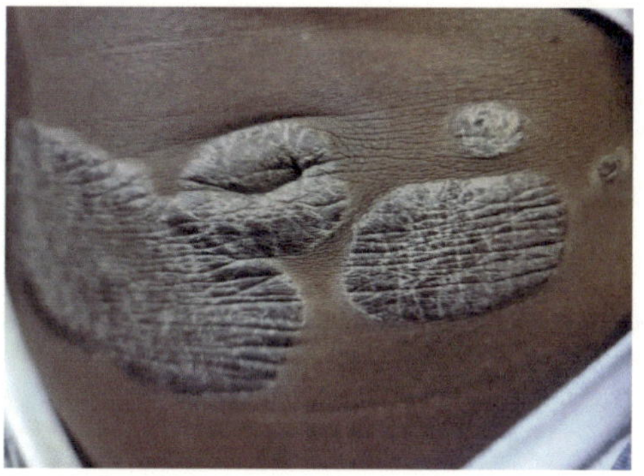

Figure 7.
Local Acanthosis Nigricans at insulin injection site.

seasons in a year as well as are from same families who earn annually. Thus, the food stored is limited and with inadequate distribution interfamily and within the family. At lease every client is able to feed unrefined food but is limited in terms of other sources of food like proteins, minerals, and vitamins.

The independents are either spending time outside to hang with friends with unstandardized meal or skip both meals and take insulin on trial to adjust his or her day.

Fuels may be a problem in early morning; thus, leftovers may be used if well kept. And majority do not have cooling methods to keep big share of raw foods, and the distance to the market or butchers is long (**Figure 7**).

4.2 Healthcare providers

There is inadequate number of healthcare providers for comprehensive management of type 1 diabetes patients in Africa. It is known that in Africa the doctor–patient ratio is low as compared to the Western countries, and the ratio is unacceptably low for the number of pediatric endocrinologists in Africa. So, the available healthcare providers are overwhelmed with work. The few available healthcare providers lack/have less knowledge about the management of diabetes, specifically type 1 diabetes.

An infectious disease burden is still on the rise; hence, there is the double burden of communicable and non-communicable diseases. Unworthy to some workers as a rare disease or unclear management brings a message of difficulty to learn and retain the knowledge. This is comparable to the emergency and outpatient conditions.

4.3 Guidelines

The continent lacks adequate guidelines with local evidence to run diabetes care. Hence, most of the guidelines used are European oriented and hence difficult to adopt and apply to the African environment. The continent still uses the acute care model; however, the chronic care model is still difficult in a setting where most of the conditions are infectious. The existing models are childhood oriented but not for adolescents, and they focus on children's pictures. The young medics prefer electronic ones, which are difficult to use when there is no electricity, and limited digital office infrastructure deploys the use.

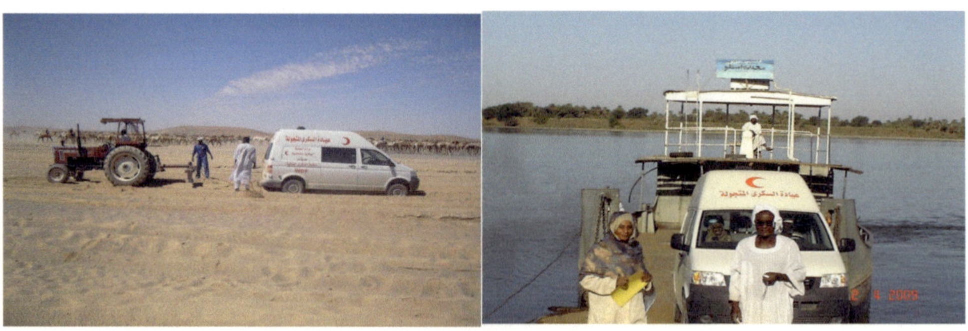

Figure 8.
Challenges in reaching out diabetic children in remote areas.

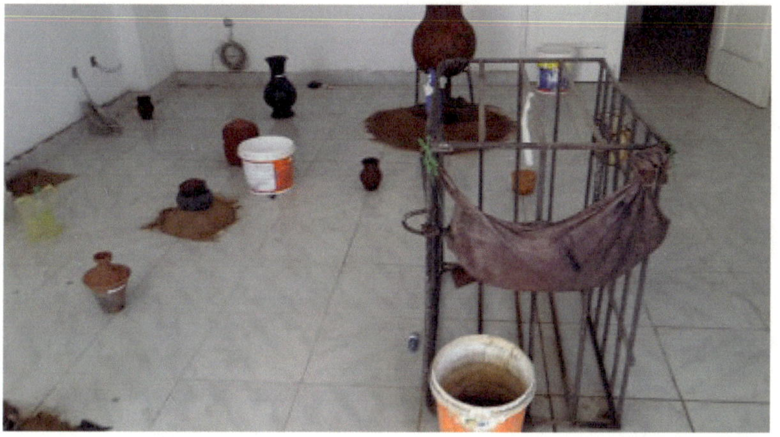

Figure 9.
Clay pot Olympics in Sudan 2016.

4.4 Diagnostic tools and medication

There is lack of diagnostic tools to diagnose, manage, and follow up patients with diabetes, as well as tools to screen for complications; hence, patients are managed poorly. There is generally poor laboratory support especially at the secondary and primary care levels coupled with high cost of supplies such as glucometers, strips, lancets, and insulin.

Despite all these challenges, there are efforts being taken in different countries to manage T1DM, including establishment of clinics specific for T1DM, training of healthcare providers in management of T1DM even if they are not diabetologists, improvement of public–private partnership in order to get support from different organizations, and public awareness campaigns.

Glycated hemoglobin test performed when the supporting programmes deliver of supplies and medicines and few clients are health insured to have this done.

4.5 Distance to healthcare facility

Most African villages are very far from the services, so it takes a long time for a client to reach hospital; they may take two or three days to reach a clinic. Some of the countries have managed to assist with mobile clinic, but most of the countries cannot afford this (**Figure 8**).

4.6 Storage challenges

Lack of fridges and electricity have forced people to use local pots, which is a challenge in temperature control (**Figure 9**).

5. Poor glycemic control

Despite the provision of insulin for those who are being supported by different organizations, their HbA1C is still very high (**Figure 10a** and **10b**).

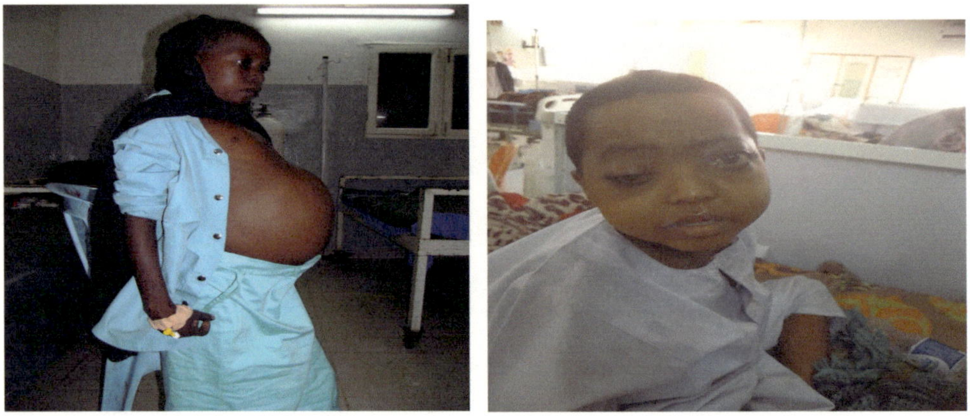

(a) (b)

Figure 10.
(a) Mauriac syndrome and coeliac disease, (b) Mucormycosis of the eyes in a poorly controlled diabetic.

6. Conclusion

Diagnosis and management of type 1 diabetes has improved over the past decade, but there are still challenges. More than a hundred pediatric endocrinologist have been trained from Nairobi, Lagos and Khartoum for the African sub-region, but the continent needs more pediatric endocrinologists for comprehensive care of type 1 diabetes mellitus. More education about type 1 diabetes is needed to improve awareness so that early diagnosis and management can be made.

Author details

Edna S. Majaliwa[1*], Emmanuel Ameyawak[2], Janet Bulemela[3] and Asmahan T. Abdalla[4,5]

1 Paediatric Endocrinologists Muhimbili National Hospital, Dar es Salaam, Tanzania

2 Paeditaric Endocrinologist, Komfo Anokye Teaching Hospital, Kumasi, Ghana

3 St Francis Hospital, Ifakara, Tanzania

4 Sudan Childhood Diabetes Centre, Sudan

5 International University of Africa, Khartoum, Sudan

*Address all correspondence to: ednasiima07@gmail.com

References

[1] Daneman D. Type 1 diabetes. Lancet. 2006;**367**(9513):847-858

[2] Mayer-Davis EJ, Kahkoska AR, Jefferies C, et al. ISPAD Clinical Practice Consensus Guidelines 2018: Definition, epidemiology, and classification of diabetes in children and adolescents. Pediatric Diabetes. 2018;**19**(July):7-19. DOI: 10.1111/pedi.12773

[3] Abdulkadir J. Malnutrition related diabetes mellitus. The Journal of the Association of Physicians of India. 1987;**35**(9):671

[4] Balasubramanyam A, Garza G, Rodriguez L, et al. Accuracy and predictive value of classification schemes for ketosis-prone diabetes. Diabetes Care. 2006;**29**(12):2575-2579. DOI: 10.2337/dc06-0749

[5] Azad Khan AK, Ali L. Tropical calcific pancreatitis and fibrocalculus pancreatic diabetes in Bangladesh. Journal of Gastroenterology and Hepatology. 1997;**12**(6):175-180. DOI: 10.1111/j.1440-1746.1997.tb00458.x

[6] Elamin A, Ghalib M, Eltayeb B, Tuvemo T. High incidence of type I diabetes mellitus in Sudanese children, 1991-1995. Annals of Saudi Medicine. 1997;**17**(4):478-480. DOI: 10.5144/0256-4947.1997.478

[7] Jasem D, Majaliwa ES, Ramaiya K, Najem S, Swai ABM, Ludvigsson J. Incidence, prevalence and clinical manifestations at onset of juvenile diabetes in Tanzania. Diabetes Research and Clinical Practice. 2019:156. DOI: 10.1016/j.diabres.2019.107817

[8] Mebrahtu G, Maniam J, James S, Ogle GD. High incidence of type 1 diabetes in adolescents and young adults in Eritrea. Diabetic Medicine. 2021;**38**:e14544. DOI: 10.1111/dme.14544

[9] Marshall SL, Edidin D, Arena VC, et al. Research: Epidemiology prevalence and incidence of clinically recognized cases of type 1 diabetes in children and adolescents in Rwanda, Africa. Diabetic Medicine. 2015;**32**:1186-1192. DOI: 10.1111/dme.12701

[10] Afoke AO, Ejeh NM, Nwonu EN, Okafor CO, Udeh NJ, Ludvigsson J. Prevalence and clinical picture of IDDM in Nigerian Igbo schoolchildren. Diabetes Care. 1992;**15**(10):1310-1312. DOI: 10.2337/diacare.15.10.1310

[11] Agbre-Yace ML, Oyenusi EE, Oduwole AO, Ake MD, Abodo JR. Prevalence of diabetes mellitus among children and adolescents in the district of Abidjan in Cote d'Ivoire: A population-based study. Journal of Diabetes and Metabolic Disorders. 2016;**15**(1):1-9. DOI: 10.1186/s40200-016-0261-7

[12] Levitt NS. Diabetes in Africa: Epidemiology, management and healthcare challenges. Heart. 2008;**94**(11):1376-1382. DOI: 10.1136/hrt.2008.147306

[13] Hall V, Thomsen R, Henriksen O, Lohse N. Diabetes in Sub Saharan Africa 1999-2011: Epidemiology and public health implications. A systematic review. BMC Public Health. 2011;**11**(564):1-12. DOI: 10.1186/1471-2458-11-564

[14] Alberti G, Zimmet P, Shaw J, Bloomgarden Z, Kaufman F, Silink M. Type 2 diabetes in the Young. Diabetes Care. 2004;**27**(7):1798-1811

[15] Matsha TE, Raghubeer S, Tshivhase AM, et al. Incidence of hnf1a

and gck mody variants in a South African population. The Application of Clinical Genetics. 2020;**13**:209-219. DOI: 10.2147/TACG.S281872

[16] Piñero-Piloña ARP. Idiopathic Type 1 diabetes. Journal of Diabetes and its Complications. 2001;**15**(6):8727

[17] Mauvais-Jarvis F, Sobngwi E, Porcher R, et al. Ketosis-prone Type 2 diabetes in patients of Sub-Saharan African origin. Diabetes. 2004;**53**(3): 645-653. DOI: 10.2337/diabetes.53.3.645

[18] Umpierrez GE, Jones S, Smiley D, et al. Insulin analogs versus human insulin in the treatment of patients with diabetic ketoacidosis: A randomized controlled trial. Diabetes Care. 2009;**32**(7):1164-1169. DOI: 10.2337/dc09-0169

[19] Umpierrez GE, Casals MMC, Gebhart SSP, Mixon PS, Scott Clark W, Phillips LS. Diabetic ketoacidosis in obese African-Americans. Diabetes. 1995;**44**(7):790-795. DOI: 10.2337/diab.44.7.790

[20] Ahren B, Corrigan CB. Intermittent need for insulin in a subgroup of diabetic patients in Tanzania. Diabetic Medicine. 1985;**2**(4):1985

[21] Dodu SRA. Current practice diabetes in the tropics. British Medical Journal. 1967;**2**(June):747-749

[22] Oli JMBG, Tropical DD. Islet cell antibodies and diabetes in. Tropical and Geographical Medicine. 1981;**33**(2):161-164

[23] Battelino T, Danne T, Bergenstal RM, et al. Clinical targets for continuous glucose monitoring data interpretation: Recommendations from the international consensus on time in range. Diabetes Care. 2019;**42**(8):1593-1603. DOI: 10.2337/dci19-0028

[24] Edelman SV, Argento NB, Pettus J, Hirsch IB. Clinical implications of real-time and intermittently scanned continuous glucose monitoring. Diabetes Care. 2018;**41**(11):2265-2274. DOI: 10.2337/dc18-1150

[25] Šoupal J et al. Glycemic outcomes in adults with T1D are impacted more by continuous glucose monitoring than by insulin delivery method: 3 years of follow-up from the comisair study. Diabetes Care. 2020;**43**(1):37-43. DOI: 10.2337/dc19-0888

[26] Ahmed H, Elshaikh T, Abdullah M. Early diabetic nephropathy and retinopathy in patients with type 1 diabetes mellitus attending Sudan childhood diabetes Centre. Journal Diabetes Research. 2020;**2020**:1-8. DOI: 10.1155/2020/7181383

[27] Abuelwafaa N, Ahmed H, Omer I, Abdullah M, Ahmed A, Musa A. Electrophysiological characterization of neuropathy complicating type 1 diabetes mellitus. Journal of Diabetes Research. 2019;**2019**:11. DOI: 10.1155/2019/2435261

Chapter 3

Medical Nutrition Therapy for Type I Diabetes Mellitus

Om Prakash Sah

Abstract

Diabetes mellitus is described by high blood glucose level resulting from deficiencies in insulin secretion, insulin action, or both. Type 1 diabetes is a condition in which pancreatic beta-cell get destructed and leads to absolute insulin deficiency. Lack of insulin causes hyperglycemia, polyuria, polydipsia, polyphagia, body mass loss, dehydration, electrolyte disturbance, and ketoacidosis. MNT necessitates an individualized tactic and effective nutrition self-management education, recommendation, and support. A key component of MNT is the provision of adequate calories for normal growth and development for children and adolescents with T1DM. The patient should monitor their saccharide intake either through saccharide counting or meal planning exchange lists for flexibility and variety in meals. Saccharide intake from whole grains, vegetables, fruits, legumes, and dairy products, with an emphasis on foods higher in fiber and lower in glycaemic load, should be advised over other sources, especially those containing sugars. Saccharide counting is helpful for people with diabetes in managing blood glucose level by tracking the grams of saccharide consumed at meals. All persons with T1DM need a substitute of insulin that mimics normal insulin action. An insulin-to-saccharide ratio can be established for an individual that will guide determinations on the amount of mealtime insulin to infuse.

Keywords: type 1 Diabetes, medical nutrition therapy, carbohydrates counting, glycemic index, glycemic load, insulin, insulin regimens, exchange lists, serving sizes

1. Introduction

Diabetes mellitus is described by high blood glucose level resulting from deficiencies in insulin secretion, insulin action, or both. Insulin is a hormone that is essential for the use or storage of body fuels that are Saccharide, protein, and fat. Beta-cells of the pancreas produce insulin. Persons with diabetes do not produce sufficient insulin; hyperglycemia (elevated blood glucose) occurs with insulin shortage [1] This chapter provides nutritional information regarding nutrients requirement, glycemic content of several foods, adjusting food's saccharide according to the insulin doses, medical nutrition therapy, idea about saccharide count for type 1 diabetic persons, management of blood glucose during exercise, and management of type 1 patient during sick days. This chapter would be helpful for type 1 patients and their caretaker, nutritionist, nurses, and doctors.

1.1 Type 1 diabetes

Type 1 diabetes is a condition in which pancreatic beta-cell get destructed and leads to absolute insulin deficiency. Lack of insulin causes hyperglycemia, polyuria, polydipsia, polyphagia, body mass loss, dehydration, electrolyte disturbance, and ketoacidosis [1].

T1DM has two varieties: immune-mediated and idiopathic.

1. Immune-mediated diabetes mellitus is outcome from an autoimmune devastation of the beta-cells of the pancreas.

2. Idiopathic T1DM states to forms of the disease that have no recognized etiology. Although only a marginal of individuals with T1DM fall into this category. Most of them are of African or Asian origin [2].

At this time there are no known means to thwart T1DM. Persons with T1DM are reliant on exogenous insulin to inhibit ketoacidosis and death. T1DM can develop at any age. Although more cases are diagnosed in people earlier than the age of 30 years, it also occurs in older individuals [1].

Around 17–30% of persons with T1DM have autoimmune thyroid disease., and celiac disease happens in 1–16% of persons contrasted with 0.3–1% in the common population [2]. Children with T1DM should be screened for celiac disease soon after diagnosis. If celiac disease is biopsy-confirmed, children should be placed on a gluten-free diet by a registered dietitian nutritionist (RDN) experienced in managing diabetes and celiac disease [1].

There are two types of normal physiological insulin secretion: continuous basal insulin secretion and incremental prandial insulin secretion, controlling meal-related glucose excursions. Individuals with type 1 and insulin-requiring type 2 diabetes lack both basal and meal-related prandial secretion. Historically, conventional treatment included predetermined or "fixed" insulin doses and following a rigid calorie- and saccharide-controlled meal plan based on the insulin regimen. Some individuals with type 1 and insulin-requiring diabetes still use this method for a variety of reasons, such as age, cost, fewer required injections, lack of access to insulin analogs, personal preference, or prescribing habits of the health care provider [3].

2. Medical nutrition therapy (MNT)

MNT necessitates an individualized tactic and effective nutrition self-management education, recommendation, and support. It is essential for total diabetes care and management. Supervising glucose, HbA1C and lipid level, blood pressure, body mass, and quality-of-life issues is essential in assessing the success of nutrition-related recommendations [1].

The goals of MNT are usually stated as:

- Stabilizing specific dietary suggestions with the limits of insulin therapy

- Minimizing hypoglycemia

- Conforming to ideal growth and development in young people

- Decreasing adverse metabolic and cardiovascular effects of acquired insulin resistance
- Diminish the risks of microvascular problems by maintaining the lowest practicable and safe HbA1C and glucose level.
- Empowering the person having diabetes along with their family members with the right food choices and options to maintain the pleasure of eating.
- Providing practical tools for developing healthy eating patterns rather than focusing on individual macronutrients, micronutrients, or single foods and emphasizing nutrient-dense foods rather than calorie-dense foods.
- Emphasizing the importance of chew count, saccharide count, and portion control to achieve good glycemic control.
- Developing meal planning with patients and sharing plan with the medical team so an insulin regimen could be integrated into the patient's usual lifestyle.

2.1 Energy requirements for T1DM

A key component of MNT is the provision of adequate energy for normal growth and development for children and adolescents with T1DM. Therefore it is important to screen growth by assessing height and body mass every 3 months and recording it on growth charts. Usual energy intake can be adjusted to accommodate growth or to prevent excessive body mass (**Table 1**) [4].

3. Macronutrients distribution and eating patterns

The macronutrients distribution should be based on individualized assessment of current eating patterns and preferences, while keeping total calorie and metabolic goals in mind.

3.1 Saccharide

Evidence is inconclusive for an ideal amount of saccharide intake for an individual with diabetes. The type and amount of saccharide are both important. The patient should monitor their saccharide intake either through saccharide counting or meal planning exchange lists for flexibility and variety in meals.

Guidelines for daily Energy Requirement in Children
4184 KJ + 418.4KJ/year age (for 0–12 years old)
6276–8368 KJ + 418.4KJ/year age > 12 (for females 12–15)
8368–10,460 KJ + 8368KJ/year age > 12 (for males 12–15)
source: [5].

Table 1.
Calculation of energy requirements in T1DM.

Saccharide intake from whole grains, vegetables, fruits, legumes, and dairy products, with an emphasis on foods higher in fiber and lower in glycaemic load, should be advised over other sources, especially those containing sugars. Regulated saccharide at each meal and snack should be provided, with set doses of insulin in diabetics receiving insulin. Visible sugar can be restricted to <10% of total energy intake [5].

Evidence exists that the amount and type of saccharide eaten affect blood glucose level; however, the total amount of saccharide eaten is the primary interpreter of glycemic response. Day-to-day steadiness in the number of saccharide eaten at meals is reported to improve glycemic control, especially in persons on fixed insulin regimens. Whereas in persons with T1DM who adjust their mealtime insulin doses or who are on insulin therapy, insulin doses should be regulated to match saccharide intake [3].

Saccharide counting is an eating plan technique based on the theory that all types of saccharide (except fiber) are digested with the majority being absorbed into the bloodstream and that the total amount of saccharide consumed has a greater outcome on blood glucose elevations than the specific type. Saccharide counting is helpful for people with diabetes in managing blood glucose level by tracking the grams of saccharide consumed at meals. Persons are encouraged to keep protein and fat food sources as steady as possible because they do not importantly disturb blood glucose level even though they require insulin for metabolism.

$$\text{One saccharide count/choice or serving} = \text{Approx. } 10 = -15 \text{ grams of saccharide} \quad (1)$$

Counting saccharide servings provides an accurate 'guess' of how the blood glucose will rise after a meal or a snack. Monitoring total grams of Saccharide by use of saccharide counting remains the key strategy in achieving glycemic control for people with T1DM.

Choice and quality of saccharide depends on Glycemic index (GI) and Glycemic Load (GL) of the food.

3.1.1 Glycemic index and glycemic load

The glycemic index (GI) of food was developed to compare the physiologic influences of Saccharide on glucose. The GI is a method used to categorize food based on how they impact blood glucose. The GI measures the relative area under the postprandial glucose curve of 50 g of digestible Saccharide compared with 50 g of a reference food, either glucose or white bread. The GI does not measure how rapidly blood g lucose level increase. The peak glucose response for individual foods and meals, either high or low GI, occurs at approximately the same [6]. It is the ranking of foods from 0 to 100 based on their immediate effect on blood glucose level (**Table 2**).

Glycemic load (GL) is a ranking system that corrects the glycemic index for the number of saccharide in a typical serving size. We cannot deliberate a food's glycemic

High	(70 and above)
Medium	(56–69)
Low	(55 and under)
source: [5].	

Table 2.
The common classification of GI of foods is as follows:

High	≥ 20
Medium	11 to 19
Low	≤ 10
source: [5].	

Table 3.
Classification of GL.

index without taking the glycemic load into account. The GL takes the GI one step further and quantifies the rise in blood sugar based on the number of saccharide the food contains in a typical serving. The estimated GL of foods is calculated by multiplying the GI by the amount of digestible saccharide and divided by 100 in each food (digestible saccharide = total saccharide – Dietary Fiber)

$$GL = (\text{Digestible saccharide per serving} \times GI)/100 \tag{2}$$

The study found that watermelon has a high GI that is 76 but it is mostly holding water; a typical 100-gram serving of watermelon has 7-gram digestible saccharide. Now the GL of watermelon is 5.32 (76 × 7/100 = 5.32). This categorizes watermelon as a low GL food. So, a typical serving size will not cause a huge spike in blood glucose. Overall the GL is a better reflection of expected blood glucose responses to foods based on how much we usually eat in a serving makes it more useful than the GI (**Table 3** and **Figure 1**).

3.1.2 Fiber and whole grains

The suggestions for fiber intake for people with diabetes are similar to the suggestions for the common public. Diets containing 44 to 50 g of fiber daily improve glycemia; It is unknown if free-living individuals can daily consume the amount of fiber needed to improve glycemia. However, eating foods containing 25 g fiber per

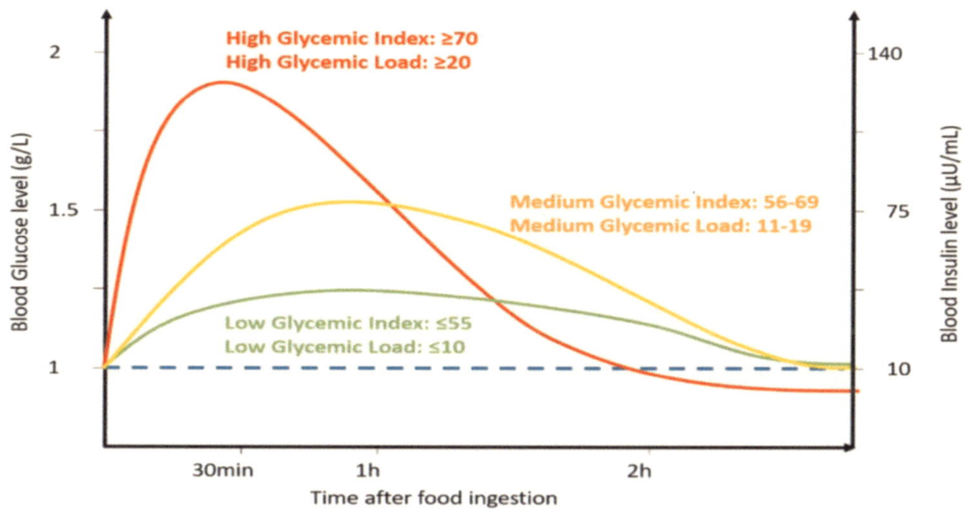

Figure 1.
Schematic diagram of the influence of GI or GL on blood glucose (left axis) or insulin (right axis). Low vs. medium vs. high GI or GL and their corresponding value range are indicated [7].

day for adult female and 38 g per day for adult male is expectant. As with the common people, individuals with diabetes should eat at least half of all grains as whole grains [1].

3.1.3 Saccharide distribution across meals

There are two main Eating tactics for using saccharide counting; using insulin-to-saccharide ratios to regulate premeal insulin doses for variable saccharide intake, or following constant saccharide eating plan when using fixed insulin regimens. Testing pre and post-meal blood glucose level is significant for making regulations in either food intake or medication to achieve blood glucose goals.

Depending on the type of insulin prescribed, mid-meal and bedtime snacks may or may not be necessary. For example, if the patient is on a combination of long-acting and rapid-acting analog insulin, a mid-meal, and a bedtime snack are not necessary. However, if a patient is on conventional premix insulin or regular insulin before meals and intermediate-acting insulin pre-dinner, a mid-meal and a bedtime snack are important.

For patients on rapid-acting insulin, low saccharide-containing foods should be prescribed at mid-meals or the patient must take rapid-acting insulin for a saccharide-containing snack based on his insulin to saccharide ratio [5].

3.2 Protein

Protein intake goals should be individualized based on current eating patterns as well as the presence of other comorbidities.

3.2.1 Recommendations for protein intake

The amount of protein usually consumed by persons with diabetes (15–20% of energy intake) has the smallest acute effects on glycemic response, lipids, and hormones, and no long-term effect on insulin supplies. For people with diabetes, evidence is indecisive to recommend an ideal amount of protein intake for enhancing glycemic control or improving CVD risk factors; therefore aims should be individualized [3]. 20–25% of the total calories from protein sources is recommended by the International Society for Pediatric and Adolescents with diabetes [8]. Prefer 50% of protein intake from high biological value protein. Protein intake with every meal is suggested to reduce the glycaemic response. For those with diabetic kidney disease, dietary protein should be kept at 0.8 g/kg body mass/day. Individualization is the key.

Although nonessential amino acids go through gluconeogenesis, in well-controlled diabetes, the glucose generated does not appear in the general circulation; the glucose generated is likely stored in the liver as glycogen. When glycolysis occurs, it is unknown if the primary source of glucose was saccharide or protein. Although protein is just as potent a stimulant of acute insulin proclamation as saccharide, it has no long-term outcome on insulin needs. Totaling protein to the treatment of hypoglycemia does not stop subsequent hypoglycemia and the addition of protein only adds up unnecessary and usually annoying calories. Furthermore, protein does not lengthy the absorption of Saccharide and should not be added to snacks (or meals) to counteract hypoglycemia [1].

3.3 Fats

Fats are an essential part of a healthy diet and they should not be evaded they should be consumed daily. Evidence is uncertain for an ideal amount of total fat intake for people with diabetes. Therefore, goals should be individualized. Fat quality appears to be far more imperative than quantity.

The amount of dietary fat, cholesterol, and trans-fat recommended for people with diabetes is the same as that recommended for the general population, i.e. >10% of Total energy intake (TEI) from monounsaturated fatty acid (MUFA), of TEI from polyunsaturated fatty acid (PUFA), of TEI from saturated fatty acid (SFA) and nil Trans-fats. Besides glycaemic index and glycaemic load, saccharide counting does not take into account protein or fat content but, stimulation of insulin release is multifactorial [5].

Protein and fat, if consumed in large amounts can slow down the breakdown of Saccharide from the meal causing the blood glucose level to rise gradually. Fat delays gastric emptying releasing glucose slowly and hence does not cause an immediate spike in blood glucose level.

3.4 Alcohol

Risks related to alcohol intake include hypoglycemia (particularly for those using insulin or insulin secretagogue therapies), body mass gain, and hyperglycemia (for those consuming excessive amounts). In adults with diabetes, intake should be limited to one drink per day or less for women and two drinks per day or less for men. One standard drink is equal to 12 ounces of regular beer, 5 ounces of wine, and 1.5 ounces of distilled spirits [5].

3.5 Micronutrients

There is no clear evidence of benefit from vitamin or mineral supplementation in people with diabetes who do not have an underlying deficiency. In limited groups such as the elderly, pregnant or lactating women, strict vegetarians, or those on calorie-restricted diets, a multivitamin supplement may be needed. A diet that is low in sodium (less than 2300 mg per day) can help manage blood pressure [5].

4. Insulin

Insulin is a hormone produced in the β-cells of the pancreas, which are part of the Islets of Langerhans. β-cells release insulin, with each meal and help the body use or store the blood glucose. In type 1 diabetes, the pancreas no longer secrets insulin. The β-cells have been destroyed and they need insulin shots to use glucose from meals.

4.1 Types of insulin

4.1.1 Rapid-acting insulin

Insulin lispro (Humalog), insulin aspart (Novolog), and insulin glulisine (Apidra) are rapid-acting insulins. They are used as bolus (premeal or prandial) insulins. They are insulin analogs that contrast with human insulin in amino acid sequence. It binds to insulin receptors and thus functions like human insulin (**Table 4**).

Rapid-Acting	Onset of Action	Peak Action	Usual Effective Duration
Insulin lispro (Humalog)	<0.25–0.5 hr	0.5–2.5 hr	3–6.5 hr
Insulin aspart (NovoLog)	<0.25 hr	0.5–1.0 hr	3–5 hr
Insulin glulisine (Apidra)	<0.25 hr	1–1.5 hr	3–5 hr

Adapted from Kaufman FR editor: Medical management of type 1 diabetes, ed 6, Alexandria, Va, 2012, American Diabetes Association.

Table 4.
Rapid-acting insulin.

4.1.2 Regular insulin

Short-acting insulin with a gentler onset of action and later activity peak. For the greatest outcomes, the slow onset of regular insulin requires it to be taken 30 to 60 minutes before meals (**Table 5**).

4.1.3 Intermediate-acting insulin

The only available intermediate-acting insulin is NPH and is cloudy in form (**Table 6**).

4.1.4 Long-acting insulins

Insulin glargine (Lantus) and insulin detemir (Levemir) are long-acting insulins. Insulin glargine is slow dissolution at the injection site, resulting in a relatively constant and peakless delivery over 24 hours. it is usually given at bedtime. However, it can be given before any meal, but, whichever time is chosen, it must be given constantly at that time. Insulin determir is absorbed relatively quickly from the subcutaneous tissue and then binds to albumin in the bloodstream, resulting in a lengthy action time of approximately 17 hours. Generally, it is given twice a day. It decreases the chances of nocturnal hypoglycemia (**Table 7**).

Short-Acting	Onset of Action	Peak Action	Usual Effective Duration
Regular (Humulin R and Novolin R)	0.5–1 hr	2–3 hr	3–6 hr

Adapted from Kaufman FR editor: Medical management of type 1 diabetes, ed 6, Alexandria, Va, 2012, American Diabetes Association.

Table 5.
Regular insulin.

Intermediate-Acting	Onset of Action	Peak Action	Usual Effective Duration
NPH	2–4 hr	4–10 hr	10–16 hr

Adapted from Kaufman FR editor: Medical management of type 1 diabetes, ed 6, Alexandria, Va, 2012, American Diabetes Association.

Table 6.
Intermediate-acting insulin.

Long-Acting	Onset of Action	Peak Action	Usual Effective Duration
Insulin glargine (Lantus)	2–4 hr	Peakless	20–24 hr
Insulin determir (Levemir)	0.8–2 hr. (dose dependent)	Peakless	12–24 hr. (dose dependent)

Adapted from Kaufman FR editor: Medical management of type 1 diabetes, ed 6, Alexandria, Va, 2012, American Diabetes Association.

Table 7.
Long-acting insulin.

Mixtures	Onset of Action	Peak Action	Usual Effective Duration
70/30 (70% NPH, 30% regular)	0.5–1 hr	Dual	10–16 hr
Humalog Mix 75/25 (75% neutral protamine lispro [NPL], 25% lispro)	<0.25 hr	Dual	10–16 hr
Humalog Mix 50/50 (50% protamine lispro, 50% lispro)	<0.25 hr	Dual	10–16 hr
NovoLog Mix 70/30 (70% neutral protamine aspart [NPA], 30% aspart)	<0.25 hr	Dual	15–18 hr

Adapted from Kaufman FR editor: Medical management of type 1 diabetes, ed 6, Alexandria, Va, 2012, American Diabetes Association.

Table 8.
Premixed insulin.

4.1.5 Premixed insulin

Premixed insulins are fixed component preparations of rapid or short-acting and intermediate- or long-acting insulins for both fasting and postprandial glycemic control [9]. Persons using premixed insulins must eat at specific times and be consistent in saccharide intake to prevent hypoglycemia (**Table 8**).

4.1.6 Insulin regimens

All persons with T1DM need a substitute of insulin that mimics normal insulin action. To mimic normal insulin action, rapid-acting (or short-acting) insulin is given before meals, and this is meant as bolus insulin. Bolus insulin doses are corrected based on the number of saccharide in the meal.

An insulin-to-saccharide ratio can be established for an individual that will guide determinations on the amount of mealtime insulin to infuse. Basal (Long-acting) insulin dose is the amount of insulin required in the post absorptive state to control endogenous glucose output primarily from the liver. Basal insulin also limits lipolysis and the surplus flux of free fatty acids to the liver. These physiologic insulin regimens allow added flexibility in the type and timing of meals.

For normal persons with T1DM, the required insulin dosage is about 0.5 to 1 unit/kg of body mass per day. About half percentage of the total daily insulin dose is used to provide for basal insulin needs. The remainder (rapid-acting insulin) is divided among the meals by giving about 1 to 1.5 units of insulin per 10 to 15 g of saccharide consumed. As a result of the presence of higher level of counterregulatory hormones in the morning, many individuals may require larger doses of mealtime insulin for saccharide consumed at breakfast than for meals later in the day. The type and timing of insulin regimens should be customized based on eating and exercise habits and blood glucose level [1].

4.2 Insulin guidelines

It is often necessary to regulate insulin dosage to prevent hypoglycemia. This occurs most often with moderate to energetic activity lasting more than 45 to 60 minutes. For most persons, a modest decrease (of about 1 to 2 units) in the rapid- (or short-) acting insulin during the period of exercise is a suitable starting point. For lengthy vigorous exercise, a larger decrease in the total daily insulin dosage may be essential. After exercise, insulin dosing also may have to be reduced [1].

4.3 Insulin substitution therapy

Insulin replacement therapy, also referred to as intensive insulin therapy or basal-bolus therapy, is a comprehensive approach to helping patients achieve optimal blood glucose control by mimicking the physiologic delivery of insulin. This approach uses current understanding of factors affecting glucose homeostasis to permit patients to use flexible insulin dosing to match their lifestyles and preferences.

For Type 1 diabetes, a basal-bolus regimen with a long-acting analog and a short- or rapid-acting insulin analog is the most physiologic insulin regimen and the best option for optimal glycemic control [10].

4.3.1 Diabetes technology

Diabetes technology is described as the hardware, devices, and software that people with diabetes use to help manage their condition, from lifestyle to blood glucose levels. Traditionally, diabetes technology has been divided into two main classes: insulin administered by syringe, pen, or pump, and continuous glucose monitor (CGM). More recently, diabetes technology has gotten bigger to include hybrid devices that both monitor glucose and deliver insulin, some automatically, as well as software that serves as a medical device, providing diabetes self-management support [11].

I. Self-Monitoring of Blood Glucose (SMBG)

People who are on insulin using SMBG should be inspired to test when appropriate based on their insulin regimen. This may include testing when fasting, preceding meals and snacks, at bedtime, before exercise, when low blood glucose is suspected, after treating low blood glucose until they are normoglycemic, and earlier and while performing critical tasks.

When suggesting SMBG, ensure that patients gather ongoing instruction and regular evaluation of technique, results, and their ability to use data, including uploading/sharing data (if applicable), from SMBG devices to adjust therapy. SMBG is especially significant for insulin-treated patients to monitor for and avoid hypoglycemia and hyperglycemia. A database study on children and adolescents with type 1 diabetes presented that, after adjustment for multiple confounders, increased daily frequency of SMBG was significantly associated with lower A1 [11].

II. Continuous Glucose Monitoring Devices (CGM)

People using CGM devices need to have the ability to perform self-monitoring of blood glucose to calibrate their monitor and/or verify readings if discordant with their symptoms. For optimal CGM device operation and ongoing use, robust

Type of CGM	Description
Real-time CGM (rtCGM)	CGM systems that measure and display glucose levels continuously
Intermittently scanned CGM (isCGM)	CGM systems that measure glucose levels continuously but only display glucose values when swiped by a reader or a smartphone
Professional CGM	CGM devices that are placed on the patient in the provider's office (or with remote instruction) and worn for a discrete period of time (generally 7–14 days). Data may be blinded or visible to the person wearing the device. The data are used to assess glycemic patterns and trends. These devices are not fully owned by the patient - they are a clinic-based device, as opposed to the patient-owned rtCGM/isCGM devices.

Table 9.
Continuous glucose monitoring (CGM) devices.

diabetes education, training, and support are required. There are two basic types of CGM devices: those that are owned by the user, un-blinded, and intended for frequent/continuous use, and those that are owned and applied in/by the clinic, which provides data that is blinded or unblended for a discrete period (professional CGM). **Table 9** provides the definitions for the types of CGM devices [11].

When used properly, real-time continuous glucose monitors in conjunction with multiple daily injections and continuous subcutaneous insulin infusion, and other forms of insulin therapy is a valuable tools to lower and/or retain A1C levels and/or reduce hypoglycemia in adults and youth with diabetes.

When used properly, intermittently scanned continuous glucose monitors in conjunction with multiple daily injections and continuous subcutaneous insulin infusion and other forms of insulin therapy can be useful and may drop A1C levels and/or decrease hypoglycemia in adults and youth with diabetes to replace self-monitoring of blood glucose.

The use of professional CGM and/or intermittent real-time or intermittently scanned CGM can be helpful in identifying and correcting patterns of hyper- and hypoglycemia and improving A1C levels in people with diabetes on noninsulin as well as basal insulin regimens [11].

5. Diet-planning strategies

Dietitians offer several diet planning stratagems to help diabetic people for maintaining glycemic control. These stratagems emphasize control of saccharide intake and portion sizes. People using intensive insulin therapy must learn to match insulin injections with meals and to match insulin dosages to saccharide intake.

The first step is to determine an appropriate saccharide intake and suitable distribution pattern; an example is shown in **Table 9**. With the help of nutrition assessment, a person's usual energy and saccharide intake are estimated. Frequent monitoring of blood glucose levels can help determine whether additional saccharide restriction would be helpful [12]. We cannot consider a food's glycemic index without taking the glycemic load into account (**Table 10**).

The sample given in **Table 9** illustrates a meal pattern for a person consuming 8373.6 KJ (2000 Kcal) daily with a saccharide allowance of 50% of KJ.

Meals	Saccharide Allowance	
	Grams	**Portions(15 g carbohydrate)**
Breakfast	60	4
Lunch	60	4
Afternoon snack	30	2
Evening snack	30	2
Dinner	75	5
Totals	**255 g**	**17**

Table 10.
Sample saccharide distribution for 8373.6 KJ.

$$\text{Calculation}: \ 50\% \times 2000 \ \text{Kcal} = 250\text{g saccharide per day}$$

$$1000\text{Kcal of saccharide} \div 4\text{kcal/g saccharide} = 250\text{g saccharide per day}$$

$$250\text{g saccharide} \div 15\text{g} \left(1 \text{ saccharide portion} = 16.7 \text{ saccharide portions per day}\right)$$

Secondly, in type 1 diabetes, the insulin regimen must manage with the individual's dietary and lifestyle choices. People using conventional insulin treatment must maintain a consistent saccharide intake from day to day to tally their particular insulin prescription, whereas those using intensive therapy can adjust insulin dosages when carbohydrate intakes change.

Saccharide counting can be done either by counting the grams of saccharide provided by foods or by counting saccharide portions, expressed in terms of servings that contain approximately 15gm each. **Appendix 1** shows the serving size of different foods group containing 15gm saccharide, which is one saccharide count. One person

Sample menu	
Foods	**Carbohydrate Portions**
Breakfast: **Carbohydrate goal = 4 portions or 60 g**	
3/4c unsweetened, ready-to-eat cereal	1
1/2 c low-fat milk	½
1 scrambled egg	–
1 slice whole-wheat toast (with margarine or butter)	1
170 g orange juice	1 ½
Lunch: **Carbohydrate goal = 4 portions or 60 g**	
2/3 c cooked rice	2
Red gram, dal (raw wt. 30 g)	1
vegetables combination (including carrots, broccoli, and/or dark green leafy) cooked, made with oil; 125 g	1/2
Cucumber salad; 100 g	1/2

Sample menu	
Foods	**Carbohydrate Portions**
Afternoon snack: **Carbohydrate goal = 2 portions or 30 g**	
2 sandwich cookies	1
1 medium apple	1
Dinner: **Carbohydrate goal = 5 portions or 75 g**	
3 chapati (Raw weight flour = 70 g)	3
Palak-paneer (Paneer-50 g; Spinach-100 g)	½
Red gram, dal (raw wt. 30 g)	1
½ small baked potato (with margarine or butter)	½
Bed-time snack: **Carbohydrate goal = 2 portions or 30 g**	
1 c low-fat millk	1
1 slice whole-wheat toast	1

Table 11.
Translating saccharide portions into a Day's meals.

learned the basic saccharide counting method, individuals can select whatever foods they wish as long as they do not exceed their saccharide goals.

Sample menu for type 1 diabetic people done by translating saccharide portions into day's meals (**Table 11**).

6. Sick day guidelines/enteral feeds

It is extremely important to educate individuals with type 1 diabetes and their caretakers about the signs and symptoms of a sick day and its management. If sick days are neglected or not managed well it can result in hyperglycemia, hypoglycemia, diabetic ketoacidosis (DKA), hyperosmolar hyperglycaemic state (HHS), or any adverse effect leading to hospital admission. More than hypoglycemia, hyperglycemia and diabetic ketoacidosis are the major causes of hospital admissions during acute illness.

6.1 Principles for sick day management for individuals with type 1 diabetes

- Diabetes medications (insulin/oral agents) must never be stopped. However, it needs to be adjusted based on blood glucose level.

- It is advisable to frequently monitor blood glucose level every two or three hours including at night.

- If blood glucose is >14 mmol/L, check ketones.

- If blood glucose is 15–20 mmol/L with or without ketosis, it is advisable to give 10–20% of the total daily insulin dose (or 0.1 units/kg body mass) as short-or rapid-acting insulin analogue every 2 to 4 hours until blood glucose falls to <15 mmol/L.

- Eating and drinking can be a challenge during sick days. Include food that is easy on the stomach such as rice and curd, and khichdi. If these foods are also difficult to digest, include liquids that contain Saccharide. Aim for 15 grams of saccharide every three to four hours. This may include food containing saccharide like fruit juice, pudding, and fruit-flavored yogurt to prevent hypoglycemia and also maintain some caloric intake.

- In case of hypoglycemia i.e. blood glucose <3.88 mmol/L, reduce insulin dosage by 20 to 50%. In case of severe hypoglycemia where a child is also unconscious or having fits or completely incapable of taking glucose orally, glucagon injection may be useful in reversing the symptoms of hypoglycemia.

- A standard enteral formula (50% saccharide) or a lower-saccharide (33—40% saccharide) formula may be used in individuals with diabetes. At least 30% of total energy should be given as lipid. Drinking adequate amounts of fluids and ingesting saccharide are important [5].

7. Non-nutritive sweeteners

Lowered calorie sweeteners permitted by the Food and Drug Administration (FDA) include sugar alcohols (erythritol, sorbitol, mannitol, xylitol, isomalt, lactitol, and hydrogenated starch hydrolysates) and tagatose. They deliver a lower glycemic response and contain, on average, 2 calories per gram. Sugar alcohols produce a decreased postprandial glucose response than sucrose or glucose and have lower accessible energy but need to be used with carefulness in TIDM children since they can lead to osmotic diarrhea. Sugar alcohols are partly absorbed, hence only half of the Saccharide from sugar alcohols contributes to total saccharide intake [5]. FDA approved sweeteners list is listed in **Table 12**.

FDA approved Sweeteners	Accepted daily intake (ADI) (mg/kg body mass)
Sucralose	5 mg/kg body mass/day
Aspartame	50 mg/kg body mass/day
Acesulfame K (Contraindicated in hyperkalemia)	15 mg/kg body mass/day
Saccharin (Contraindicated in Pregnancy)	5 mg/kg body mass/day
Steviol glycosides	4 mg/kg body mass/day
Siraitia grosvenorii Swingle (Luo Han Guo) fruit extracts (SGFE)	Not Specified
Advantame	32.8 mg/kg body mass/day
Neotame	0.3 mg/kg body mass/day

Source: Adapted from U. S Department of Health and Human Services (2015).

Table 12.
Common artificial sweeteners.

8. Physical activity/exercise

The physical activity comprises bodily movement fabricated by the tightening of skeletal muscles that requires energy expenditure in surplus of resting energy expenditure. Exercise is a subsection of physical activity: planned, structured, and repetitive bodily movement executed to improve or maintain one or more components of physical fitness.

Physical activity should be a vital part of the treatment plan for persons with diabetes. Exercise aids all persons with diabetes improve insulin sensitivity, diminishing cardiovascular risk factors, controlling body mass, and improving well-being.

In persons with T1DM, the glycemic response to exercise varies, contingent on overall diabetes control, plasma glucose, and insulin level at the start of exercise; timing, intensity, and duration of the exercise; previous food intake; and previous conditioning. A significant variable is the level of plasma insulin during and after exercise. Hypoglycemia can arise because of insulin-enhanced muscle glucose uptake by the exercising muscle.

Hypoglycemia is a possible problem associated with exercise in persons taking insulin or insulin secretagogues. Hypoglycemia can ensue during, immediately after, or many hours after exercise. This is because of increased insulin sensitivity after exercise and the need to supply liver and muscle glycogen, which can take up to 24 to 30 hours.

Hyperglycemia also can consequence from the exercise of high intensity, likely because of the effects of counterregulatory hormones. When a person exercises at what for him or her is a high level of exercise strength, there is a greater-than-normal increase in counterregulatory hormones. As a result, hepatic glucose release beats the rise in glucose use. The raised glucose level also may spread into the post-exercise state. Hyperglycemia and worsening ketosis also can consequence in persons with T1DM who are deprived of insulin for 12 to 48 hours and are ketotic. Vigorous activity should be escaped in the presence of ketosis [2]. It is not, however, necessary to delay exercise based simply on hyperglycemia, provided the individual senses well and urine and/or blood ketones are negative. High-intensity exercise is more likely to be the reason for hyperglycemia than insulin deficiency.

8.1 Exercise guidelines

8.2 Saccharide for insulin or insulin Secretagogue users

Through moderate-intensity exercise, glucose uptake is increased by 8 to 13 g/hr.; this is the basis for the suggestion to add 15 g of saccharide for every 30 to 60 minutes of activity (depending on the intensity) over and above normal practices. Moderate exercise for less than 30 minutes usually does not need any additional saccharide or insulin adjustment, unless the individual is hypoglycemic earlier than the start of exercise. Added Saccharide should be consumed if pre-exercise glucose level are less than 5.6 mmol/L.

For the exerciser with diabetes whose blood glucose level may plunge sooner and lower than the exerciser without diabetes, feeding saccharide after 40 to 60 minutes of exercise is significant and also may support in preventing hypoglycemia. Drinks comprising 6% or less of saccharide empty from the stomach as quickly as water and have the advantage of providing both needed fluids and Saccharide. Consuming Saccharide immediately after exercise improves the repletion of muscle and liver glycogen stores. For the exerciser with diabetes, this takes on added value because of the increased risk for late-onset hypoglycemia [1].

9. Exchange lists for diabetes

The exchange system sorts foods into groups by their proportions of carbohydrate, fat, and protein. Each food list comprises foods grouped together because they have similar nutrient content and serving sizes. Then any food on a list can be "exchanged" for any other on that same list. Foods on the Starch list, Fruits list, Milk list, and Sweets, Desserts, and Other Carbohydrates list are similar because they contain 12 to 15 grams of carbohydrate per serving.

9.1 Serving sizes

The serving sizes have been carefully adjusted and defined so that a serving of any food on a given list provides roughly the same amount of carbohydrate, fat, and protein, and, therefore, total energy. Any food on a list can thus be exchanged, or traded, for any other food on the same list without significantly affecting the diet's energy-nutrient balance or total kilocalories [12]. Foods are listed with their serving sizes, which are usually measured after cooking. When you begin, measuring the size of each serving will help you learn to "eyeball" correct serving sizes [1]. The amounts of nutrients in one serving from each list are shown in **Appendix 2**.

10. Conclusion

Type 1 diabetes is a condition in which pancreatic beta-cell get destructed and leads to absolute insulin deficiency. Lack of insulin causes hyperglycemia, polyuria, polydipsia, polyphagia, body mass loss, dehydration, electrolyte disturbance, and ketoacidosis. MNT necessitates an individualized tactic and effective nutrition self-management education, recommendation, and support. A key component of MNT is the provision of adequate calories for normal growth and development for children and adolescents with T1DM. The patient should monitor their saccharide intake either through saccharide counting or meal planning exchange lists for flexibility and variety in meals. Saccharide intake from whole grains, vegetables, fruits, legumes, and dairy products, with an emphasis on foods higher in fiber and lower in glycaemic load, should be advised over other sources, especially those containing sugars. Saccharide counting is helpful for people with diabetes in managing blood glucose level by tracking the grams of saccharide consumed at meals. All persons with T1DM need a substitute of insulin that mimics normal insulin action. An insulin-to-saccharide ratio can be established for an individual that will guide determinations on the amount of mealtime insulin to infuse.

Appendices

Appendix 1.

Glycemic index and glycemic load of selected foods.

FOODS	GI	GL
Grains		
Buckwheat	54	16

DOI: http://dx.doi.org/10.5772/intechopen.108619

FOODS	GI	GL
Rice, Basmati	58	22
Rice, Brown	50	16
White bread (avg)	70	10
Whole wheat bread (avg)	77	9
Oatmeal	55	12
Vegetables		
Carrots (avg)	47	3
Peas (green, avg)	48	3
Potato, baked (avg)	85	26
Potato, boiled	88	16
Potato, French fries	75	22
Potato, microwaved	82	27
Pumpkin	75	3
Sweet corn	60	11
Sweet potato (avg)	61	17
Yam (avg)	37	13
Legumes		
Baked beans (avg)	48	7
Broad beans	79	9
Chickpeas (avg)	28	8
Kidney beans (avg)	28	7
Lentils (avg)	29	5
Soy beans (avg)	18	1
Fruit		
Apple (avg)	38	6
Apricot (dried)	31	9
Banana (avg)	51	13
Cherries	22	3
Grapes (avg)	46	8
Kiwi fruit (avg)	53	6
Mango	51	8
Orange (avg)	48	5
Papaya	59	10
Peach, fresh (avg)	42	5
Pear (avg)	38	4
Pineapple	59	7
Raisins	64	28
Watermelon	72	4

FOODS	GI	GL
Dairy Foods		
Milk, full fat	27	3
Milk, skimmed	32	4
Milk, condensed	61	33
Custard	43	7
Ice cream, regular (avg)	61	8
Yogurt, low fat	33	10
Beverages		
Apple juice	40	12
Coca Cola	63	16
Fanta	68	23
Orange juice (avg)	52	12
Snack Foods		
Fish sticks	38	7
Peanuts (avg)	14	1
Popcorn	72	8
Potato chips	57	10
Sugars		
Honey (avg)	55	10
Fructose (avg)	19	2
Glucose	100	10
Lactose (avg)	46	5
Sucrose (avg)	68	7

From Brand Miller J et al.: The new glucose revolution, New York, 2003, Avalon/Marlowe & Company.

Appendix 2.

The following chart shows the amount of nutrients in one serving from each list.

STARCH LIST
The Starch list includes bread, cereals and grains, starchy vegetables, crackers and snacks, and legumes (dried beans, peas, and lentils).
1 starch choice = 15 grams carbohydrate, 0–3 grams protein, 0–1 grams fat, and 334.72 KJ.
1 starch is:
• 1/2 cup of cooked cereal, grain, or starchy vegetable
• 1/2 cup of cooked rice or pasta
• 28.35 g of a bread product, such as 1 slice of bread
• 21.26 to 28.35 g of most snack foods (some snack foods may also have extra fat)

Note: 1 OZ equal to 28.35gm, 1cup(metric) equal to 250 ml.

Food	Serving Size	Food	Serving Size
Bread		**Cereals and Grains**	
Reduced-calorie*	2 slices, (42.5 g)	Barley, cooked	1/3 cup
White, whole-grain, pumpernickel, rye, unfrosted raisin	1 slice, (28.35 g)	Bran, dry, Oat*	1/4 cup
Chapatti, small, 6 inches across	1	Bran, dry,Wheat*	1/2 cup
Cornbread, 1 3/4 inch cube†	1, (42.5 g)	Bulgar (cooked)*	1/2 cup
English muffin	1/2	**Cereals**	
Hot dog bun or hamburger bun	1/2, (28.35 g)	Rice,milled	1/2 cup
Naan, 8 inches by 2 inches	1/4	Wheat, semolina	1/2 cup
Pancake, 4 inches across, 1/4 inch thick	1	Bran*	1/2 cup
Pita, 6 inches across	1/2	Cooked (oats, oatmeal)	1/2 cup
Roll, plain, small	1 (28.35 g)	Puffed	1 1/2 cup
Stuffing, bread†	1/3 cup	Shredded wheat, plain	1/2 cup
Taco shell, 5 inches across†	2	Sugar-coated	1/2 cup
Tortilla, corn, 6 inches across	1	Unsweetened, ready-to-eat	3/4 cup
Tortilla, flour, 6 inches across	1	Couscous	1/3 cup
Tortilla, flour, 10 inches across	1/3 tortilla		
Waffle, 4-inch square or 4 inches across†	1		
Granola		**Crackers and Snacks**	
Low-fat	1/4 cup	Animal crackers	8
Regular†	1/4 cup	**Crackers**	
Grits, cooked	1/2 cup	Round-butter type†	6
Kasha	1/2 cup	Saltine-type	6
Millet, cooked	1/3 cup	Sandwich-style, cheese or peanut butter filling† 3	3
Muesli	1/4 cup	Whole-wheat regular†	2–5 (21.26 g)
Pasta, cooked	1/3 cup	Whole-wheat lower fat or crispbreads*	2–5 (21.26 g)
Polenta, cooked	1/3 cup	Graham cracker, 21/2-inch square	3
Wheat germ, dry	3 Tbsp	Matzoh	21.26 g
Wild rice, cooked	1/2 cup	Melba toast, about 2-inch by 4-inch piece	4 pieces
Starchy Vegetables		Oyster crackers	20
Cassava	1/3 cup	Popcorn (Microwave Popped)	3 cups
Corn	1/2 cup	With butter†*	3 cups
On cob, large	1/2 cob (141.75 g)	No fat added*	3 cups
Hominy, canned*	3/4 cup	Lower fat*	3 cups

Food	Serving Size	Food	Serving Size
Mixed vegetables with corn, peas, or pasta* 1 cup	1 cup	Pretzels	21.26 g
Parsnips* 1/2 cup	1/2 cup	Rice cakes, 4 inches across	2
Peas, green* 1/2 cup	1/2 cup	**Snack Chips**	
Plantain, ripe 1/3 cup	1/3 cup	Fat-free or baked (tortilla, potato), baked pita chips	15–20 (21.26 g)
Potato		Regular (tortilla, potato)†	9–13 (21.26 g)
Baked with skin	1/4 large (85.05 g)	**Beans, Peas, and Lentils** ***The Choices on this List Count as 1 Starch + 1 lean meat.***	
Boiled, all kinds	1/2 cup or 1/2 medium (85.05 g)	Baked beans*	1/3 cup
Mashed, with milk and fat†	1/2 cup	Beans, cooked (black, garbanzo, kidney, lima, navy, pinto, white)*	1/2 cup
French fried (oven-baked)	1 cup (56.7 g)	Lentils, cooked (brown, green, yellow)*	1/2 cup
Pumpkin, canned, no sugar added*	1 cup	Peas, cooked (black-eyed, split)*	1/2 cup
Spaghetti/pasta sauce	1/2 cup	Refried beans, canned‡*	1/2 cup
Squash, winter (acorn, butternut)*	1 cup		
Succotash*	1/2 cup		
Yam, sweet potato, plain 1/2 cup	1/2 cup		

Note: 1cup(metric) equal to 250 ml.
**More than 3 grams of dietary fiber per serving.†Extra fat, or prepared with added fat. (Count as 1 starch +1 fat).‡480 milligrams or more of sodium per serving.*

FRUITS LIST

The Fruits list includes fresh, frozen, canned, and dried fruits and fruit juices. 1 fruit choice = 15 grams carbohydrate, 0 grams protein, 0 grams fat, and 251.04 KJ.

In general, 1 fruit choice is:

- 1/2 cup of canned or fresh fruit or unsweetened fruit juice
- 1 small fresh fruit (113.4 g)
- 2 tablespoons of dried fruit

NOTE: The weight listed includes skin, core, seeds, and rind; 1cup(metric) equal to 250 ml.

Food	Serving Size	Food	Serving Size
Fruit		Orange, small*	1 (184.27 g)
Apple, unpeeled, small	1 (113.4 g)	Papaya	1/2 fruit or 1 cup cubed (226.8 g)
Apples, dried	4 rings	Peaches	

Food	Serving Size	Food	Serving Size
Applesauce, unsweetened	1/2 cup	Canned	1/2 cup
Apricots		Fresh, medium	1 (170.1 g)
Canned	1/2 cup	Pears	
Dried	8 halves	Canned	1/2 cup
Fresh*	4 whole (155.92 g)	Fresh, large	1/2 (113.34 g)
Banana, extra small	1 (113.4 g)	Pineapple	
Blackberries*	3/4 cup	Canned	1/2 cup
Blueberries	3/4 cup	Fresh	3/4 cup
Cantaloupe, small	1/3 melon or 1 cup cubed (311.85 g)	Plums	
Cherries	2	Canned	1/2 cup
Sweet, canned	1/2 cup	Dried (prunes)	3
Sweet fresh	12 (85.05 g)	Small	2 (141.75 g)
Dates	3	Raspberries*	1 cup
Dried fruits (blueberries, cherries, cranberries, mixed fruit, raisins)	2 Tbsp	Strawberries*	1 1/4 cup whole berries
Figs		Tangerines, small*	2 (226.8 g)
Dried	1 1/2	Watermelon	1 slice or 11/4 cups cubes (382.72 g)
Fresh*	1 1/2 large or 2 medium (99.22 g)	Fruit Juice	
Fruit cocktail	1/2 cup	Apple juice/cider	1/2 cup
Grapefruit		Fruit juice blends, 100% juice	1/3 cup
Large	1/2 (311.85 g)	Grape juice	1/3 cup
Sections, canned	3/4 cup	Grapefruit juice	1/2 cup
Grapes, small	17 (85.05 g)	Orange juice	1/2 cup
Honeydew melon	1 slice or 1 cup cubed (283.5 g)	Pineapple juice	1/2 cup
Kiwi*	1 (99.22 g)	Prune juice	1/3 cup
Mandarin oranges, canned	3/4 cup		
Mango, small	1/2 fruit (155.9 g) or 1/2 cup		
Nectarine, small	1 (141.75 g)		

**More than 3 grams of dietary fiber per serving.*

MILK LIST
The Milk list groups milks and yogurts based on the amount of fat they have (fat-free/low fat, reduced fat, and whole).

- Cheeses are on the Meat and Meat Substitutes list (because they are rich in protein).
- Cream and other dairy fats are on the Fats list.

NOTE: In general, one milk choice is 1 cup (8 fluid ounces or ½ pint) milk or yogurt.

Food	Serving Size
Fat-free or low-fat (1%) **1 fat-free/low-fat milk choice = 12 g carbohydrate, 8 g protein, 0–3 g fat, and 418.4 KJ.**	
Milk, buttermilk, acidophilus milk, Lactaid	1 cup
Evaporated milk	½ cup
Yogurt, plain or fl avored with an artifi cial sweetener	2/3 cup (170.1 g)
Reduced-fat (2%) **1 reduced-fat milk choice = 12 g carbohydrate, 8 g protein, 5 g fat, and 502. 08 KJ.**	
Milk, acidophilus milk, kefi r, Lactaid	1 cup
Yogurt, plain	2/3 cup (170.1 g)
Whole **1 whole milk choice = 12 g carbohydrate, 8 g protein, 8 g fat, and 669.44 KJ.**	
Milk, buttermilk, goat's milk	1 cup
Evaporated milk	½ cup
Yogurt, plain	226.8 g

Note: 1cup (metric) equal to 250 ml.

Dairy-Like Foods

Food	Serving Size	Count as
Chocolate milk		
fat-free	1 cup	1 fat-free milk +1 carbohydrate
whole	1 cup	1 whole milk +1 carbohydrate
Eggnog, whole milk	½ cup	1 carbohydrate +2 fats
Rice drink		
flavored, low fat	1 cup	2 carbohydrates
plain, fat-free	1 cup	1 carbohydrate
Smoothies, flavored, regular	283.5 g	1 fat-free milk +2½ carbohydrates
Soy milk		
light	1 cup	1 carbohydrate + ½ fat
regular, plain	1 cup	1 carbohydrate +1 fat
Yogurt		
and juice blends	1 cup	1 fat-free milk +1 carbohydrate
low carbohydrate (less than 6 grams carbohydrate per choice)	2/3 cup (170.1 g)	½ fat-free milk

Dairy-Like Foods		
Food	**Serving Size**	**Count as**
with fruit, low-fat	2/3 cup (170.1 g)	1 fat-free milk +1 carbohydrate

Note: 1cup(metric) equal to 250 ml.

Author details

Om Prakash Sah
Independent Researcher, Nepal

*Address all correspondence to: omsahcnd@gmail.com

References

[1] Franz JM, Evert BA. Krause's food & the nutrition care process (14 ed.). St. Louis, Missouri: Elsevier Inc.; 2017. p. 586

[2] American Diabetes A. Standards of medical Care in Diabetes—2014. Diabetes Care. 2014;**37**(Supplement_1): S14-S80

[3] Evert BA, Boucher JL, Crypress M, Dunbar SA, Franz JM, Nwankwo R, Verdi CL. Nutrition therapy recommendations for the management of adults with diabetes. Diabetes Care, 2014;**37**. DOI: 10.2337/dc14-S120

[4] Chiang JL, Kirkman MS, Laffel LM, Peters AL. Type 1 diabetes through the life span: A position statement of the American Diabetes Association. Diabetes Care. 2014;**37**(7):2034-2054

[5] Bajaj M, Salis S. Diabetes Mellitus. In Clinical Dietetics Manual, Second ed.; Seth, V.; Desai, N., Eds. Elite Publishing House: New Delhi; 2018. pp. 33-50

[6] Brand-Miller JC, Stockmann K, Atkinson F, Petocz P, Denyer G. Glycemic index, postprandial glycemia, and the shape of the curve in healthy subjects: Analysis of a database of more than 1,000 foods. The American Journal of Clinical Nutrition. 2009;**89**(1):97-105

[7] Venn BJ, Green TJ. Glycemic index and glycemic load: Measurement issues and their effect on diet-disease relationships. European Journal of Clinical Nutrition. 2007;**61**(Suppl. 1):S122-S131

[8] Smart CE, Annan F, Higgins LA, Jelleryd E, Lopez M, Acerini CL. ISPAD Clinical Practice Consensus Guidelines 2018: Nutritional management in children and adolescents with diabetes. Pediatr Diabetes. 2018;**19**(Suppl. 27): 136-154. DOI: 10.1111/pedi.12738

[9] Kalra S, Czupryniak L, Kilov G, Lamptey R, Kumar A, Unnikrishnan AG, et al. Expert opinion: Patient selection for premixed insulin formulations in Diabetes care. Diabetes therapy: research, treatment and education of diabetes and related disorders. 2018; **9**(6):2185-2199

[10] Evelyne Fleury-Milfort N. Insulin replacement therapy. Diabetes CE. 2009; **16**(11):32

[11] Association AD. 7. Diabetes technology: Standards of medical Care in Diabetes—2021. Diabetes Care. 2020; **44**(Supplement_1):S85-S99

[12] Sharon RR, Kathryn P, Ellie W. Understanding Normmal and Clinical Nutrition (y. cossio Ed. 9th ed.). Wadsworth: Cengage Learning. 2012

Chapter 4

Type 1 Diabetes: Current Advances in High-Throughput Technologies and Computational Biology for Biomarker Studies

Tiffanie Leeman, Katherine P. Richardson, Paul M.H. Tran and Sharad Purohit

Abstract

Biomarkers are essential for the identification of high-risk populations as well as the monitoring of preventive and therapeutic outcomes for type 1 diabetes (T1D). In this chapter, we will discuss the progress made in T1D biomarker discovery using high throughput genomic, transcriptomic, and proteomic technologies collectively called as omic technologies. We also discuss the potential of artificial intelligence and omics data in the early prediction of T1D. Readers will gain an overview of the status of T1D biomarkers based on omic technologies. High throughput omic technologies combined with computational biology offer great opportunities for biomarker discovery. As we move forward, the utilization of a biomarker panel for the prediction and prevention of T1D is needed.

Keywords: type 1 diabetes, biomarkers, high throughput omic technology, bioinformatics, artificial intelligence, computational biology

1. Introduction

Type 1 diabetes (T1D) is an autoimmune disease that results from the immune-targeted destruction of insulin-producing β-cells in the pancreas [1, 2]. The disease does not discriminate based on age, sex, or race, making it devastating on a global scale. Public health officials approximated that in 2017, 451 million adults were treated with diabetes across the globe [3]. Estimating that by the year 2045, approximately 693 million patients globally will have diabetes; however, only half will have an official diagnosis [3]. T1D results from complex interactions between genes and the environment leading to autoimmune reactions toward pancreatic islet cells (**Figure 1**). The unchecked immune reaction reduces the beta-cell mass, thereby causing insulin insufficiency leading to T1D in these genetically susceptible individuals.

Traditional methods for diagnosis include glucose tolerance testing and monitoring of HbA1c levels in at-risk patients. However, these diagnostic techniques are only

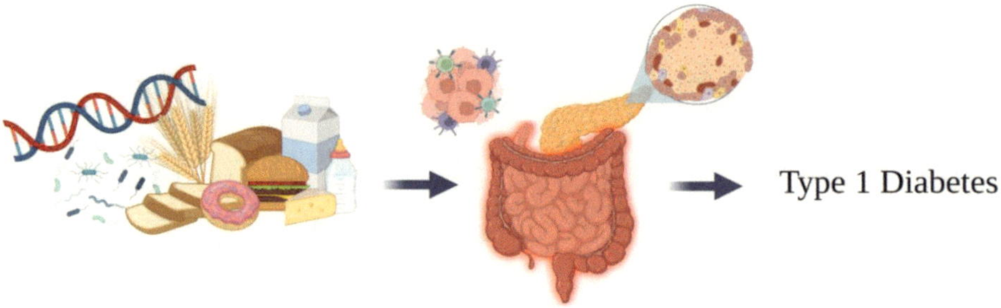

Figure 1.
Susceptibility genes and environmental triggers in development and progression of type-1 diabetes. Created using BioRender.com.

effective after the onset of diabetes has occurred. Preventative techniques for T1D are currently unavailable due to two main factors: (1) the inability to predict and accurately assess risk for the high-risk population and (2) the etiology of the disease is not well-established [4]. Although higher prevalence is seen in families with established autoimmune diseases, current screening techniques for islet autoantibodies in high-risk first-degree relatives of T1D patients are not very effective, as most cases of T1D occur spontaneously in the general population [5]. In addition, screening large populations poses challenges in both efficacy and funding. Due to these limitations, diabetes research is moving toward personalized prevention strategies, which focus on an individual's unique genetic and environmental risk factors that lead to the progression of T1D [2].

Biomarkers hold the key to unlocking diabetes preventative strategies and monitoring therapeutic outcomes. Over the past several decades, islet cell autoantibodies (ICA) have become an earlier predictor of T1D [2]. Since then, the discovery of other autoantibodies, such as those against specific islet autoantigens insulin and glutamate dehydrogenase (GAD), have continued to improve assays in their predictive value [2]. However, these islet autoantibodies still face the limitation of appearing in later stages of T1D development [2]. In addition, islet autoantibodies have not been useful for assessing therapeutic outcomes [2]. Early detection and prevention of T1D is crucial for the high-risk population and requires the discovery of new biomarkers. These biomarkers can come from metabolic pathways, DNA, RNA, glycans, lipids, and proteins (**Figure 2**). This chapter will address current biomarkers, omic technologies, computational biology, and the use of AI in identifying biomarkers in T1D research, and finally major issues with the discovery as well as validation of T1D biomarkers.

2. Current biomarkers in T1D

2.1 Autoantibodies and autoreactive T cells

The immune system develops autoantibodies (AAbs) in order to attack self-proteins. AAbs are used for T1D diagnosis, classification, and prediction of disease development. They do not play a direct role in disease pathogenesis, unlike autoreactive T cells [6]. Instead, AAbs are strong indicators of islet cell destruction [7]. They can be utilized to identify those at increased risk for T1D because they are produced during the natural history of T1D, including the stage before disease diagnosis [8].

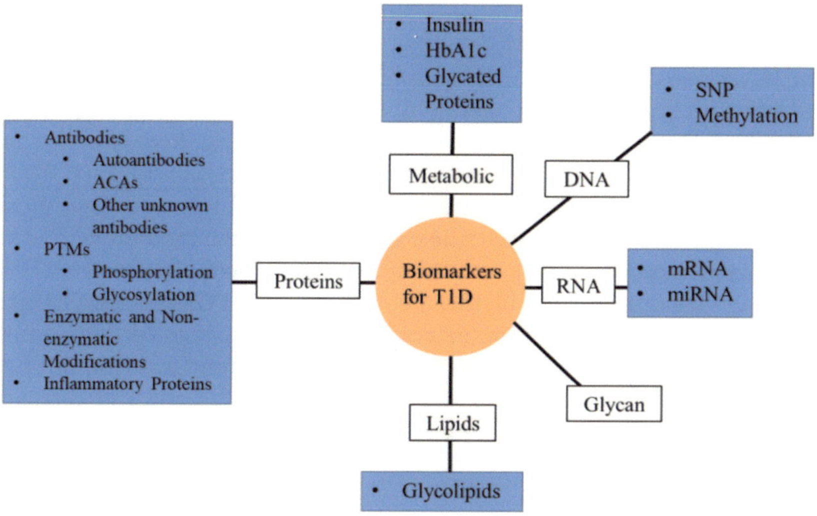

Figure 2.
Potential sources of biomarkers for T1D.

Autoantibody	Prevalence [9]	Risk of T1D
ICA	0.681	3% [10]
IAA	0.424	13.1% [11]
GADA	0.636	12.9% [11]
IA2A	0.714	40.5% [11]
ZnT8A	0.654	55%*, [11]

*ICA: Intracytoplasmic autoantibody, IAA: Insulin autoantibody, GADA: Glutamate Dehydrogenase-65 autoantibody, IA2A: Insulinoma antigen-2 autoantibody, ZnT8a: Zinc transporter 8 autoantibody. *5 year risk.*

Table 1.
Autoantibodies to pancreatic antigens, prevalence rate, and risk of developing T1D in 5 years.

There are five commonly tested AAb markers used in the diagnosis of T1D, which include ICA (islet-cell cytoplasmic AAb), GADA (glutamic acid decarboxylase (GAD) AAb), IA-2A (insulinoma 2 (IA-2)-associated AAb), IAA (insulin AAb), and ZNT8A (zinc transporter 8 AAb) (**Table 1**). At least one of the five autoantibodies is present in >95% of individuals with T1D upon hyperglycemia detection [8]. Patients with multiple autoantibody positivity are at a higher risk of developing T1D, although this risk varies depending on age, antibody type, and metabolic status [12]. However, a subset of patients who do not have any of the above AAbs at diagnosis have been found, indicating either a possibility of insensitive tests or the presence of additional T1D-associated autoantibodies in these patients.

Although AAbs appear before T1D diagnosis, they appear relatively late in the autoimmune process. T1D prevention may be more effective before the onset of the active autoimmune response and appearance of AAbs, suggesting that AAbs may not be effective markers to identify high-risk groups for T1D prevention [2]. Overall, AAbs are not useful as biomarkers for therapeutic outcomes and do not track disease progression [13]. Thus, it is crucial to investigate additional biomarkers that can serve as predictors of disease progression.

Autoreactive CD4+ and CD8+ T cells are thought to be the main mediators behind beta cell destruction in T1D [6, 14]. Insulitis, or leukocyte invasion of pancreatic islets, has been observed in mouse models and pancreatic biopsies of T1D patients, with infiltrates, predominately consisting of CD8+ cytotoxic T cells [15]. As autoreactive T cells play a direct role in beta cell destruction, T cell markers have the potential to provide unique insights into the pathogenesis and progression of T1D [6]. Despite their large potential, T cell biomarkers run into many challenges, making them difficult to use routinely. T cell quantification assays are limited by their lack of sensitivity [15, 16], as well as the low frequency of autoreactive T cells in peripheral blood and low avidity for peptide MHC ligands [17]. Avidity for TCR is hoped to increase through engineering the MHC peptide ligand into a multimer in recent studies [18]. Other advancements are being made in T cell biomarker identification, but further validation and standardization of the most promising biomarkers and assays are needed before widespread use [19, 20].

2.2 Genetics

Relatives of patients with T1D are at increased risk of developing T1D compared to the general population [21]. Human leukocyte antigen (HLA) has been shown to be a major genetic determinant in the development of T1D, accounting for approximately 50% of genetic risk [22, 23]. HLA class II alleles DR04, DR03, and homozygous DR04/DR03 genotypes increase the risk of T1D, while DR02 is highly protective against the disease [23]. Currently, genetic risk screening for T1D is performed by HLA-genotyping. However high-risk HLA genotypes are only present in 30–40% of T1D patients. Suggesting that HLA genotyping is too insufficient in sensitivity and specificity to be a useful T1D marker [6, 7]. While the HLA locus encodes for the strongest genetic susceptibility genes for T1D, there are five other non-HLA gene regions also associated with the disease: INS, CTLA-4, PTPN22, SUMO4, IL2RA, and IFIH1 (**Table 2**) [21, 27, 29].

Individually, non-HLA genes only weakly contribute to the assessment of risk for T1D. However, when used in combination, non-HLA genes may prove to have more predictive value [2]. Among the non-HLA genes, the INS VNTR has the strongest association with T1D [21]. The working theory is polymorphisms in the INS gene may lead to immune tolerance to insulin by changing the amount of insulin mRNA in the thymus during fetal development and childhood [30]. Similar polymorphisms

Gene	OR	95% CI
HLA DR3/DR4	16.59 [23]	13.7–20.1 [23]
Insulin VNTR	2.4 [24]	1.7–3.4 [24]
CTLA4	1.41 [25]	1.31–1.53 [25]
PTPN22	1.83 [26]	1.284–2.596 [26]
SUMO4	1.236 [27]	1.112–1.373 [27]
GRS	AUC 0.73 [28]	0.70–0.77 [28]

HLA: human leukocyte antigen, VNTR: variable number of tandem repeats, CTLA4: cytotoxic T-lymphocyte associated protein 4, PTPN22: protein tyrosine phosphatase 22, SUMO: small ubiquitin-like modifier, GRS: genetic risk score, AUC: area under the curve

Table 2.
Genes associated with T1D and odds ratio.

have been also associated with CTLA-4 [31]. In a recent report by Ueda et al., the CT60-A/G single nucleotide polymorphism (SNP) was suggested to produce lower amounts of sCTLA-4 mRNA in T1D patients [32]. However, a recent study found serum sCTLA-4 (protein) levels to be slightly higher in T1D patients. Although contradicting the idea that CT-60 SNP controls the expression of sCTLA-4, sCTLA-4 may still be a risk factor for T1D. These observations propose that sCTLA-4 may contribute to the development of autoimmune diseases, probably through inhibiting the B7-mCTLA-4 interaction and down-regulation of T cell activation [31]. Further characterization of these genes and disease variants requires genotyping of a large number of subjects [2].

3. Omic technologies

Several recent developments in instrumentation and protocols have enabled the evaluation of individual genotypes, gene expression, and protein expression. These developments have led to the creation of high-throughput approaches, collectively known as omics technology, that allow researchers to analyze large-scale measurements of genes, polymorphisms, and proteins in a given sample. In this section, we provide a brief description of the use of individual omics technology that are used in T1D research.

3.1 Genomics

Microarray technology allows researchers to analyze gene expression on a larger scale. The technology utilizes gene expression profiling in a number of disease states including but not limited to: various cancers, SLE, multiple sclerosis, and T1D [7]. One study using microarray analysis identified 116 differentially expressed genes between peripheral blood lymphocyte samples in T1D patients and AAb-negative controls, and many of these genes are involved in important immunoregulatory functions [7]. Microarray analysis has been performed in pancreatic tissue of T1D and healthy controls, with one study by Yip et al., identifying 48 differentially genes in human pancreata [33]. Studies also show the potential for use of miRNA microarrays in identifying biomarkers for the diagnosis of T1D [34–37] and predicting complications such as ketoacidosis [38]. Differential mRNA and miRNA expression profiles characterized by microarray analysis have helped to provide insight into the pathogenesis of T1D, as many of these genes are involved in cellular functions such as oxidative stress response, DNA repair, inflammation, and apoptosis [39]. After appropriate validation of candidate genes discovered with microarray analysis, multivariate analysis, or computational techniques can be used to identify patients at high risk of developing T1D [40].

3.2 Genome-wide association analysis (GWAS) and genetic risk scores

The polygenic risk score method summarizes multiple genetic risk elements into a single score. There are benefits to establishing successful genetic risk scores. Over the past 20 years, the advancement in technology has allowed for publicly available genetic data. Combine this with the decreased costs in genotyping processes, the T1D genetic risk score (T1D GRS) has the opportunity to demonstrate its applicability for "disease prediction, discrimination, investigation of unusual cohorts, and investigation of biology in large datasets where genetic data are available" [41]. In 2018, a group following a cohort from The Environmental Determinants of Diabetes in the Young (TEDDY) study created a genetic score based on 3 SNPs for HLA class II genotyping and 41 SNPs in other genes. The score identified newborn children, with no family history of T1D, who had a >10% risk for developing pre-symptomatic T1D, a nearly 2-fold higher risk than children identified by high-risk HLA genotypes alone [42].

GWAS previously associated the 3p21.31 locus with T1D [43]. The 3p21.31 locus encodes for many chemokine receptors including the C-C motif chemokine receptor 2 [44]. C-C motif chemokine ligand 2 (CCL2) is a pro-inflammatory chemokine that binds to CCR2 to promote T cell recruitment and macrophage activation. Tran et al analyzed CCL2 levels in the DAISY cohort and found paradoxically decreased CCL2 in T1D patients compared to controls. The proposed mechanism was that variants in the 3p21.31 genetic locus promote the development of T1D by increasing CCR2 expression, causing subsequent pancreatic islet cell destruction while simultaneously depleting the CCL2 pool [44].

The major limitation of genetic risk score development is the genetic heterogeneity among different ethnic groups and populations. This especially proves to be a challenge in identifying T1D susceptibility genes [1]. Most genetic risk score validation utilizes populations of European ancestry. Studies of genetic risk scores in African ancestry populations suggest that an ancestry-specific genetic risk score may improve the prediction of T1D [45].

3.3 Proteomics

As proteins directly carry out cellular functions and disease processes, protein biomarkers have great potential for T1D prediction and monitoring treatment outcomes. The proteomic analysis allows us to discover and quantify these proteins on a large scale. Proteomic techniques can be divided into two main types: mass spectrometry-based and array-based (**Table 3**) [54].

3.3.1 Mass spectrometry based proteomics

Mass spectrometry (MS) measures the mass charge ratio (m/z) of ions, which is used to characterize biomolecules with extremely high sensitivity and high throughput [55].

Separation techniques such as 2D and 3D polyacrylamide gel electrophoresis and 2D high performance liquid chromatography are often performed before MS to enrich

Platform	Separation	Throughput
Mass-spectrometry	HPLC [46]	↑Proteins ↓Samples
	GC [47]	
	CE [48]	
Array	96-well [49]	↓Proteins ↑Samples
	Beads [50–52]	
	NAPPA [8, 53]	

HPLC: high performance liquid chromatography, GC: gas chromatography, CE: capillary electrophoresis, Beads: Luminex bead assay, NAPPA: Nucleic Acid Programmable Protein Arrays.

Table 3.
High throughput proteomic approaches for biomarkers in T1D.

low-abundance proteins [56], Standard 2D polyacrylamide gel electrophoresis (2D PAGE) alone has several limitations for biomarker discovery including low throughput and low resolution, and is thus used in conjugation with MS analysis [7]. The two-dimensional liquid chromatography (2DLC) mass spectrometry platform has been widely used in the discovery of protein candidates that may serve as biomarkers [46]. MS and MS combined techniques have been used to identify a number of biomarkers in T1D.

3.3.2 Array based proteomics

Array-based techniques can be divided into targeted assays that measure a select number of molecules, and Nucleic Acid Programmable Protein Arrays (NAPPA) arrays (**Table 4**). Targeted array-based techniques such as Enzyme-linked immunoassays (ELISA) and Luminex bead assays involve measurement of selected molecules based on the role of the molecule in a disease process and availability of the assay. These assays are limited by the number of protein markers that can be tested at once, yet a large number of samples can be tested. Array-based assays have been used to discover many candidate cytokines, chemokines, adhesion molecules, and receptors that may play a role in the development of T1D and its complications.

In contrast, NAPPA arrays provide high throughput information on thousands of candidate proteins in a more limited number of samples. NAPPA arrays contain imprinted gene on glass slides and a wheat germ expression system that converts the DNA to RNA to protein. This protein array then detects circulating levels of antibodies against the proteins in the blood of T1D individuals [53]. Recent studies by Bian et al. utilized NAPPA and ELISA to analyze more than 50% of the human proteome in the serum of recent onset T1D patients. They discovered six novel T1D-associated autoantibodies and created a combined AAb panel that had a higher AUC and sensitivity in diagnosis compared to the conventional AAb ZnT8A (**Table 5**) [8, 61]. More studies are required to confirm the findings utilizing the NAPPA in T1D.

4. Artificial intelligence (AI) use in T1D research

Although various T1D prevention trials have been conducted, response to preventative therapies appears to be limited to only a few individuals. A major factor in this lack of response is the difficulty identifying appropriate high-risk subjects who would benefit from such trials. Personalized prevention strategies based on one's own risk and etiology may prove to be more efficient than prevention for the whole at-risk population. Therefore, a panel of multiple biomarkers is needed to identify individual risks for potential subjects in T1D prevention trials.

Protein	Technique
Single markers	ELISA [1, 49]
Multimarkers	Bead Array [4, 50–52, 56–60]
	NAPPA [8, 53]

ELISA: enzyme-linked immunosorbent assay, Array Bead: Luminex bead array, NAPPA: Nucleic Acid Programmable Protein Arrays.

Table 4.
Array-based technologies in biomarker studies in T1D.

Protein antigen	AUC	Sensitivity at 95% specificity
ZnT8A alone	0.62	38.3
Novel AAb panel (anti-PTPRN2, -MLH1, -PPIL2, and -QRFPR)	0.74	37.5
Novel AAb panel + ZnT8A	0.81	55.2

AUC: area under the curve, ZnT8A: Zn transporter 8 autoantibody, PTPRN22: protein tyrosine phosphatase receptor 22, MLH1: MutL protein homolog 1, PPIL2: Peptidylprolyl Isomerase Like 2, QRFPR: Pyroglutamylated RFamide Peptide Receptor.

Table 5.
Novel T1D AAb panel identified by NAPPA array: AUC and sensitivity compared to ZnT8A [8].

Advances in omic technology have allowed researchers to discover several potential biomarkers. Validation of these biomarkers requires thousands of samples, irrespective of the technique, and thus biomarker development is often hindered by limited availability of biological samples. Recently, T1D repositories such as TEDDY and TrialNet have addressed this problem by providing a large pool of available sample data for omic analysis. However, high computational power is required to analyze numerous biomarkers in these large data sets and identify the optimal markers for a panel.

AI machine learning has been used for a broad range of applications in cancer treatment, including diagnosis and classification of cancer as well as prediction of progression and treatment outcomes [62]. This suggests that AI may help to solve the issue of early prediction of T1D as well. The main goal of AI in T1D biomarker discovery is to combine information on the small differences in serum biomarkers between T1D and healthy patients and utilize this information to predict which patients are at high risk of developing T1D in the future.

Recent studies have utilized various machine-learning techniques to analyze large amounts of omics data (**Table 6**). Repeated Optimization for Feature Interpretation (ROFI) is one such technique that uses a repeated selection algorithm 500 times to generate important matrices for each feature [65, 67]. These matrices define the importance of a feature as the percentage of times it was selected to be included out of the 500 times the algorithm was run [65, 66]. After the feature importance values have been established, the final model is produced [65]. These studies illustrate the potential utility of machine learning in analyzing large amounts of data from diverse fields of omics data (genomics, proteomics, metabolomics, and lipidomics), clinical risk factors, and environmental factors for early prediction and prevention of T1D. Machine learning also has the potential to improve the prediction of T1D complications such as diabetic nephropathy, retinopathy, and peripheral neuropathy [11, 57]. The goal is that machine learning-derived risk scores can be used to identify T1D patients who would benefit the most from targeted preventative therapies before the development of these complications.

5. Conclusion

Currently, individuals at high risk of developing T1D are identified with multiple autoantibodies and HLA genotyping. These existing biomarkers do not fully meet the need for T1D prediction and prevention due to many issues with sensitivity and specificity, as well as the relatively late appearance of autoantibodies. Successful prevention of T1D requires the identification of high-risk populations early in the disease course before the appearance of islet autoantibodies and clinical disease onset. Due to

Computational approach	Omics platform	Omics approach	Number of features (post optimization)	Accuracy/ AUC/ Sensitivity	Ref
Model averaging	SELDITOF	Proteomics	146	90.0% sensitivity	[63]
Support Vector Machine	GWAS	Genomics	417	AUC 0.84	[28]
Repeated Optimization for feature interpretation (ROF)	HPLC-MS, Multiplex assay	Proteomics, Immunologic, Genomics, Metabolomics	76	AUC 0.92	[64]
	GC-TOF MS, Illumina ImmunoChip	Metabolomics, Genomics	42	AUC 0.74	[65]
	GC-TOF MS, genetic risk score	Metabolomics, Genomics, Immunologic	16	AUC 0.84	[66]

ROF: Repeated Optimization for Feature Interpretation, number of features presented after post-optimization of the computational method, SELDI-TOF: Surface-enhanced laser desorption/ionization time-of-flight mass spectrometry, GWAS: genome-wide association study, HPLC-MS: high performance liquid chromatography-Mass spectrometry, GC-TOF: gas chromatography time-of-flight mass spectrometry.

Table 6.
Computational approaches for biomarkers in T1D.

the multifactorial nature of T1D, no single biomarker can provide adequate power to predict the disease. Therefore, research into T1D prevention has to rely on the combination of multiple markers. Advances in high throughput omic technologies such as GWAS and NAPPA arrays have offered new opportunities to discover such biomarkers. In addition, advanced computational techniques including machine learning are being increasingly utilized to analyze numerous biomarkers in large data sets. Despite these advances, there is still an urgent need for new and improved biomarkers for T1D prediction and prevention. Surrogate biomarkers are needed to access the outcomes of preventative therapy trials in their early stages. Due to the long asymptomatic period for diabetes, it is too expensive and time-consuming for clinical trials to wait for the final clinical outcome. The lack of suitable surrogate biomarkers for T1D has severely hampered progress in clinical trials. Newer markers will also need to provide information on response to treatment in existing T1D patients. This information will aid in predicting which patients would benefit from specific therapies.

The simultaneous consideration of genomic, transcriptomic, and proteomic data, using advanced computational techniques will be required for accurate assessment of T1D risk and monitoring of therapeutic outcomes in the future.

Acknowledgements

This work was supported by JDRF awards to SP (2-2011-153, 10-2006-792, and 3-2004-195). PMHT was supported by NIH/NIDDK fellowship (F30DK12146101A1).

Conflict of interest

The authors declare no conflict of interest.

Author details

Tiffanie Leeman[1,2], Katherine P. Richardson[2], Paul M.H. Tran[1,2]
and Sharad Purohit[2,3,4]*

1 Medical College of Georgia, Augusta University, Augusta, GA, USA

2 Center for Biotechnology and Genomic Medicine, Augusta University, Augusta, GA, USA

3 Department of Gynecology and Obstetrics, Medical College of Georgia, Augusta University, Augusta, GA, USA

4 Department of Undergraduate Health Sciences, Augusta University, Augusta, GA, USA

*Address all correspondence to: spurohit@augusta.edu

References

[1] Purohit S, She JX. Biomarkers for type 1 diabetes. International Journal of Clinical and Experimental Medicine. 2008;**1**(2):98-116

[2] Carey C, Purohit S, She JX. Advances and challenges in biomarker development for type 1 diabetes prediction and prevention using omic technologies. Expert Opinion on Medical Diagnostics. 2010;**4**(5):397-410

[3] Talha Mahboob Alam MAI, Ali Y, Wahab A, Ijaz S, Baig TI, Hussain A, et al. A model for early prediction of diabetes. Informatics in Medicine Unlocked. 2019;**16**:100204. DOI: 10.1016/j.imu.2019.100204

[4] Zhi W, Purohit S, Carey C, Wang M, She J-X. Proteomic technologies for the discovery of type 1 diabetes biomarkers. Journal of Diabetes Science and Technology. 2010;**4**(4):993-1002

[5] Dayan CM, Besser REJ, Oram RA, Hagopian W, Vatish M, Bendor-Samuel O, et al. Preventing type 1 diabetes in childhood. Science. 2021;**373**(6554):506-510

[6] Mathieu C, Lahesmaa R, Bonifacio E, Achenbach P, Tree T. Immunological biomarkers for the development and progression of type 1 diabetes. Diabetologia. 2018;**61**(11):2252

[7] Collins CD, Purohit S, Podolsky RH, Zhao HS, Schatz D, Eckenrode SE, et al. The application of genomic and proteomic technologies in predictive, preventive and personalized medicine. Vascular Pharmacology. 2006;**45**(5):258-267

[8] Bian X, Wasserfall C, Wallstrom G, Wang J, Wang H, Barker K, et al. Tracking the antibody immunome in type 1 diabetes using protein arrays. Journal of Proteome Research. 2017;**16**(1):195-203

[9] Ziegler AG, Rewers M, Simell O, Simell T, Lempainen J, Steck A, et al. Seroconversion to multiple islet autoantibodies and risk of progression to diabetes in children. JAMA. 2013;**309**(23):2473-2479

[10] Ross C, Ward ZJ, Gomber A, Owais M, Yeh JM, Reddy C-L, et al. The prevalence of islet autoantibodies in children and adolescents with type 1 diabetes mellitus: A global scoping review. Frontiers in Endocrinology. 2022;**13**:815703. DOI: 10.3389/fendo.2022.815703

[11] Purohit S, Tran PMH, Tran LKH, Satter KB, He M, Zhi W, et al. Serum levels of inflammatory proteins are associated with peripheral neuropathy in a cross-sectional type-1 diabetes cohort. Frontiers in Immunology. 2021;**12**:654233. DOI: 10.3389/fimmu.2021.654233

[12] Jacobsen LM, Bocchino L, Evans-Molina C, DiMeglio L, Goland R, Wilson DM, et al. The risk of progression to type 1 diabetes is highly variable in individuals with multiple autoantibodies following screening. Diabetologia. 2020;**63**(3):588-596

[13] Yi L, Swensen AC, Qian W-J. Serum biomarkers for diagnosis and prediction of type 1 diabetes. Translational Research: The Journal of Laboratory and Clinical Medicine. 2018;**201**:13

[14] Gomez-Tourino I, Arif S, Eichmann M, Peakman M. T cells in type 1 diabetes: Instructors, regulators and effectors: A comprehensive review. Journal of Autoimmunity. 2016;**66**:7

[15] Varela-Calvino R, Calviño-Sampedro C, Gómez-Touriño I, Cordero OJ. Apportioning blame: Autoreactive CD4+ and CD8+ T cells in type 1 diabetes. Archivum Immunologiae et Therapiae Experimentalis. 2017;**65**(4):275-284

[16] Schloot NC, Meierhoff G, Karlsson Faresjö M, Ott P, Putnam A, Lehmann P, et al. Comparison of cytokine ELISpot assay formats for the detection of islet antigen autoreactive T cells: Report of the third immunology of diabetes society T-cell workshop. Journal of Autoimmunity. 2003;**21**(4):365-376

[17] Trudeau JD, Kelly-Smith C, Verchere CB, Elliott JF, Dutz JP, Finegood DT, et al. Prediction of spontaneous autoimmune diabetes in NOD mice by quantification of autoreactive T cells in peripheral blood. The Journal of Clinical Investigation. 2003;**111**(2):217-223

[18] Eisenbarth GS, Kotzin BL. Enumerating autoreactive T cells in peripheral blood: A big step in diabetes prediction. The Journal of Clinical Investigation. 2003;**111**(2):179-181

[19] Ahmed S, Cerosaletti K, James E, Long SA, Mannering S, Speake C, et al. Standardizing T-cell biomarkers in type 1 diabetes: Challenges and recent advances. Diabetes. 2019;**68**(7):1366-1379

[20] Brooks-Worrell B, Warsen A, Palmer JP. Improved T cell assay for identification of type 1 diabetes patients. Journal of Immunological Methods. 2009;**344**(1):79-83

[21] Redondo MJ, Steck AK, Pugliese A. Genetics of type 1 diabetes. Pediatric Diabetes. 2018;**19**(3):346-353

[22] Davies JL, Kawaguchi Y, Bennett ST, Copeman JB, Cordell HJ, Pritchard LE, et al. A genome-wide search for human type 1 diabetes susceptibility genes. Nature. 1994;**371**(6493):130-136

[23] Noble JA, Valdes AM, Cook M, Klitz W, Thomson G, Erlich HA. The role of HLA class II genes in insulin-dependent diabetes mellitus: Molecular analysis of 180 Caucasian, multiplex families. American Journal of Human Genetics. 1996;**59**(5):1134-1148

[24] Pietropaolo M, Yu S, Libman IM, Pietropaolo SL, Riley K, LaPorte RE, et al. Cytoplasmic islet cell antibodies remain valuable in defining risk of progression to type 1 diabetes in subjects with other islet autoantibodies. Pediatric Diabetes. 2005;**6**(4):184-192

[25] Bjørnvold M, Undlien DE, Joner G, Dahl-Jørgensen K, Njølstad PR, Akselsen HE, et al. Joint effects of HLA, INS, PTPN22 and CTLA4 genes on the risk of type 1 diabetes. Diabetologia. 2008;**51**(4):589-596

[26] Chen Z, Fei M, Fu D, Zhang L, Ma Y, Wang Y, et al. Association between cytotoxic T lymphocyte antigen-4 polymorphism and type 1 diabetes: A meta-analysis. Gene. 2013;**516**(2):263-270

[27] Song GG, Choi SJ, Ji JD, Lee YH. Association between the SUMO4 M55V (A163G) polymorphism and susceptibility to type 1 diabetes: A meta-analysis. Human Immunology. 2012;**73**(10):1055-1059

[28] Wei Z, Wang K, Qu HQ, Zhang H, Bradfield J, Kim C, et al. From disease association to risk assessment: An optimistic view from genome-wide association studies on type 1 diabetes. PLoS Genetics. 2009;**5**(10):e1000678

[29] Howson JM, Walker NM, Smyth DJ, Todd JA. Analysis of 19 genes

for association with type I diabetes in the Type I diabetes genetics consortium families. Genes and Immunity. 2009;**10**(Suppl. 1):S74-S84

[30] Pugliese A, Zeller M, Fernandez A, Zalcberg LJ, Bartlett RJ, Ricordi C, et al. The insulin gene is transcribed in the human thymus and transcription levels correlate with allelic variation at the INS VNTR-IDDM2 susceptibility locus for type 1 diabetes. Nature Genetics. 1997;**15**(3):293-297

[31] Purohit S, Podolsky R, Collins C, Zheng W, Schatz D, Muir A, et al. Lack of correlation between the levels of soluble cytotoxic T-lymphocyte associated antigen-4 (CTLA-4) and the CT-60 genotypes. Journal of Autoimmune Diseases. 2005;**2**:8

[32] Ueda H, Howson JM, Esposito L, Heward J, Snook H, Chamberlain G, et al. Association of the T-cell regulatory gene CTLA4 with susceptibility to autoimmune disease. Nature. 2003;**423**(6939):506-511

[33] Yip L, Fuhlbrigge R, Alkhataybeh R, Fathman CG. Gene expression analysis of the pre-diabetic pancreas to identify pathogenic mechanisms and biomarkers of type 1 diabetes. Frontiers in Endocrinology (Lausanne). 2020;**11**:609271

[34] Paula Takahashi DJX, Evangelista AF, Manoel-Caetano FS, Macedo C, Collares CVA, Foss-Freitas MC, et al. MicroRNA expression profiling and functional annotation analysis of their targets in patients with type 1 diabetes mellitus. Gene. 2014;**539**(2):213-223

[35] Snowhite IV, Allende G, Sosenko J, Pastori RL, Messinger Cayetano S, Pugliese A. Association of serum microRNAs with islet autoimmunity, disease progression and metabolic impairment in relatives at risk of type 1 diabetes. Diabetologia. 2017;**60**(8):1409-1422

[36] Liu L, Yan J, Xu H, Zhu Y, Liang H, Pan W, et al. Two novel MicroRNA biomarkers related to beta-cell damage and their potential values for early diagnosis of type 1 diabetes. The Journal of Clinical Endocrinology and Metabolism. 2018;**103**(4):1320-1329

[37] Zurawek M, Dzikiewicz-Krawczyk A, Izykowska K, Ziolkowska-Suchanek I, Skowronska B, Czainska M, et al. miR-487a-3p upregulated in type 1 diabetes targets CTLA4 and FOXO3. Diabetes Research and Clinical Practice. 2018;**142**:146-153

[38] Shi R, Dai F, He Y, Sun L, Xu M, Deng D, et al. Comprehensive analyses of type 1 diabetes ketosis- or ketoacidosis-related genes in activated CD56(+) CD16(+) NK Cells. Front Endocrinol (Lausanne). 2021;**12**:750135

[39] Takahashi P, Xavier DJ, Lima J, Evangelista AF, Collares CVA, Foss-Freitas MC, et al. Transcript expression profiles and MicroRNA regulation indicate an upregulation of processes linked to oxidative stress, DNA repair, cell death, and inflammation in type 1 diabetes mellitus patients. Journal Diabetes Research. 2022;**2022**:3511329

[40] Jin Y, Sharma A, Bai S, Davis C, Liu H, Hopkins D, et al. Risk of type 1 diabetes progression in islet autoantibody-positive children can be further stratified using expression patterns of multiple genes implicated in peripheral blood lymphocyte activation and function. Diabetes. 2014;**63**(7):2506-2515

[41] Sharp SA, Weedon MN, Hagopian WA, Oram RA. Clinical and research uses of genetic risk scores in type 1 diabetes. Current

Opinion in Genetics & Development. 2018;**50**:96-102

[42] Bonifacio E, Beyerlein A, Hippich M, Winkler C, Vehik K, Weedon MN, et al. Genetic scores to stratify risk of developing multiple islet autoantibodies and type 1 diabetes: A prospective study in children. PLoS Medicine. 2018;**15**(4):e1002548-e

[43] Onengut-Gumuscu S, Chen W-M, Burren O, Cooper NJ, Quinlan AR, Mychaleckyj JC, et al. Fine mapping of type 1 diabetes susceptibility loci and evidence for colocalization of causal variants with lymphoid gene enhancers. Nature Genetics. 2015;**47**(4):381-386

[44] Tran PMH, Purohit S, Kim E, bin Satter K, Hopkins D, Waugh K, et al. The 3p21.31 genetic locus promotes progression to type 1 diabetes through the CCR2/CCL2 pathway. Journal of Translational Autoimmunity. 2021;**4**:100127

[45] Onengut-Gumuscu S, Chen W-M, Robertson CC, Bonnie JK, Farber E, Zhu Z, et al. Type 1 diabetes risk in african-ancestry participants and utility of an ancestry-specific genetic risk score. Diabetes Care. 2019;**42**(3):406-415

[46] Zhi W, Sharma A, Purohit S, Miller E, Bode B, Anderson SW, et al. Discovery and validation of serum protein changes in type 1 diabetes patients using high throughput two dimensional liquid chromatography-mass spectrometry and immunoassays. Molecular & Cellular Proteomics. 2011;**10**(11):M111

[47] Bottini N, Musumeci L, Alonso A, Rahmouni S, Nika K, Rostamkhani M, et al. A functional variant of lymphoid tyrosine phosphatase is associated with type I diabetes. Nature Genetics. 2004;**36**(4):337-338

[48] Curovic VR, Suvitaival T, Mattila I, Ahonen L, Trost K, Theilade S, et al. Circulating metabolites and lipids are associated to diabetic retinopathy in individuals with type 1 diabetes. Diabetes. 2020;**69**(10):2217-2226

[49] Maahs DM, Siwy J, Argiles A, Cerna M, Delles C, Dominiczak AF, et al. Urinary collagen fragments are significantly altered in diabetes: A link to pathophysiology. PLoS One. 2010;**5**(9):0013051. DOI: 10.1371/journal.pone.0013051

[50] Soedamah-Muthu SS, Chaturvedi N, Schalkwijk CG, Stehouwer CDA, Ebeling P, Fuller JH, et al. Soluble vascular cell adhesion molecule-1 and soluble E-selectin are associated with micro- and macrovascular complications in Type 1 diabetic patients. Journal of Diabetes and its Complications. 2006;**20**(3):188-195

[51] Sharma A, Purohit S, Sharma S, Bai S, Zhi W, Ponny SR, et al. IGF-binding proteins in type-1 diabetes are more severely altered in the presence of complications. Front Endocrinol (Lausanne). 2016;**7**:2

[52] Purohit S, Sharma A, Zhi W, Bai S, Hopkins D, Steed L, et al. Proteins of TNF-α and IL6 pathways are elevated in serum of type-1 diabetes patients with microalbuminuria. Frontiers in Immunology. 2018;**9**:154

[53] Diez P, Gonzalez-Gonzalez M, Lourido L, Degano RM, Ibarrola N, Casado-Vela J, et al. NAPPA as a real new method for protein microarray generation. Microarrays (Basel). 2015;**4**(2):214-227

[54] Tyers M, Mann M. From genomics to proteomics. Nature. 2003;**422**(6928):193-197

[55] Lane CS. Mass spectrometry-based proteomics in the life sciences. Cellular and Molecular Life Sciences. 2005;**62**(7-8):848-869

[56] Purohit S, Sharma A, Hopkins D, Steed L, Bode B, Anderson SW, et al. Large-scale discovery and validation studies demonstrate significant reductions in circulating levels of IL8, IL-1Ra, MCP-1, and MIP-1β in patients with type 1 diabetes. The Journal of Clinical Endocrinology and Metabolism. 2015;**100**(9):E1179-E1187

[57] Al-Sari N, Kutuzova S, Suvitaival T, Henriksen P, Pociot F, Rossing P, et al. Precision diagnostic approach to predict 5-year risk for microvascular complications in type 1 diabetes. eBioMedicine. 2022;**80**:104032

[58] Sharma S, Purohit S, Sharma A, Hopkins D, Steed L, Bode B, et al. Elevated serum levels of soluble tnf receptors and adhesion molecules are associated with diabetic retinopathy in patients with type-1 diabetes. Mediators of Inflammation. 2015;**2015**:279393

[59] Wedrychowicz A, Dziatkowiak H, Nazim J, Sztefko K. Insulin-like growth factor-1 and its binding proteins, IGFBP-1 and IGFBP-3, in adolescents with type-1 diabetes mellitus and microalbuminuria. Hormone Research. 2005;**63**(5):245-251

[60] Guan R, Purohit S, Wang H, Bode B, Reed JC, Steed RD, et al. Chemokine (C-C motif) ligand 2 (CCL2) in sera of patients with type 1 diabetes and diabetic complications. PLoS One. 2011;**6**(4):e17822

[61] Gan WZ, Ramachandran V, Lim CSY, Koh RY. Omics-based biomarkers in the diagnosis of diabetes. Journal of Basic and Clinical Physiology and Pharmacology. 2019;**31**(2):0120. DOI: 10.1515/jbcpp-2019-0120

[62] Bhinder B, Gilvary C, Madhukar NS, Elemento O. Artificial intelligence in cancer research and precision medicine. Cancer Discovery. 2015;**11**(4):900-915

[63] Purohit S, Podolsky R, Schatz D, Muir A, Hopkins D, Huang Y-H, et al. Assessing the utility of SELDI-TOF and model averaging for serum proteomic biomarker discovery. Proteomics. 2006;**6**(24):6405-6415

[64] Frohnert BI, Webb-Robertson BJ, Bramer LM, Reehl SM, Waugh K, Steck AK, et al. Predictive modeling of type 1 diabetes stages using disparate data sources. Diabetes. 2020;**69**(2):238-248

[65] Webb-Robertson BM, Bramer LM, Stanfill BA, Reehl SM, Nakayasu ES, Metz TO, et al. Prediction of the development of islet autoantibodies through integration of environmental, genetic, and metabolic markers. Journal of Diabetes. 2021;**13**(2):143-153

[66] Webb-Robertson BM, Nakayasu ES, Frohnert BI, Bramer LM, Akers SM, Norris JM, et al. Integration of infant metabolite, genetic, and islet autoimmunity signatures to predict type 1 diabetes by age 6 years. The Journal of Clinical Endocrinology and Metabolism. 2022;**107**(8):2329-2338

[67] Webb-Robertson B-JMB, Lisa M, Reehl SM, Metz TO, Zhang Q, Rewers MJ, et al. ROFI - The use of repeated optimization for feature interpretation. In: 2016 International Conference on Computational Science and Computational Intelligence (CSCI). Las Vegas, NV, USA: Institute of Electrical and Electronics Engineers; 2016. pp. 29-33. DOI: 10.1109/CSCI.2016.0013

Chapter 5

Benefits of Implementation of Insulin Pump in People with Type 1 Diabetes: 10 Case Reports

Noemi Nováková, Martin Nezval and Marie Anna Robenková

Abstract

Ten people with type 1 diabetes (T1D), aged 28 to 57 years, with a duration of diabetes from 8 months to 47 years, attending an urban diabetes center, were retrospectively observed to assess the effects of intensive insulin treatment using continuous subcutaneous insulin infusion (insulin pump) for a period ranging from 2 months to 30 years, controlled either by glucometer-strips systems or using sensors for continuous glucose monitoring (CGM). Retinopathy, neuropathy, and nephropathy were present in some of them. An assessment of changes in HbA_{1c}, body mass, insulin requirements per day (INS/d), blood pressure, lipoproteins, and estimated glomerular filtration rate (eGFR) was used to determine treatment efficiency. In conclusion, a combination of adequate education, long-term therapy with an insulin pump, and early implementation of CGM appear to be the optimal approach to T1D management, resulting in improved diabetes control and/or enhanced quality of life for the users.

Keywords: type 1 diabetes, continuous subcutaneous insulin infusion (CSII), insulin pump, insulin pen, continuous glucose monitoring (CGM), case report, MiniMed 780G

1. Introduction

According to American Diabetes Association (ADA), immune-mediated diabetes, also known as "insulin-dependent diabetes," caused by cellular-mediated autoimmune destruction of the pancreatic β-cells, accounts for 5–10% of diabetes, making it the major of the two subcategories of type 1 diabetes. Islet cell autoantibodies and autoantibodies to GAD (glutamic acid decarboxylase, GAD65), insulin, the tyrosine phosphatases islet antigen 2 (IA-2) and Ia-2β, and zinc transporter 8, represent autoimmune markers. Only a minority of people with diabetes fall into the second subcategory, idiopathic T1D, with no evident β-cell autoimmunity, higher susceptibility to ketoacidosis, and permanent insulinopenia [1, 2]. The ADA's clinical practice recommendations in "Standards of Medical Care in Diabetes—2022" state that the ideal HbA_{1c} concentration should be lower than 53 mmol/mol (7%) as it correlates to a 50–76% decrease in microvascular complications (retinopathy, neuropathy, and diabetic kidney disease), development, and progression [3]. However, for many people with T1D, despite the availability of the latest innovative technology in insulin therapy, achieving the recommended target remains challenging [4–6].

When considering methods of treatment, insulin pumps should be made accessible to all people with insulin-deficient diabetes, nonetheless, specific circumstances, desires, and needs of the patient should be brought into account [6, 7]. Offering the latest available technology to all patients is one of many priorities in our hospital, including sensor-augmented pumps from Medtronic MiniMed in T1D.

The latest MiniMed 780G (**Figure 1**) system, the successor to MiniMed 640G and 670G, is equipped with advanced hybrid closed-loop (AHCL) [8–10]. The AHCL system is composed of CGM and an insulin pump. The continual administration of self-adjusting basal insulin delivery and correctional boluses every 5 minutes is based on glycemia measured in real-time. This may prevent hypoglycemia, while also making it safe, effective, and more comfortable to use [5, 8–11]. Even CGM alone has proven to be more effective than manual self-monitoring with a glucometer [12–14]. Insulin delivery *via* this system represents a near-physiological mechanism; it mimics endogenous insulin secretion to the extent of minimal need for manual user intervention [15–18]. For optimal results, in the traditional "Manual mode," the number of saccharides should be entered and the bolus calculator ("bolus Wizard") may be used as an advisor. In the "Smart Guard" mode the user needs to enter only the number of saccharides [9, 18]. The CareLink system creates person-related graphs (**Figure 2**) depicting CGM, saccharide intake, and insulin infusions, providing an organized overview for the user and their healthcare provider. Time in range (TIR) is the amount of time spent in target glycemia, represented as a percentage, in the course of defined period.

Based on previous data, the algorithm may predict glycemia and the body's reaction to insulin delivery. Therefore, it can be expected that with a longer period of use comes better control of glycaemic targets. Some other factors that play a role in optimal results include; correct application and fixation of the cannula and infusion set; turning off insulin delivery when taking off the pump (for example during showers, sports, and sex). At night, the algorithm controls glycemia according to the automatic basal rate, regardless of evening glycemia. This enables users to stay in range without any active intervention for the duration of their sleep [18]. Anyone

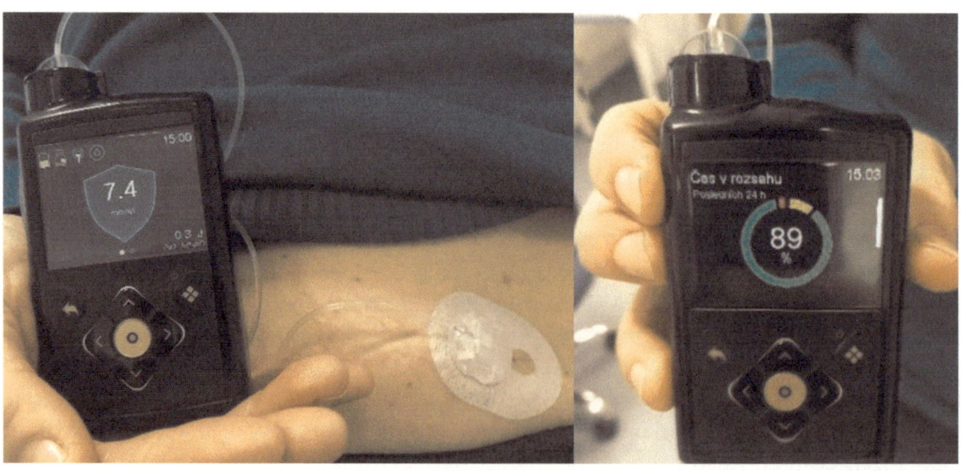

Figure 1.
Insulin pump MiniMed 780G: the SmartGuard mode showing glycaemia 7.4 mmol/l (on the left), and time in range (TIR) 89% (on the right).

DOI: http://dx.doi.org/10.5772/intechopen.110073

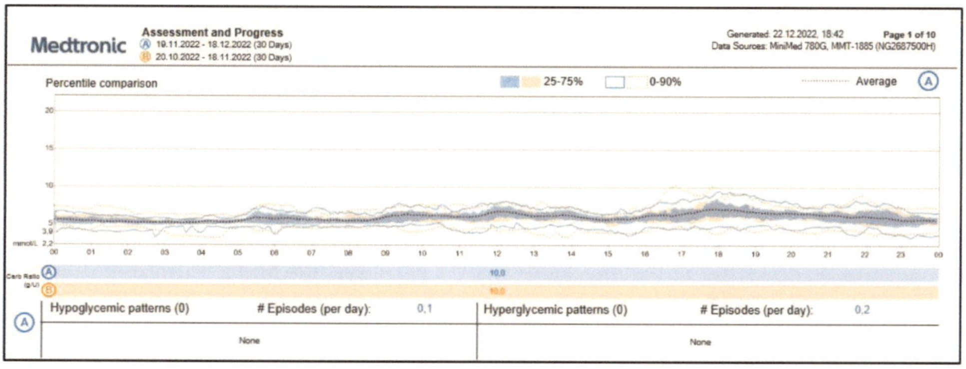

Figure 2.
This CareLink graph depicts two shaded areas of data: blue and orange, each area representing information about glycemia from a date range (A and B), (see left corner). The black dotted line in the middle represents average glycemia from the last date range (A). The darker shaded blue area represents 25–75% of all sensor readings, meaning this is where the majority of glucose readings have been. The remainder of the data is in the 0–90% range presented within the solid blue line. Data from the date range (B) are colored orange behind the blue plot. This report should be reviewed with one's healthcare professional to see progress from the last visit or the last device settings change [19]. The internet address specified for each user is www.carelink.minimed.eu.

using the technology should be well informed on how AHCL algorithms work, and most importantly how to use it to get the maximum benefit out of it [20].

2. Case reports

To demonstrate different challenges and aspects of insulin pump therapy, four men and six ladies were chosen out of 20 people with T1D registered in an urban diabetes center. They were 28 to 57 years old (y/o), with a duration of diabetes from 8 months to 47 years, and insulin pumps were implemented for a period ranging from 2 months to 30 years.

Each of the following case reports consists of a **Focus** (the reason for demonstration); a short **Medical history**; a **Current goal** (an objective for further management); a **Table** with important clinical and laboratory parameters; two **Figures**: a graph with absolute values illustrating the progress of HbA_{1c}, BMI, and INS/d in time; a graph with relative values, where 100% of HbA_{1c}, BMI, and INS/d corresponds to the highest value of a respective physiological range. Later, the effectiveness of the pump was assessed based on clinical and laboratory parameters as well as its subjective impression on the user.

Providing the user with the proper knowledge, skills and attitudes ensure the possibility that the health benefits, convenience, and comforts that the AHCL algorithm offers are utilized to their full potential. Therefore, everyone was familiarized with: physiological insulin function, prandial boluses, basal rate, the effects of physical activity, nutrition, energy intake and expenditure, and how all the above effects the parameters of therapeutic efficiency (HbA_{1c}, body mass, glycemia, and INS/d) [21]. Additionally, they were taught how to use glucometer-strips system for self-monitoring (such as Calla, Galileo Glu/Ket, Contour plus, and ambulatory glycaemic profiles), insulin pens, and most importantly, insulin pumps. Specifically, this entails refilling the insulin reservoir, catheter insertion and replacement in 3-day intervals, sensor insertion, entering saccharide information before and during meals, and overall maintenance of the pump. Education on the insulin pump was provided after implementation either within a two-week hospitalization period or in an outpatient alternative mode.

2.1 Case report Anna

Focus: 30 years lasting management of T1D using various insulin pumps, and eventually improved quality of life along with a subtle reduction in HbA_{1c} after the sensor-augmented insulin pump, MiniMed 780G, was implemented.

History: At 9 years of age (1975), Anna (today 57 y/o) was admitted to the emergency department for a hyperglycaemic coma. Based on history, clinical, and laboratory findings, T1D was diagnosed. From 1975 to 1983, treatment was done with animal insulin consisting of insulin delivery by a glass syringe and a blunt metal needle. At that time self-monitoring was not available apart from a urinalysis. Anna's description of her medical care from 1983 to 1991 is vague. In 1992, she was referred to a diabetes center and received MADI (manual insulin dispenser) [22]. In 1993, she obtained her first glucometer, which Anna describes as a milestone in her life as a person with T1D. In 1993, she obtained her first insulin pump (Dahedi Elektroniks), which reduced the INS/d day from 34 to 29 IU. Next, the pump Dahedi was replaced by a pump H-Tron V100, Disetronic (1994–2008). In 1996, she became pregnant with twins. Both children (boy and girl) were born on January 10, 1997, healthy, by planned Cesarean section (indicated by a breech position of one of the children) with body mass at births of 2.6 and 2.7 kg. In the following period of 25 years, Anna's clinical condition was stable. She performed intensive selfmonitoring (SMPG) using glucometer-strips system 5 to 12 times a day and adopted the insulin boluses according to plasma glucose, food, and exercise. In 2009 insulin pump Paradigm 722 was implemented, followed by Paradigm Veo 554. In 2010, hypothyroidism was diagnosed and treated further on.

In 2021, the hybrid insulin pump MiniMed 780G was put in motion. Anna has been continuously employing the SmartGuard mode (**Figures 3** and **4**). The important clinical and laboratory findings can be seen in **Table 1**. Current TIR: 89%.

Parameters	Units	Refer	1.12.1994	26.10.2004	13.07.2012	29.04.2015	21.09.2022
T1D duration	Years	N/A	19	29	37	40	47
Heart rate	BPM	60–90	76	—	72	78	72
Blood pressure	Torr	<130/85	110/70	—	125/70	150/80	168/89
fvS-glucose	mmol/	3.3–5.5	—	—	5.6	6.7	8.8
fvS-C-peptide	pmol/l	>300	—	500	<300*	—	—
fvS-GADA	kU/I/	0–5	—	—	0.2	—	—
fvS-HDL	mmol/l	1.2–2.7	1.26	1.74	2	1.84	2.12
fvS-LDL	mmol/l	1.2–2.6	4.19	2.23	2.72	2.83	3.25
fvS-TAG	mmol/l	0.5–1.7	1.53	1.9	0.91	0.6	0.8
fvS-creatinine	μmol/l	< 108	—	—	78	67	69
eGFR	ml/s	1.0–1.3	—	—	1.15	—	1.55
fvS-CRP	mg/l	< 10	—	—	0.7	0.6	0.7

*fvS – fasting venous serum, *since 2004 repeated five times.*

Table 1.
Anna's clinical and laboratory parameters over 28 years.

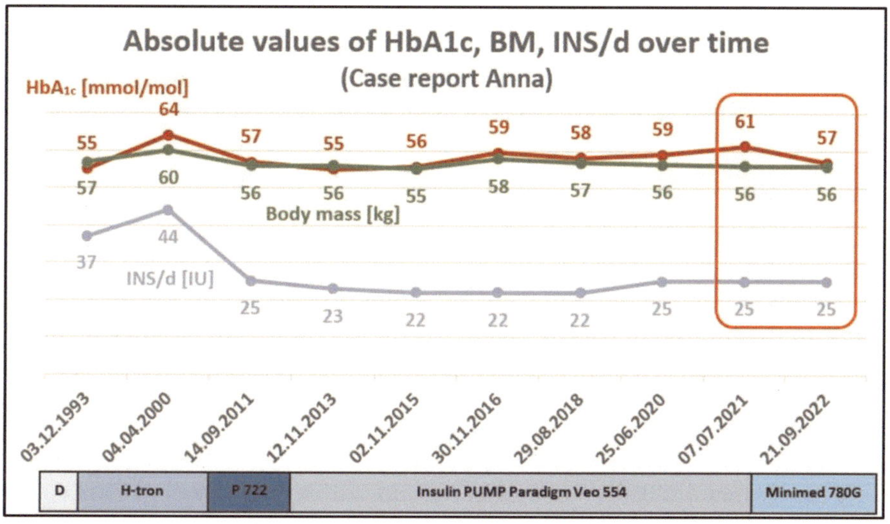

Figure 3.
Anna's absolute values of HbA_{1c}, BM, and INS/d since her first pump D (Dahedi Elektroniks) was implemented. Insulin pump H-tron (1994–2008) was followed by pumps paradigm (without CGM). Since the therapy with a sensor-augmented insulin pump MiniMed 780G with SmartGuard auto mode was applied in 2022, there is a subtle improvement in HbA_{1c} concentration (red box). See also red box in ***Figure 4****.*

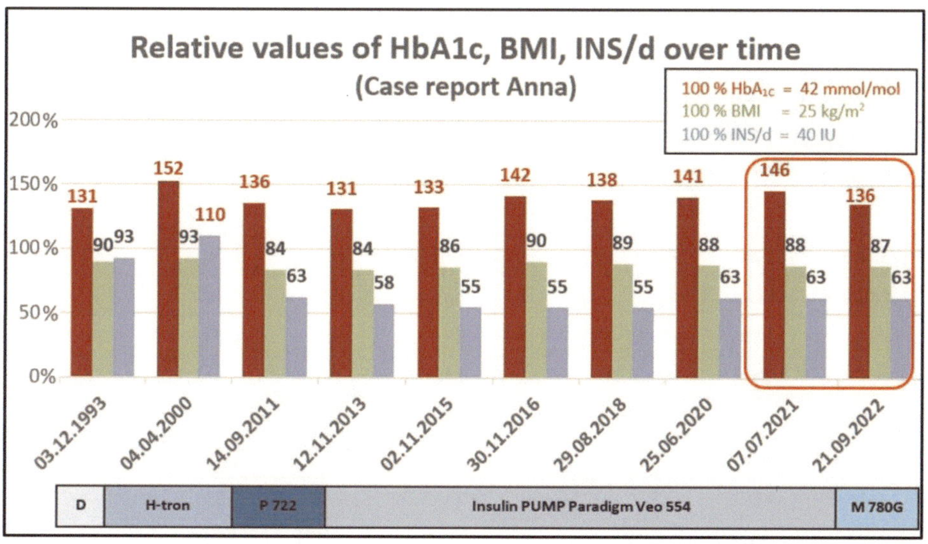

Figure 4.
Anna's relative values of HbA_{1c}, BMI, and INS/d from 1993 to 2022 indicate an extended period of HbA_{1c} at 30% above the norm with slight fluctuation and a 10% decrease within 1 year after CGM implementation. Over the entirety of 29 years, BMI remains stable in the high 80s and low 90s. There is no difference in INS/d before and after MiniMed 780G. D – Dahedi Elektroniks, P – Paradigm, M – MiniMed.

Current goal: To reduce LDL below 2.6 mmol/l and HbA_{1c} below 50 mmol/mol without hypoglycemia, therapy of hypoglycemia with glucagon; screening for macroangiopathy (**Table 1**).

2.2 Case report Betty

Focus: influence of pregnancy on HbA_{1c}, INS/d, and BMI in a lady with T1D using a pump without CGM, and effects of hybrid MiniMed 780G implemented after pregnancy.

History: Betty (today 33 y/o) was diagnosed with T1D at the age of 14 years in September 2004 in pediatric department of regional hospital. She was immediately treated by means of an insulin pen with insulin aspart and detemir, a maximum dose of insulin was 20 IU/d. In 2007, insulin pump Animas was implemented as the main form of insulin therapy. In 2015 the pump Animas was replaced by MiniMed 640G. In the course of the first pregnancy, a decrease in HbA_{1c} and marked increase in INS/d could be seen. She gave birth to a boy (delivery July 8, 2015 by Cesarean section, 4.48 kg, 54 cm). The parameters from August 31, 2015 demonstrated improved compensation (lower values of HbA_{1c}), however, the amount of insulin per day was nearly doubled (**Table 2**, **Figures 5** and **6**). Betty had a second pregnancy in 2019 (delivery November 1, 2019 by Cesarean section, girl 4.75 kg, 53 cm). During this second pregnancy, there was an apparent decrease in HbA_{1c} concentration and an increased supply of exogenous insulin (161 IU/d). To explain these similar changes in HbA_{1c} and INS/d it is worth noting that placenta is permeable to glucose but impermeable to insulin [23, 24]. Therefore, the insulin from fetal pancreas may create new fetal adipose tissue by converting the glucose crossing through placental barrier from mother's plasma. These pathways may result in fetal macrosomia (which is a known complication associated with raised HbA_{1c} concentration in the last trimester of pregnancy). Only a minority of pregnant women were able to optimize their glycemic control. This makes CGM and hybrid insulin pumps all the more favorable for treatment during pregnancy [25, 26]. However, Betty could receive the hybrid pump MiniMed 780G as late as in April 2021. Current TIR: 96% (January 5, 2023).

Parameters	Units	Refer	21.4.2014	12.10.2016	30.4.2019	16.12.2020	10.06.2022
T1D duration	years	N/A	9	12	14	16	18
Heart rate	BPM	60–90	94	89	98	94	97
Bl. pressure	Torr	<130/85	130/80	140/85	121/82	134/95	175/97
fvS-glucose	mmol/	3.3–5.5	9.9	7.0	9.0	6.0	6.8
fvS-C-peptide	pmol/l	>300	—	—	—	<7	—
fvS-GADA	kU/I/	0–5	—	—	—	33	—
fvS-HDL	mmol/l	1.2–2.7	1.29	2.04	1.55	1.17	1.17
fvS-LDL	mmol/l	1.2–2.6	2.89	3.53	2.7	3.31	3.31
fvS-TAG	mmol/l	0.5–1.7	1.26	0.88	2.7	1.39	1.39
fvS-creatinine	µmol/l	< 108	47.1	58	48	65	59
eGFR	ml/s	1.0–1.3	—	—	—	1.9	1.93
fvS-CRP	mg/l	< 10	1.9	1.8	7.9	3.6	5.1

fvS – fasting venous serum.

Table 2.
Betty's clinical and laboratory parameters over the last 8 years.

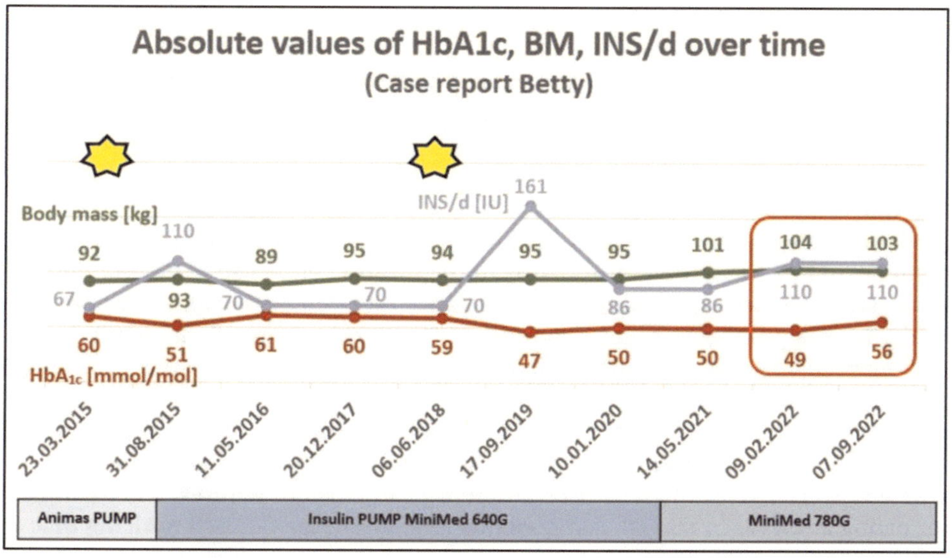

Figure 5.
Betty's absolute values of HbA_{1c}, BMI, and INS/d from 2015 to the last check-up. The Animas insulin pump was implemented in 2007. The two peaks on the blue line (INS/d) in the years 2015 and 2019 correlate to Betty's pregnancies when the insulin dosage nearly doubled and lowered HbA_{1c}, indicating better metabolic control. Pregnancy is symbolized by yellow stars. The last two check-ups show high INS/d (110 U/d) and increased body mass with no sustainable effect on HbA_{1c} (red box).

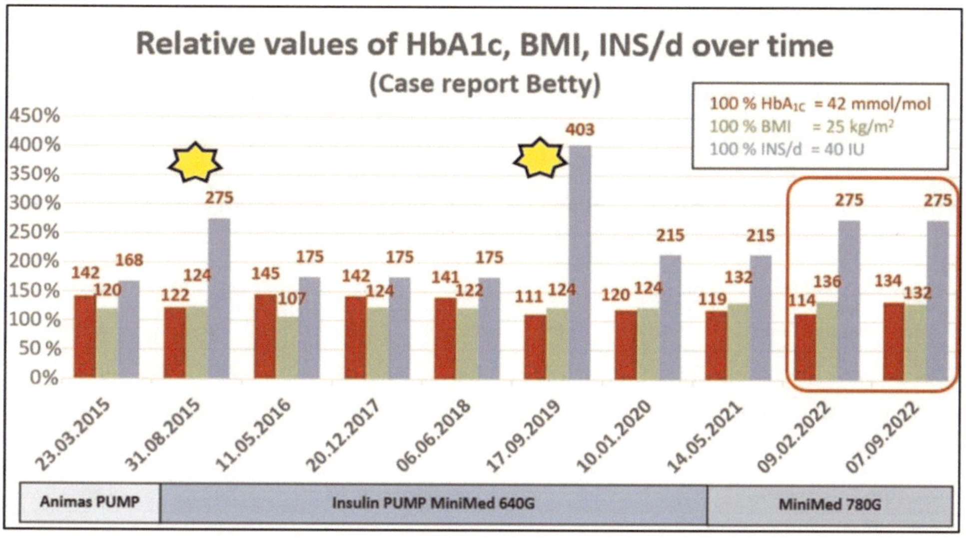

Figure 6.
Betty's relative values of HbA_{1c}, BMI, and INS/d from 2015 to 2022. HbA_{1c} has exceeded the desired reference value for a long period of time, which is illustrated by all the red percentages. Two peaks, with 275% (=110 IU/d) value INS/d during her first pregnancy in 2015, and 403% (=161 IU/d) value INS/d during her second pregnancy in 2019 (yellow stars). The last two check-ups show high insulin delivery and increased BMI with no sustainable effect on HbA_{1c} (red box). TIR was 62% (February 9, 2022).

Current goal: examine the methods for managing her increased appetite, management of hyperlipoproteinemia, hypertension, and hypoglycemia; selfmonitoring of ketones.

2.3 Case report Clark

Focus: continuously increased INS/d, and body mass along with near-optimal HbA_{1c} concentration and hypoglycaemia when using insulin pump without CGM and followed by hybrid pump with SmartGuard.

History: At 20 years of age, Clark (today 46 y/o) was diagnosed with T1D. Education and treatment by means of insulin pen and multiple daily injections resulted in improvement in clinical and laboratory findings. Clark was compliant and had no problem adjusting to the insulin boluses according to meals and physical exercise at that time. In 2009, Clark received his first insulin pump. In 2013, insulin pump Paradigm Veo (without CGM) was implemented and, in 2017, replaced with MiniMed 640G. INS/d was high (routinely adopted according to intake of saccharides), but otherwise no other issues, in clinical and laboratory parameters (**Table 3** and **Figures** 7 and **8**). In 2022 a hybrid insulin pump MiniMed 780G was introduced. Since that time Clark had troubles with his adaptation to the new algorithms dealing with saccharide ratio and insulin boluses. For example: after eating a roll for breakfast that contains 25 g of saccharides and noticing that the pump gives him only one unit of insulin, he would enter additional saccharides that he did not consume, until it would give him 2.5 units of insulin as he was used to. (Essentially ignoring that the pump gives him exactly what he needs at that moment.) This approach resulted in reoccurring hypoglycemia followed by increased food intake and growing body mass. Therefore, lower insulin doses resulting in reduced risk of hypoglycemia, lower body mass, and lower HbA_{1c} may be reached provided Clark creates a deeper understanding of the algorithm behind MiniMed 780G. At the time he is able to manage MiniMed 780G. Current TIR: 87% (January 5, 2023).

Besides T1D, Clark also has hyperlipoproteinemia (diagnosed in 2014), treated with rosuvastatin, and unstable hypertension.

Parameters	Units	Refer	21.05.2014	02.05.2015	05.09.2018	29.01.2020	23.11.2022
T1D duration	years	N/A	17	18	21	23	25
Heart rate	BPM	60–90	68	73	81	76	87
Blood pressure	Torr	<130/85	120/70	120/80	133/89	149/96	164/99
fvS-glucose	mmol/	3.3–5.5	4.9	6.4	5.3	7.5	4.9
fvS-C-peptide	pmol/l	>300	—	30	—	—	—
fvS-GADA	kU/I/	0–5	—	32.5	—	—	—
fvS-HDL	mmol/l	1.2–2.7	1.6	2.07	1.63	1.42	1.85
fvS-LDL	mmol/l	1.2–2.6	3.2	2.52	3.42	1.92	1.91
fvS-TAG	mmol/l	0.5–1.7	0.6	0.76	0.92	1.62	0.86
fvS-creatinine	µmol/l	< 108	90	121.6	95.7	83.6	77.7
eGFR	ml/s	1.0–1.3	—	—	—	1.7	1.7
fvS-CRP	mg/l	< 10	0.1	0.5	0.2	0.2	0.5

fvS – fasting venous serum.

Table 3.
Clark's clinical and laboratory parameters from the diagnosis of T1D over the last 8 years.

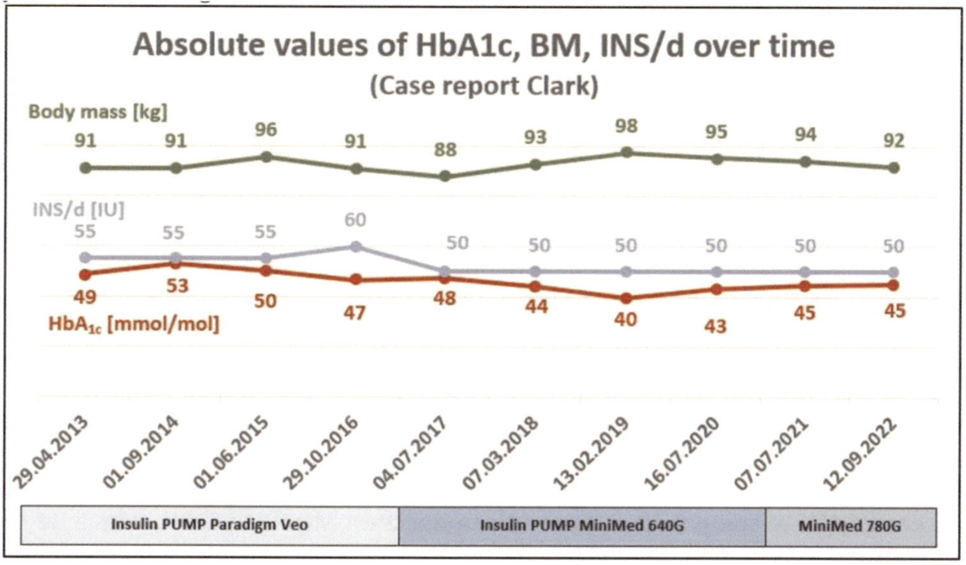

Figure 7.
Clark's absolute values of HbA_{1c}, BM, and INS/d show relatively constant values of HbA_{1c} and INS/d over 9 years of time, while his body mass changed within a range of 88 kg and 98 kg. Treatment with an insulin pump was initiated in 2009. Followed by the insulin pump Paradigm Veo 554 implemented in April 2013, MiniMed 640G in April 2017, and MiniMed 780G in January 2022. Using CGM could potentially improve HbA_{1c} concentration with a lower number of insulin units needed.

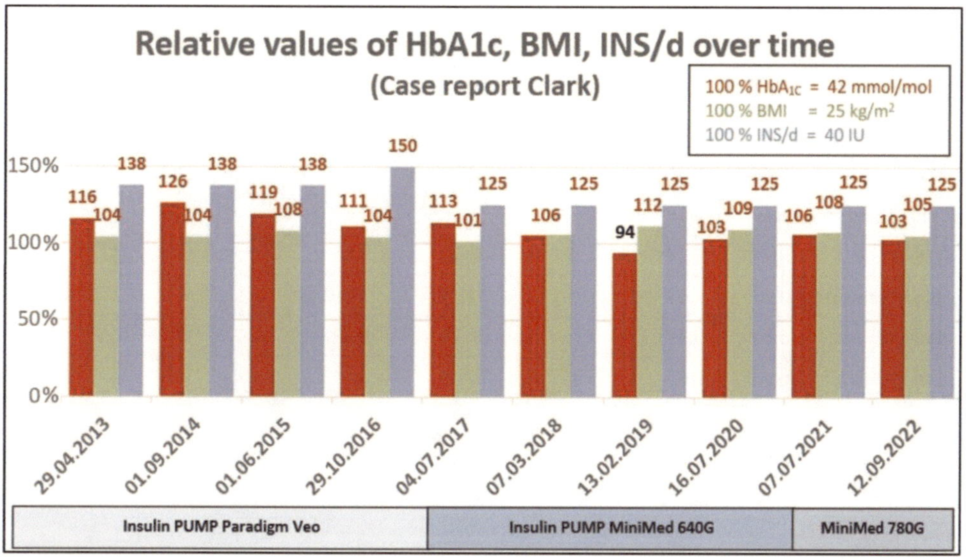

Figure 8.
Clark's relative values of HbA_{1c}, BMI, and INS/d from 2013 until the last check-up. Red values of INS/d in columns indicate the overuse of insulin to lower glycemia. Nevertheless, there is an apparent difference between the needed insulin dose during the use of the Paradigm Veo 554, MiniMed 640G, and MiniMed 780G.

Current goal: reeducation on the use of MiniMed 780G with SafeGuard mode: input of saccharides, temporary targets, reassurance that the pump delivers the optimal doses without manual intervention, and management of high blood pressure and hypoglycemia.

2.4 Case report Daniel

Focus: long-term inadequate compensation during therapy by insulin pump with an improvement after switching to a hybrid pump with CGM and SmartGuard.

History: Daniel (today 51 y/o) was diagnosed with T1D in 2000. Primarily, he experienced polydipsia (drinking almost ten liters per day). Upon examination, glycemia was 30 mmol/l. Insulin therapy was initiated, however, glycated hemoglobin HbA_{1c} (70 mmol/mol) and unexpected hypoglycemia (twice a month) persisted. After 13 years (December 3, 2013), Daniel was given the Paradigm Veo 554 insulin pump (without CGM). Despite this, glycated hemoglobin showed no improvement. He was diagnosed with retinopathy in his left eye in 2015. It was recommended to regularly measure glycemia and learn to recognize hypoglycemia. The implementation of continuous monitoring with a new hybrid insulin pump MiniMed 780G made this easier and showed immediate improvement in glycated hemoglobin and a decrease in INS/d (**Figures 9** and **10**).

When asked to compare Paradigm Veo to the latest MiniMed 780G, which he started using in September of 2022, he stated that it is easy to work with especially thanks to its ability to connect to a mobile phone. Besides T1D, Daniel is also treated for hypertension (ramipril), nephropathy with interstitial and glomerular damage, hypercholesterolemia (rosuvastatin), and neuropathy (**Table 4**). In 2021, he developed a dental defect. Daniel received a glucometer Galileo Glu/Ket, in order to use it in circumstances such as vomiting, nausea, fever, etc. Namely, some of these symptoms were recently present without apparent explanation. Current TIR: 87% (January 5, 2023).

Parameters	Units	Refer	29.11.2013	07.05.2015	04.05.2018	28.04.2021	05.10.2022
T1D duration	years	N/A	13	15	18	21	22
Heart rate	BPM	60–90	—	64	74	79	86
Blood pressure	torr	<130/85	—	130/80	161/105	147/88	157/98
fvS-glucose	mmol/	3.3–5.5	10.9	21.7	13.7	7.0	6.2
fvS-C-peptide	pmol/l	>300	Neg.	30	—	—	—
fvS-GADA	kU/I/	0–5	14	17	—	—	—
fvS-HDL	mmol/l	1.2–2.7	1.22	1.66	1.27	1.55	1.58
fvS-LDL	mmol/l	1.2–2.6	2.62	3.9	2.24	2.42	1.97
fvS-TAG	mmol/l	0.5–1.7	2.95	1.06	1.8	1.23	0.76
fvS-creatinine	μmol/l	< 108	69.6	67.4	64	71.9	62.4
eGFR	ml/s	1.0–1.3	—	—	—	1.73	1.81
fvS-CRP	mg/l	< 10	3.3	0.6	0.4	1.4	4.5

fvS – fasting venous serum.

Table 4.
Daniel's clinical and laboratory parameters over 9 years.

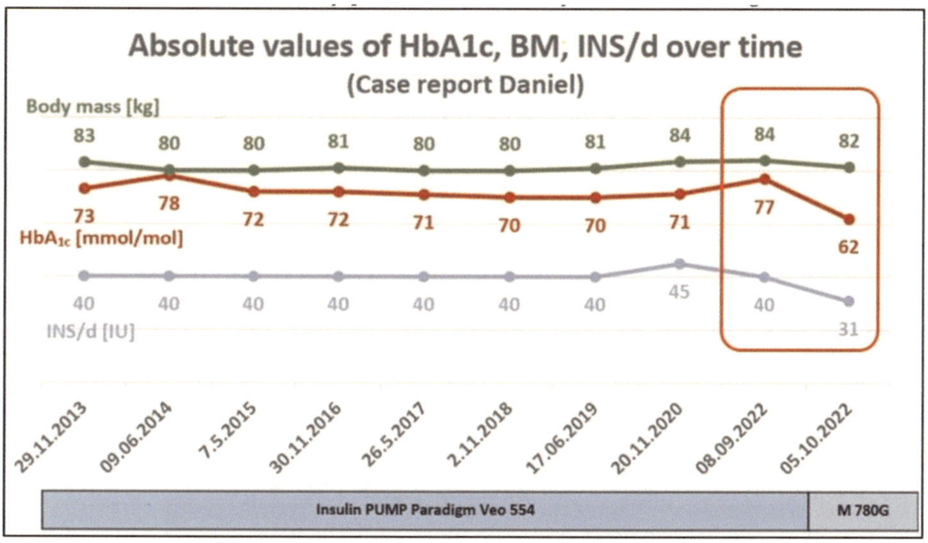

Figure 9.
Daniel's absolute values of HbA_{1c}, BM, and INS/d over 9 years. Since he has been diagnosed with T1D in 2000, he has been treated with insulin by delivering it via an insulin pen. His first insulin pump, Paradigm Veo 554, was implemented on December 3, 2013. Laboratory values were constant until the application of a sensor-augmented insulin pump in September 2022, when the HbA_{1c} concentration decreased alongside a lower insulin dosage is needed (red box).

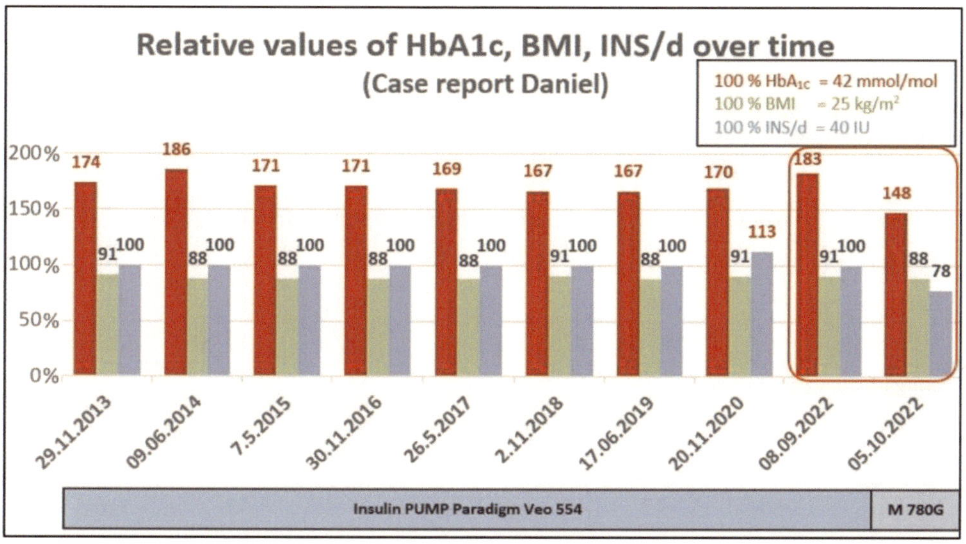

Figure 10.
Daniel's relative values of HbA_{1c}, BMI, and INS/d from 2013 to 2022. Red values of HbA_{1c} indicate a long-lasting period in which the respective parameters exceeded the upper limit of the reference range. HbA_{1c} was constant until the application of a sensor-augmented insulin pump (MiniMed 780G) in September 2022, when the HbA_{1c} concentration decreased (to 148% = 62 mmol/mol) alongside a lower insulin dosage (78% = 31 IU/d) needed (red box).

Current goal: education in the use of the glucometer Galileo Glu/Ket as means of measurement of glycemia and ketone bodies, management of hypertension, and regular dental and eye exams.

2.5 Case report Edward

Focus: insulin pump implementation in 2014 led to post-initial remission until 2018, which was followed by an increase in HbA_{1c}, body mass, and IU/d needed.

History: Edward (today 46 y/o) was diagnosed with T1D at 27 years of age, in 2014. The diagnosis was made based on the abrupt onset of clinical symptoms such as polydipsia, polyuria, fatigue, and eventually loss of body mass (2 kg/month). He was given insulin in the form of Novopen (insulin aspart and detemir). After 6 weeks, an insulin pump, Paradigm Veo (**Figure 11**), was implemented while doing intensive self-monitoring of plasma glucose (SMPG) using glucometer Contour plus. Initially, Edward was skeptical about the insulin pump; due to his physical activity and sports, he was not sure if the pump would be an obstruction during his activities (**Table 5**). After education, when seeing the last parameters (**Figures 12** and **13**), he agreed to try MiniMed 780G.

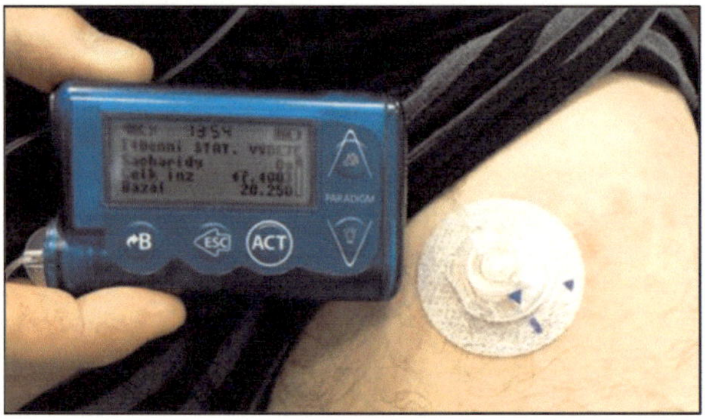

Figure 11.
Paradigm Veo 554 and a subcutaneous cannula on the front of the thigh.

Parameters	Units	Refer	11.2.2014	21.09.2016	20.07.2020	14.04.2021	21.09.2022
T1D duration	Months	N/A	0	32	78	87	104
Heart rate	BPM	60–90	64	88	84	67	80
Blood pressure	Torr	<130/85	130/70	130/70	156/86	136/89	135/80
fvS-glucose	mmol/	3.3–5.5	5.6	6.8	9.5	7.8	7.5
fvS-C-peptide	pmol/l	>300	258	—	142	—	—
fvS-GADA	kU/I/	0–5	47	—	12	—	—
fvS-HDL	mmol/l	1.2–2.7	1.3	1.3	1.3	1.2	1.4
fvS-LDL	mmol/l	1.2–2.6	4.2	3.6	2	2.7	2.8
fvS-TAG	mmol/l	0.5–1.7	0.9	1.4	0.8	0.9	0.9
fvS-creatinine	µmol/l	< 108	71.1	65.2	79.3	80.5	84.9
eGFR	ml/s	1.0–1.3	—	—	—	1.71	1.65
fvS-CRP	mg/l	< 10	0.4	0.3	1.2	0.6	0.7

fvS – fasting venous serum.

Table 5.
Edward's clinical and laboratory parameters over 8 years from the diagnosis of T1D in 2014 to the last check-up.

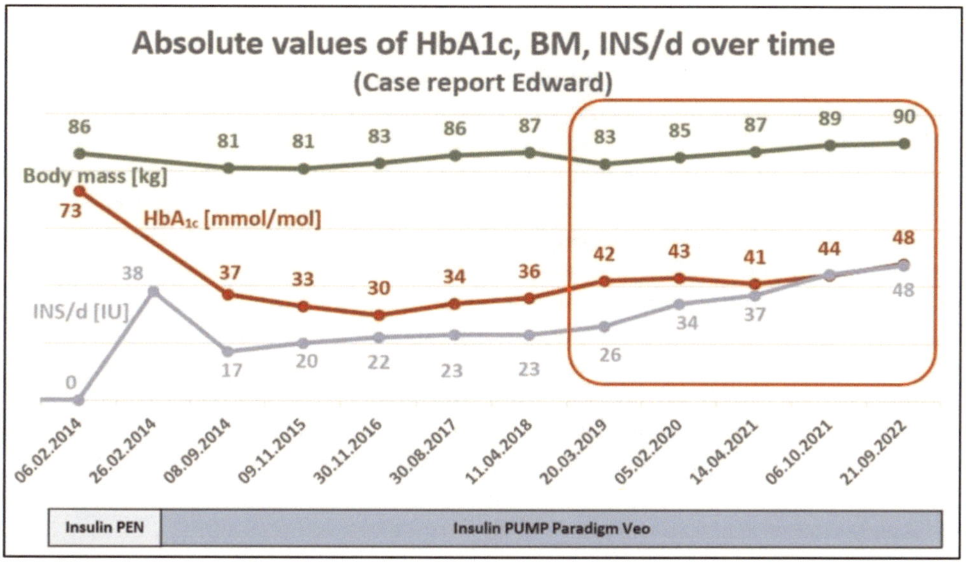

Figure 12.
Edward's absolute values of HbA_{1c}, BM, and INS/d reflect a rapid decrease in HbA_{1c} (from 73 mmol/mol to 37 mmol/mol) after insulin therapy was started with an insulin pen. After the implementation of an insulin pump, Paradigm Veo 554, in April 2014, HbA_{1c} concentration continued to decrease even further while fewer insulin units were needed for better compensation. After the year 2018 (red box), INS/d started to increase alongside HbA_{1c}, which may be due to the end of supposed post-initial remission period that lasted about 4 years (2014-2018).

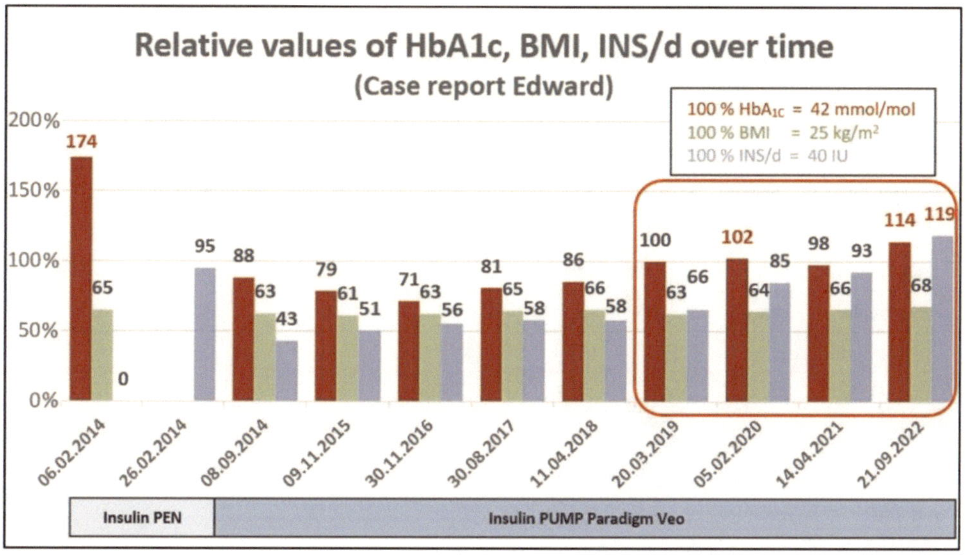

Figure 13.
Edward's relative values of HbA_{1c}, BMI, and INS/d illustrate long-lasting satisfactory metabolic compensation. The most recent result shows an increase in both HbA_{1c} from 86–114% and INS/d from 58–119% (red box). His BMI varies between 61% and 68% of its reference range.

Current goal: acknowledging Edward's reluctance as valid, while also motivating him to use CGM, as his worsening compensation can be attributed to the lack thereof.

2.6 Case report Fiona

Focus: insulin pump implementation can result in subjective improvement, without effect in laboratory parameters.

History: The first signs of T1D appeared in 2014 so Fiona (today 48 y/o) was treated with an insulin pen for 15 months. The HbA_{1c} concentration has been increasing during this treatment, thus the insulin pump MiniMed 640G was implemented and she was trained in selfmonitoring on glucometer-strips system Contour (**Figure 14**). Up until the beginning of the year 2017, her clinical and laboratory findings were improving. Since then, her HbA_{1c} concentration has been increasing (**Table 6**, **Figures 15** and **16**). The reason for this rise is multifactorial: difficult life situations, struggling to keep a constant regime of glycemia monitoring, etc. Fiona is satisfied with the insulin pump as it improved the quality of her everyday life; she does not need to prick herself a few times per day as she works on shifts. Fiona is not convinced to use CGM, although she is aware of insufficient compensation and low frequency of self-monitoring: two times per day, sometimes only once a week.

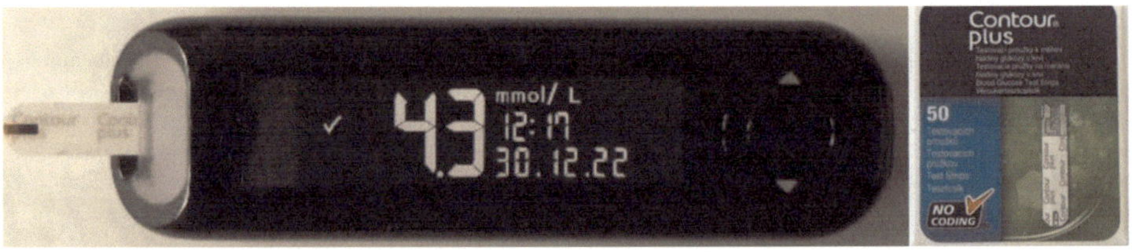

Figure 14.
Glucometer Contour plus one showing glycaemia 4.3 mmol/l. Box with test strips (on the right).

Parameters	Units	Refer	06.10.2014	15.06.2016	15.07.2019	18.10.2021	9.11.2022
T1D duration	Months	N/A	1	21	58	85	98
Heart rate	BPM	60–90	62	66	70	60	105
Blood pressure	torr	<130/85	120/80	161/72	116/82	138/90	149/101
fvS-glucose	mmol/	3.3–5.5	—	8.4	14.7	10.3	11.9
fvS-C-peptide	pmol/l	>300	235	—	—	—	—
fvS-GADA	kU/I/	0–5	>250	>250	—	—	—
fvS-HDL	mmol/l	1.2–2.7	1.9	2.18	1.83	1.78	2.03
fvS-LDL	mmol/l	1.2–2.6	2.03	3.15	2.18	2.8	3.39
fvS-TAG	mmol/l	0.5–1.7	0.8	0.4	0.58	0.76	0.71
fvS-creatinine	μmol/l	< 108	52.9	60	56	56.3	56
eGFR	ml/s	1.0–1.3	—	—	1.77	1.77	1.76
fvS-CRP	mg/l	< 10	0.9	1	1.8	1.7	1.5

fvS – fasting venous serum.

Table 6.
Fiona's clinical and laboratory parameters from T1D start over 8 years.

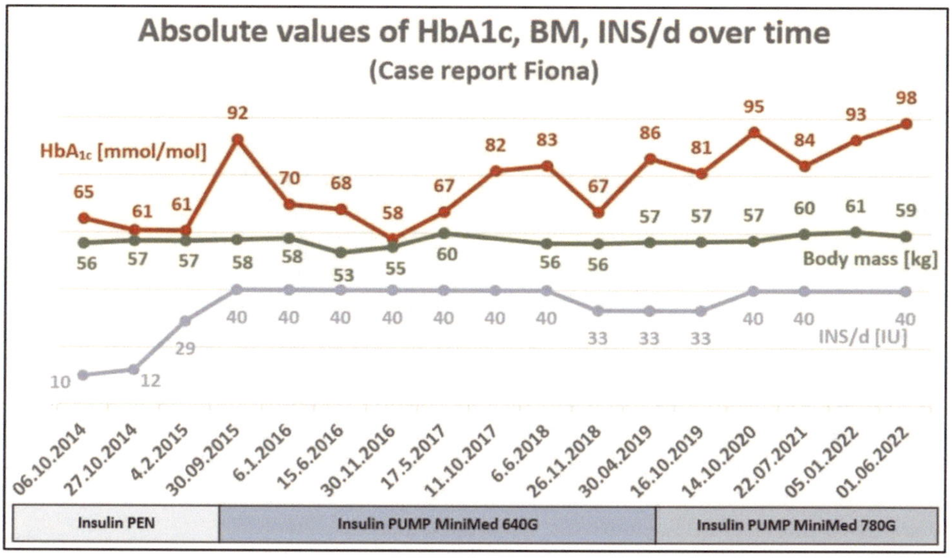

Figure 15.
Fiona's absolute values of HbA_{1c}, BM, and INS/d from 2014 to 2022. HbA_{1c} concentrations were increasing during the treatment with an insulin pen, thus insulin pump MiniMed 640G was implemented. The last seven values show a systematic increase in HbA_{1c}, which is a result of a lack of compensation.

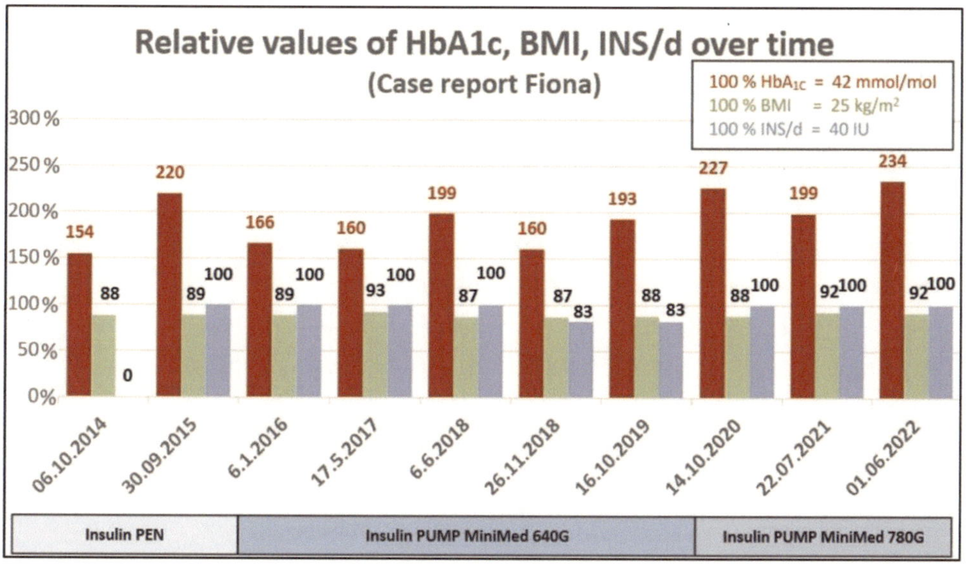

Figure 16.
Fiona's relative values of HbA_{1c}, BMI, and INS/d over an 8-year-long period. All red HbA_{1c} digits illustrate long-term unsatisfactory results with average values 190% of the reference range, although more insulin could be used for better correction. Her BMI has fluctuated between 88 and 93% of the upper limit of its reference range.

Her glycemia is mostly high, and she is afraid to deliver an additional bolus because of an unpleasant experience with hypoglycaemia.

Current goal: to motivate Fiona to use CGM.

2.7 Case report George

Focus: growing body mass and INS/d in a man using SmartGuard mode and TIR 100%.

History: George (today 32 y/o) was diagnosed with T1D in April 2021 and treated with insulin *via* an insulin pen, immediately resulting in an initial decrease in HbA_{1c}. By September of the same year, a hybrid insulin pump MiniMed 780G was implemented. George is compliant and has been achieving excellent compensation in terms of HbA_{1c} and time in range (TIR). However, instead of entering data about the amount of consumed saccharides, which would have allowed the pump to automatically infuse the right insulin dose, tailored to his metabolism, glycemia, and remaining function of beta-cells, he has been entering the order for a bolus in insulin units (**Figure 17**). This order tends to be less effective, resulting in higher insulin intake and a gradual increase in body mass (**Figures 18** and **19**). Even though the conversion of saccharides to IU could be appropriate for the use of an insulin pen or pump without AHCL, it lowers the efficiency of pumps with AHCL. Current TIR: 100% (November 16, 2022).

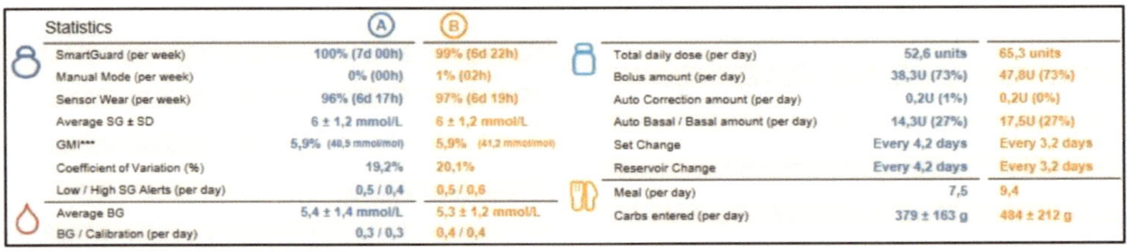

Statistics	A	B
SmartGuard (per week)	100% (7d 00h)	99% (6d 22h)
Manual Mode (per week)	0% (00h)	1% (02h)
Sensor Wear (per week)	96% (6d 17h)	97% (6d 19h)
Average SG ± SD	6 ± 1,2 mmol/L	6 ± 1,2 mmol/L
GMI***	5,9% (40,5 mmol/mol)	5,9% (41,2 mmol/mol)
Coefficient of Variation (%)	19,2%	20,1%
Low / High SG Alerts (per day)	0,5 / 0,4	0,5 / 0,6
Average BG	5,4 ± 1,4 mmol/L	5,3 ± 1,2 mmol/L
BG / Calibration (per day)	0,3 / 0,3	0,4 / 0,4
Total daily dose (per day)	52,6 units	65,3 units
Bolus amount (per day)	38,3U (73%)	47,8U (73%)
Auto Correction amount (per day)	0,2U (1%)	0,2U (0%)
Auto Basal / Basal amount (per day)	14,3U (27%)	17,5U (27%)
Set Change	Every 4,2 days	Every 3,2 days
Reservoir Change	Every 4,2 days	Every 3,2 days
Meal (per day)	7,5	9,4
Carbs entered (per day)	379 ± 163 g	484 ± 212 g

Figure 17.
*CareLink Statistics: A comparison between date range A (blue) and B (orange). Progress between both date ranges, blood glucose (BG), insulin usage, and saccharides consumed (**Table 7**).*

Parameters	Units	Refer	12.08.2021	29.11.2021	16.02.2022	25.05.2022	16.11.2022
T1D duration	months	N/A	4	8	11	14	19
Heart rate	BPM	60–90	104	104	104	107	110
Blood pressure	torr	<130/85	152/94	152/94	152/94	155/92	131/87
fvS-glucose	mmol/l	3.3–5.5	6.2	—	5.1	4.6	4.5
fvS-C-peptide	pmol/l	>300	632	—	>600	—	—
fvS-GADA	kU/l	0–5	58.8	—	—	—	—
fvS-HDL	mmol/l	1.2–2.7	1.16	—	1.04	1.04	1.16
fvS-LDL	mmol/l	1.2–2.6	3.31	—	2.75	2.75	3.31
fvS-TAG	mmol/l	0.5–1.7	1.4	1.38	1.63	1.63	1.4
fvS-creatinine	µmol/l	< 108	78.6	79	68.9	77.9	78.6
eGFR	ml/s	1.0–1.3	1.99	—	1.99	1.89	1.87
fvS-CRP	mg/l	< 10	1.1	—	4.7	0.5	0.7

fvS – fasting venous serum.

Table 7.
George's clinical and laboratory parameters from the diagnosis of T1D over 14 months.

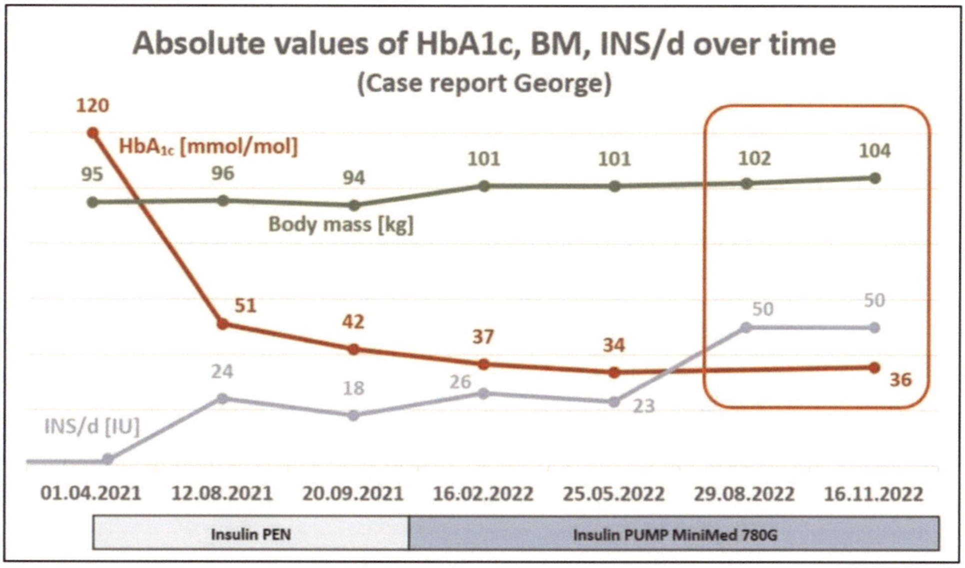

Figure 18.
George's absolute values of HbA_{1c}, BM, and INS/d over 19 months illustrate the initial rapid correction of HbA_{1c} (from 120 to 51 mmol/mol) after initiation of insulin treatment by insulin pen. Later, there is sufficient HbA_{1c} control, at the expense of the high insulin delivery, up to 50 IU/d (red box), and thus an increase in body mass (from 94 to 104 kg). HbA_{1c} concentration was not measured on August 29, 2022.

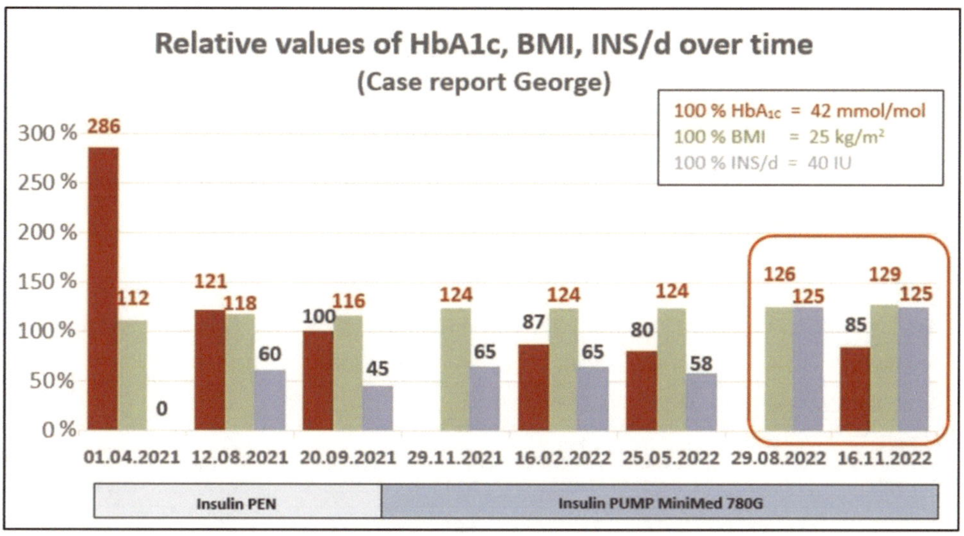

Figure 19.
George's relative values of HbA_{1c}, BMI, and INS/d over 19 months. Rising BMI (up to 129%) is probably due to an increase in INS/d (to 125% of the upper limit of its reference range), highlighted in the red box, which enables glucose to enter cells through the insulin-dependent glucose transporter GLUT4 [27]. His HbA_{1c} concentration is under control. HbA_{1c} concentration was not measured on August 8, 2022.

Current goal: adequate education about the correct use of the hybrid pump when using the SmartGuard mode and management of hypertension and hyperlipoproteinemia.

2.8 Case report Helen

Focus: swift correction of HbA_{1c} attributed to immediate insulin treatment and implementation of hybrid insulin pump MiniMed 780G 3 weeks after T1D diagnosis.

History: Helen's (today 53 y/o) issues began when she experienced blurry vision while on holiday. In combination with losing 8 kg over 2 weeks, polydipsia and polyuria led her to seek out medical attention with reason to suspect diabetes. Helen was diagnosed with T1D on September 23, 2021; her HbA_{1c} concentration was 115 mmol/mol. She began treatment with an insulin pen (28 IU/d). After three weeks (October 10, 2021), Helen was indicated to implement the insulin pump MiniMed 780G with a reduced total insulin dose per day (20 ID/d), (**Figures 20** and **21**). She claims that it took her approximately one week to fully understand how to use the insulin pump, how to connect sensor Guardian 4, and how to switch the manual or SmartGuard mode. When asked to compare insulin treatment by means of pen vs. pump, Helen prefers the insulin pump unhesitatingly for its comfortability and lesser frequency of multiple needle pricks.

The biggest challenge for Helen, considering using the pump, is visiting the pool area. Helen called the Medtronic helpline to get information on how to make her summer holiday more comfortable and stay well compensated at the same time. At the time, she was told that her insulin pump is waterproof for up to 24 hours and that the sensor with a transmitter is water resistant for up to 30 minutes. According to Medtronic, although MiniMed 780G is waterproof, it is recommended to remove it before bathing or swimming, because the wear and tear that comes from regular use can increase the risk of water damage [8]. Besides T1D, there is hypertension, transient atrial fibrillation, treated hypothyroidism, and hyperlipoproteinemia in her medical history (**Table 8**). Current TIR: 75% (December 14, 2022).

Parameters	Units	Refer	29.09.2021	12.01.2022	21.06.2022	29.09.2022	14.12.2022
T1D duration	Months	N/A	0	4	9	12	15
Heart rate	BPM	60–90	84	79	82	73	75
Blood pressure	Torr	<130/85	150/96	146/92	149/93	123/81	149/73
fvS-glucose	mmol/	3.3–5.5	16.6	6.3	6.6	5.3	6.5
fvS-C-peptide	pmol/l	>300	166	—	—	—	—
fvS-GADA	kU/I	0–5	>250	—	—	—	—
fvS-HDL	mmol/l	1.2–2.7	0.82	1.24	1.12	1.27	1.14
fvS-LDL	mmol/l	1.2–2.6	3.23	3.05	2.67	2.82	3.34
fvS-TAG	mmol/l	0.5–1.7	1.81	0.94	1.18	0.92	0.8
fvS-creatinine	μmol/l	< 108	52.1	52.4	56.7	62.1	57.2
eGFR	ml/s	1.0–1.3	1.76	1.75	1.7	1.65	1.69
fvS-CRP	mg/l	< 10	3.4	1.2	0.7	1	1.8

fvS – fasting venous serum.

Table 8.
Helen's clinical and laboratory parameters from the diagnosis of T1D over 15 months.

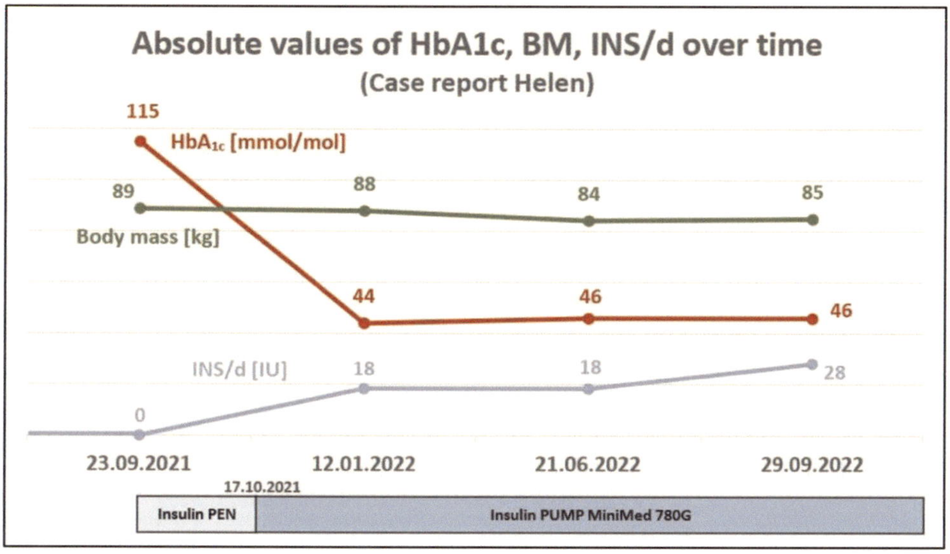

Figure 20.
Helen's absolute values of HbA1c, BM, and INS/d over 12 months show a decrease in HbA1c concentration after the initiation of insulin therapy, when using an insulin pen at the beginning for 24 days, and followed by MiniMed 780G (manual/SmartGuard mode).

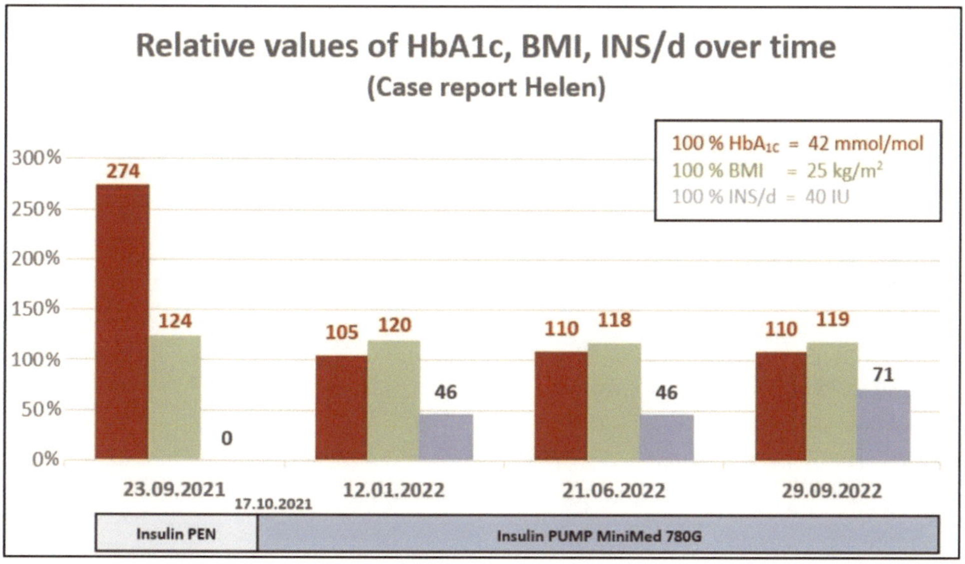

Figure 21.
Helen's relative values of HbA_{1c}, BMI, and INS/d over 12 months show a rapid HbA_{1c} decrease after the initiation of insulin therapy. BMI values indicate an irregular, subtle fluctuation in the range of no larger than 6%. Considering the alternative use of manual/SmartGuard/manual mode, changes in INS/d, body, HbA_{1c}, and increased satisfaction with the pump one can assume gradual but adequate metabolic compensation based on successful education and flexible management of the hybrid insulin pump.

Current goal: to reduce HbA_{1c} below 42 mmol/mol, management of hypertension and hyperlipoproteinemia, and monitoring of ketones by means of Galileo Glu/Ket.

2.9 Case report Isabella

Focus: a person who found professional care shortly after the first signs of T1D and received hybrid insulin pump MiniMed 780G within 6 weeks.

History: Isabella (today 38 y/o) experienced a long period of illness before presenting with hyperglycemia on Easter in 2022. Due to her untimely diagnosis before a four-day-long holiday, she was given only an insulin pen (28 IU/d), glucometer Galileo Glu/Ket, and short instructions *via* mobile phone. Within 10 days, detailed education was initiated and, ultimately, in 6 weeks, she was given an insulin pump MiniMed 780G, to which she adapted and has shown exemplary cooperation (**Figures 22–24**).

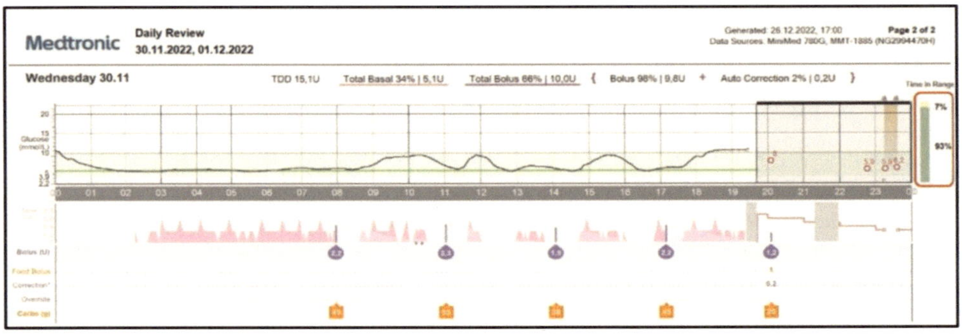

Figure 22.
*There are two modes shown in the CareLink graph: SmartGuard mode (00,00–19,45) and manual mode (19,45–00,00), depicted by the gray area. In SmartGuard mode, pink waves represent basal insulin over the span of four meals (orange boxes) and insulin boluses are indicated by purple drops. Manual mode: the basal rate is indicated with a pink descending line, and glycemia is measured manually. Current TIR: 93% (red box) (**Table 9**).*

Parameters	Units	Refer	16.04.2022	29.06.2022	15.08.2022	02.11.2022	—	—	—
T1D duration	Months	N/A	0	2	4	7	—	—	—
Heart rate	BPM	60–90	—	—	82	86	—	—	—
Blood pressure	Torr	<130/85	—	—	114/63	124/81	—	—	—
fvS-glucose	mmol/	3.3–5.5	13.67	6.3	—	5.4	—	—	—
fvS-C-peptide	pmol/l	>300	420	—	—	—	—	—	—
fvS-GADA	kU/l	0–5	>250	—	—	—	—	—	—
fvS-HDL	mmol/l	1.2–2.7	1.35	1.53	—	1.32	—	—	—
fvS-LDL	mmol/l	1.2–2.6	5.09	3.4	—	3.36	—	—	—
fvS-TAG	mmol/l	0.5–1.7	0.9	1	—	0.84	—	—	—
fvS-creatinine	µmol/l	< 108	72.7	69.9	—	60.7	—	—	—
eGFR	ml/s	1.0–1.3	1.75	1.76	—	1.85	—	—	—
fvS-CRP	mg/l	< 10	1.9	0.6	—	0.5	—	—	—

fvS – fasting venous serum.

Table 9.
Isabella's clinical and laboratory parameters from the diagnosis of T1D over 6 months.

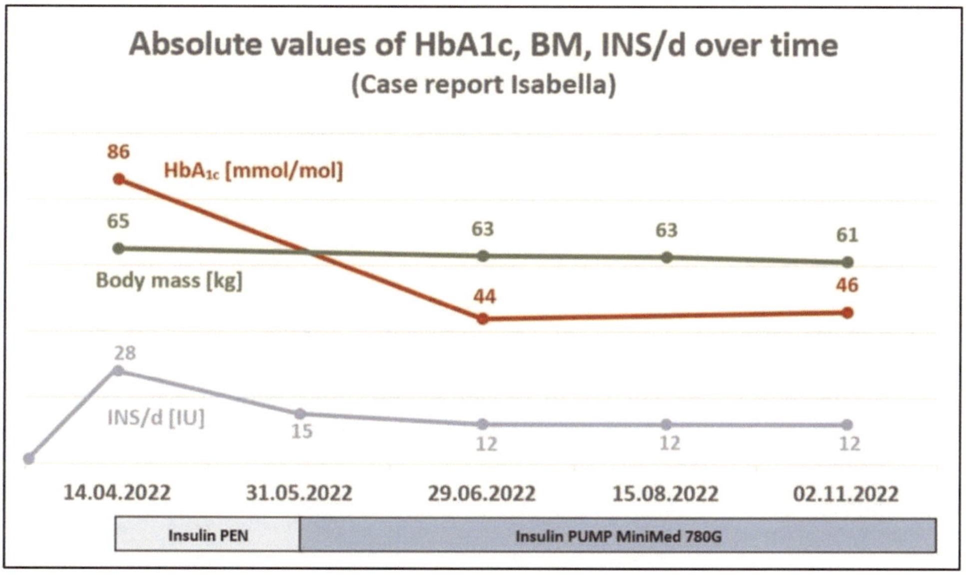

Figure 23.
Isabella's absolute values of HbA_{1c}, BM, and INS/d show rapid glycemic control (from 86 to 44 mmol/mol) after the beginning of insulin therapy. For the last 6 months, we see a stable amount of insulin (12 INS/d) requirement, decreasing body mass, but slightly rising HbA_{1c}.

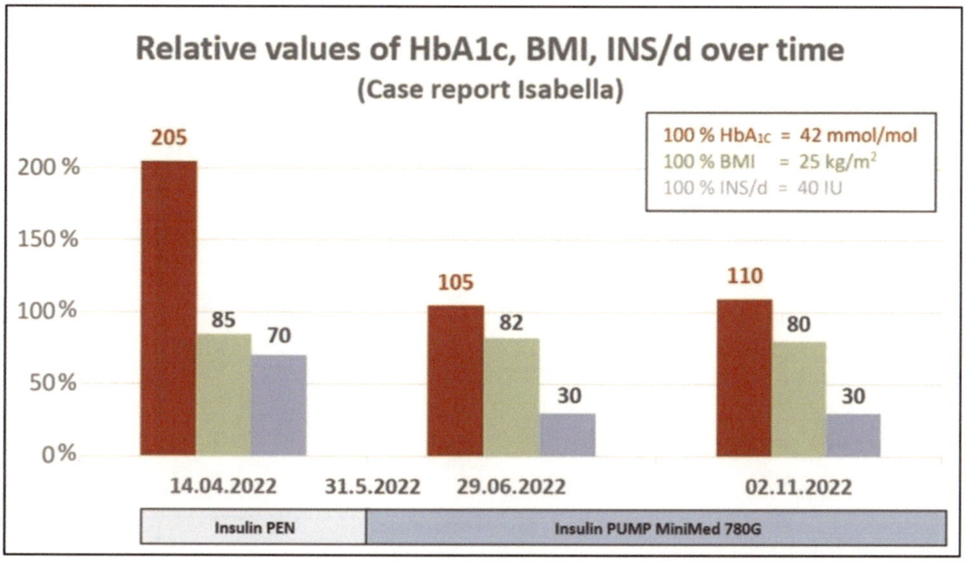

Figure 24.
Isabella's relative values of HbA_{1c} BMI, INS/d show apparent glycemic control after the beginning of insulin therapy, currently, with INS/d 12 IU, that is, 30% of upper limit of its reference range. HbA_{1c} decreased to nearly half of its previous concentration from period with insulin pen. There is also a slight decrease in BMI. This highlights the impact of swift implementation of MiniMed780G as well as continuous education on postinitial remission of insulin secretion.

Current goal: to continue education, reduce HbA_{1c} below 42 mmol/mol, management of hypoglycemia, and hyperlipoproteinemia; monitoring ketones (Galileo Glu/Ket).

2.10 Case report Jane

Focus: implementation of MiniMed 780G 5 months after T1D diagnosis.

History: Jane (today 28 y/o) was initially diagnosed with gestational diabetes during her third pregnancy. Till delivery (in the 34th week, November 22, 2021, girl, 1840 g, 43 cm) she was treated with insulin detemir 8 IU/d. Discharged without any antidiabetic medication [28]. In April 2022, she started to experience polydipsia, polyuria, nausea without vomiting, and anorexia with a loss of 10 kg in body mass. On May 31st, 2022 she was admitted to hospital and diagnosed with T1D (HbA_{1c} 146 mmol/mol), put on insulin aspart, and trained in selfmonitoring by means of glucometer-strips system Galileo Glu/Ket (**Figure 25**). Although it was questionable if Jane would adapt well to having an insulin pump, the implementation of MiniMed 780G on October 31, 2022 at an out-patient clinic (with a basal insulin rate of 12.35 IU/d) proved to be a reliable method of therapy (**Table 10**, **Figures 26** and **27**).

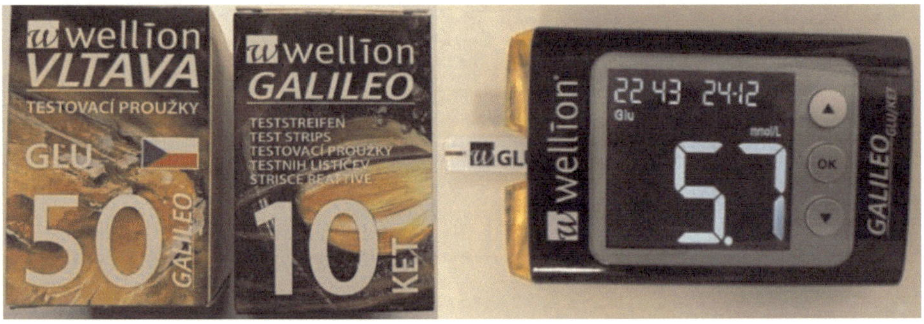

Figure 25.
Strips for glucose (on the left) and beta-hydroxybutyrate (in the middle) glucometer Galileo Glu/Ket showing glycaemia 5.7 mmol/l (on the right).

Parameters	Units	Refer	01.06.2022	14.07.2022	17.10.2022	16.12.2022	—	—	—
T1D duration	months	N/A	0	1	4	6	—	—	—
Heart rate	BPM	60–90	82	96	99	101	—	—	—
Blood pressure	Torr	<130/85	110/78	105/69	126/85	122/72	—	—	—
fvS-glucose	mmol/	3.3–5.5	10.6	7.8	—	5.6	—	—	—
fvS-C-peptide	pmol/l	>300	263	—	—	264	—	—	—
fvS-GADA	kU/I	0–5	>250	>250	—	—	—	—	—
fvS-HDL	mmol/l	1.2–2.7	1.09	1.63	—	1.77	—	—	—
fvS-LDL	mmol/l	1.2–2.6	2.41	2.02	—	2.00	—	—	—
fvS-TAG	mmol/l	0.5–1.7	1.98	1.09	—	0.63	—	—	—
fvS-creatinine	μmol/l	< 108	52.4	52.7	—	66.3	—	—	—
eGFR	ml/s	1.0–1.3	2.09	2.08	—	1.93	—	—	—
fvS-CRP	mg/l	< 10	—	0.5	—	0.5	—	—	—

fvS – fasting venous serum.

Table 10.
Clinical and laboratory parameters of Jane from T1D start over 6 months.

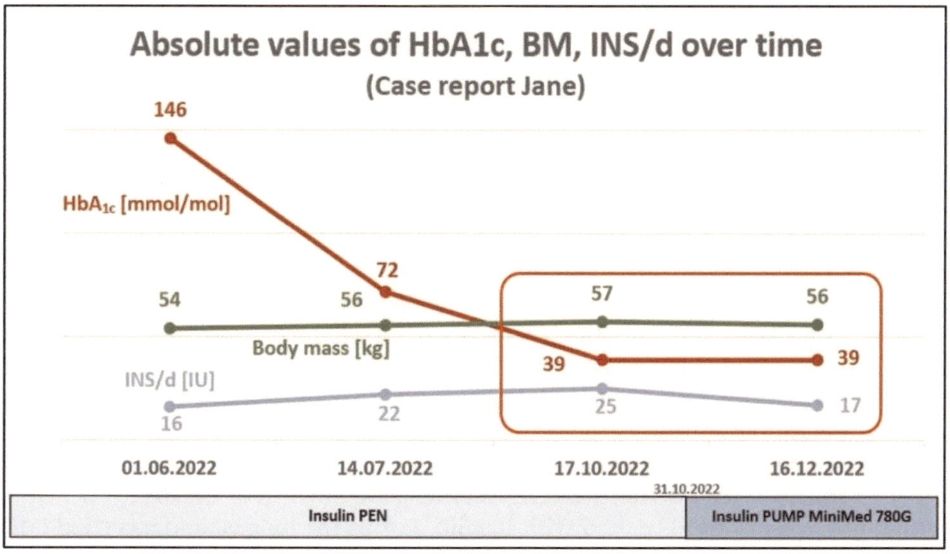

Figure 26.
Jane's absolute values of HbA_{1c}, BM, and INS/d over 6 months showed an intense decrease in HbA_{1c} concentration, an overall stable body mass, and a slight fluctuation in INS/d. After the implementation of a sensor-augmented insulin pump, MiniMed 780G, on October 31, 2022, the INS/d decreased from 25 IU/d to 17 IU/d while maintaining the same HbA_{1c} concentration (see the red box).

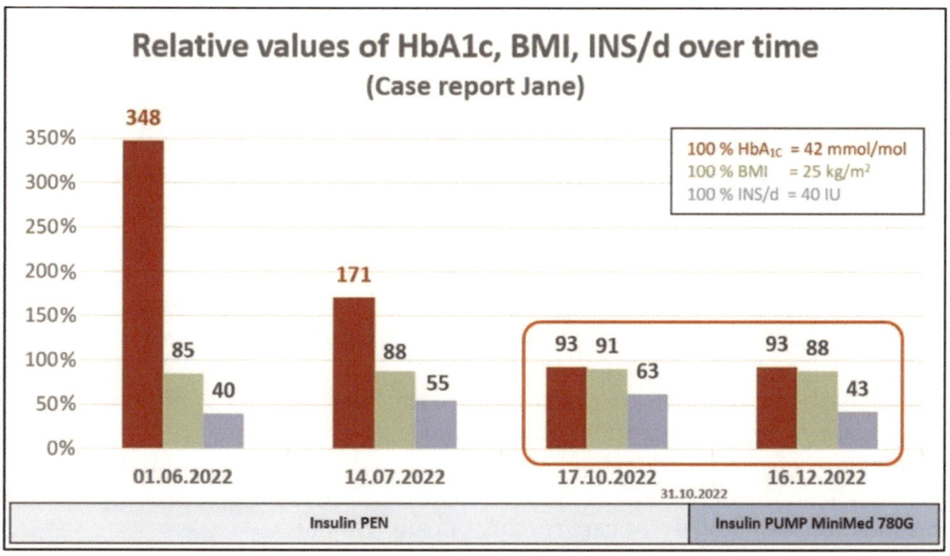

Figure 27.
Jane's relative values of HbA1c, BMI, and INS/d from June 2022 to December 2022. Since the beginning of treatment, HbA1c decreased from 348% of the upper limit of the acceptable value to 171%, and although insulin requirement was increasing, it was still in the reference range. Post implementation of a sensor-augmented insulin pump, MiniMed 780G, the trend of rising required insulin declined to 43% of physiological insulin needs.

Jane expected difficulties in learning how to use the pump, however, today is satisfied with the device. Continuously on SmartGuard, current TIR: 91% (January 5, 2023).

Current goal: to continue the management of T1D, hypoglycemia, and ketosis.

3. Discussion

In this chapter, 10 people with T1D using insulin pumps were observed from a clinical and laboratory medical perspective. Eight of them were given a pump during hospitalization and the remaining two had their pump implemented at an outpatient clinic. When being given an insulin pump, their subjective needs, and opinions were considered.

The case reports are arranged according to the duration of treatment with an insulin pump from 29 years to 2 months. Each case report represents a unique progression, with specific individual complications, and challenges for the insulin pump user, educator, physician, and other members of the diabetes team. All subjects were given the appropriate knowledge, skills, and attitudes during a systematic education. It was shown that the insulin pump did not pose a hindrance to their occupation and everyday life. MiniMed 780G is used by eight individuals, while two are still not convinced to use CGM.

Anna's collected data demonstrates glycemic control without drastic fluctuations. She has been treated with insulin pumps the longest and has tried out several different devices. After being provided with the newest technology in CGM, her compensation improved even further. This trend is not unlike the one observed with Daniel, where there was a noticeable increase in control after implementing AHCL.

Betty's case report was apparent in her lack of glycemic control, despite having an insulin pump, even during pregnancy, which is likely the cause of the elevated body mass at birth in her children. In contrast, Jane, who previously had gestational diabetes, developed T1D as late as 6 months after delivery and had favorable results after the implementation of the insulin pump.

Another common issue encountered was a lack of understanding and "trust" in the AHCL algorithm. Clark tended to deliver extra boluses to achieve the dose he was used to, instead of allowing the pump to function how it was supposed to. Similarly, George, instead of entering data about the number of saccharides he consumed, has been entering the order for a bolus in insulin units. In both scenarios, the increased insulin worsens the risk of recurrent hypoglycemia.

The case reports of Clark, George, Fiona, and Edward highlight the importance of systematic education on the use of CGM, saccharide ratio, and SmartGuard.

Helen, Isabella, and Jane are comparable in the identification of diabetes symptoms, pursuit of medical attention, almost immediate implementation of a hybrid insulin pump, successful education, and metabolic compensation (probably due to "honeymoon recovery" of endogenous insulin secretion). Ideally, swift implementation should be the standard of care for any person with T1D.

4. Conclusions

Presented case reports imply that the hybrid insulin pump, supported with a professional education program, appears to be an effective first option for insulin substitution in people with insulin-deficient diabetes, nonetheless, specific circumstances, desires, and needs of a person with T1D should be brought into account.

Acknowledgements

We extend our sincerest gratitude to the Department of Internal Medicine II - Gastroenterology and Geriatrics at the University Hospital Olomouc, and the Department of Physiology at the Faculty of Medicine and Dentistry, Palacký University Olomouc, Czech Republic, as well as to Bc. Hana Zálešáková, MUDr. Blanka Doubravová, Ondřej Cienciala, and Bc. Marie Libichová (diabetes educator). Furthermore, we would like to express our special thanks to Tereza Nezvalová, Rachel, Petr, and Laura Novákovi, Dhanuka Sammu, Jakub Olejko, and Viktória Molnárová for their unwavering support.

Dedication

This chapter is dedicated to the memory of professor MUDr. Antonín Mores (1908-1997), in tempore Head, Department of Pediatrics, Faculty of Medicine, Palacký University Olomouc, for his empathy for all children and introduction of liberalized diet for boys and girls with T1D [29].

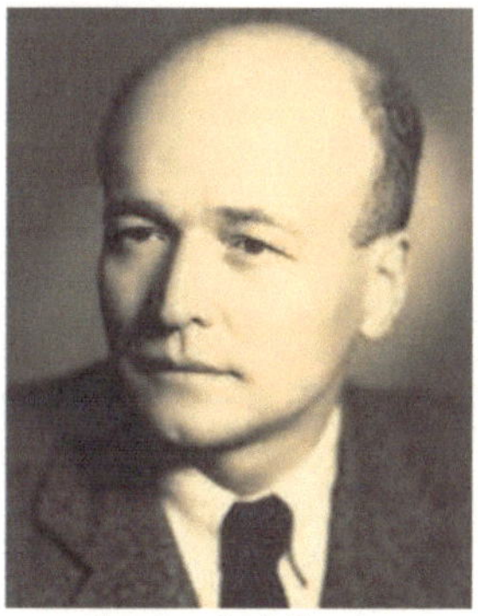

Antonín Mores

Author details

Noemi Nováková[1,2]*, Martin Nezval[1,2] and Marie Anna Robenková[1,2]

1 Department of Internal Medicine II - Gastroenterology and Geriatrics, University Hospital Olomouc, Czech Republic

2 Faculty of Medicine and Dentistry, Department of Physiology, Palacký University Olomouc, Czech Republic

*Address all correspondence to: noemkak@gmail.com

References

[1] American Diabetes Association Professional Practice Committee. 2. Classification and diagnosis of diabetes: Standards of medical care in diabetes-2022. Diabetes Care. 2022;**45**(Suppl. 1): S17-S38. DOI: 10.2337/dc22-S002

[2] Catarino D, Silva D, Guiomar J, Ribeiro C, Ruas L, Cardoso L, et al. Non-immune-mediated versus immune-mediated type 1 diabetes: Diagnosis and long-term differences-retrospective analysis. Diabetology & Metabolic Syndrome. 2020;**12**:56. DOI: 10.1186/s13098-020-00563-x

[3] American Diabetes Association Professional Practice Committee, Draznin B, Aroda VR, Bakris G, Benson G, Brown FM, et al. 6. Glycemic targets: Standards of medical care in diabetes-2022. Diabetes Care. 2022;**45** (Suppl. 1):S83-S96. DOI: 10.2337/dc22-S006

[4] Collyns OJ, Meier RA, Betts ZL, Chan DSH, Frampton C, Frewen CM, et al. Improved glycemic outcomes with medtronic minimed advanced hybrid closed-loop delivery: Results from a randomized crossover trial comparing automated insulin delivery with predictive low glucose suspend in people with type 1 diabetes. Diabetes Care. 2021;**44**(4):969-975. DOI: 10.2337/dc20-2250

[5] Bruttomesso D. Toward automated insulin delivery. The New England Journal of Medicine. 2019;**381**(18): 1774-1775. DOI: 10.1056/NEJMe1912822

[6] Matejko B, Juza A, Kieć-Wilk B, Cyranka K, Krzyżowska S, Chen X, et al. Transitioning of people with type 1 diabetes from multiple daily injections and self-monitoring of blood glucose directly to minimed 780G advanced hybrid closed-loop system: A two-center, randomized, controlled study. Diabetes Care. 2022;**45**(11):2628-2635. DOI: 10.2337/dc22-0470

[7] American Diabetes Association Professional Practice Committee, Draznin B, Aroda VR, Bakris G, Benson G, Brown FM, et al. 7. Diabetes technology: Standards of medical care in diabetes-2022. Diabetes Care. 2022;**45** (Suppl. 1):S97-S112. DOI: 10.2337/dc22-S007

[8] MiniMed 780G, advanced hybrid closed loop system. [Internet] 2021. Available from: https://www.medtronic-diabetes.co.uk/insulin-pump-therapy/MiniMed-780g-system. [Accessed: 2022-12-2024]

[9] Silva JD, Lepore G, Battelino T, Arrieta A, Castañeda J, Grossman B, et al. Real-world performance of the minimed™ 780g system: First report of outcomes from 4120 users. Diabetes Technology and Therapeutics. 2022;**24**(2):113-119. DOI: 10.1089/dia.2021.0203

[10] O'Neill S. Update on technologies, medicines and treatments including Libre 3, MiniMed 780G and Glucomen Day continuous glucose monitoring. Diabetic Medicine. Jan 2021;**38**(1): e14451. DOI: 10.1111/dme.14451

[11] Carlson AL, Sherr JL, Shulman DI, Garg SK, Pop-Busui R, Bode BW, et al. Safety and glycemic outcomes during the minimed™ advanced hybrid closed-loop system pivotal trial in adolescents and adults with type 1 diabetes. Diabetes Technology & Therapeutics. 2022;**24**(3): 178-189. DOI: 10.1089/dia.2021.0319

[12] Carr ALJ, Evans-Molina C, Oram RA. Precision medicine in type 1 diabetes. Diabetologia. 2022;**65**(11):

1854-1866. DOI: 10.1007/s00125-022-05778-3

[13] Šoupal J, Petruželková L, Grunberger G, Hásková A, Flekač M, Matoulek M, et al. Glycemic outcomes in adults with T1D are impacted more by continuous glucose monitoring than by insulin delivery method: 3 years of follow-up from the COMISAIR study. Diabetes Care. 2020;**43**(1):37-43. DOI: 10.2337/dc19-0888

[14] Cohen O, Körner A, Chlup R, Zoupas C, Ragozin A, Wudi K, et al. Improved glycemic control through continuous glucose sensor – Augmented insulin pump therapy: Prospective results from a community and academic practice patient registry. Journal of Diabetes Science and Technology. 2009;**3**(4):804-811

[15] Stechova K. Insulin pump therapy: Education and its goals. Vnitřní Lékařství. 2019;**65**(4):248-255. English. DOI: 10.36290/vnl.2019.042

[16] McAdams BH, Rizvi AA. An overview of insulin pumps and glucose sensors for the generalist. Journal of Clinical Medicine. 2016;**5**(1):5. DOI: 10.3390/jcm5010005

[17] Chlup R, Krystyník O, Mlčák P, Zapletalová J, Bartek J. Intensive management of type 1 diabetes in adults: One centre experience 1970–2022. In: Chlup R, editor. Type 1 Diabetes Mellitus [Internet]. London: IntechOpen; 2022. [Accessed: 2022-12-17 . DOI: 10.5772/intechopen.108032. Available from: https://www.intechopen.com/online-first/84607

[18] Obermannova B. Edukace při MiniMedu 780G (User's education on MiniMed 780G, Czech.), Česká diabetologie Speciál. 2021 (Czech Diabetology special, Czech.). ISBN: 978-80-88400-15-8

[19] Medtronic, Understanding the Assessment and Progress Report [internet]. 2017. Available from: https://www.medtronicdiabetes.com/CareLinkPDF/CareLink-System-Assessment-and-Progress-Report.pdf. [Accessed: 2022-12-23]

[20] Berget C, Thomas SE, Messer LH, Thivener K, Slover RH, Wadwa RP, et al. A clinical training program for hybrid closed loop therapy in a pediatric diabetes clinic. Journal of Diabetes Science and Technology. 2020;**14**(2):290-296. DOI: 10.1177/1932296819835183

[21] American Diabetes Association Professional Practice Committee, Draznin B, Aroda VR, Bakris G, Benson G, Brown FM, et al. 9. Pharmacologic approaches to glycemic treatment: Standards of medical care in diabetes-2022. Diabetes Care. 2022;**45** (Suppl. 1):S125-S143. DOI: 10.2337/dc22-S009

[22] Menzel R, Chlup R, Jutzi E, Hildmann W. "Catheter-pens"–An alternative to insulin pump treatment? Experimental and Clinical Endocrinology. 1990;**95**(1):157-169. DOI: 10.1055/s-0029-1210948

[23] Illsley NP, Baumann MU. Human placental glucose transport in fetoplacental growth and metabolism. Biochimica et Biophysica Acta - Molecular Basis of Disease. 2020; **1866**(2):165359. DOI: 10.1016/j.bbadis.2018.12.010

[24] Menon RK, Cohen RM, Sperling MA, Cutfield WS, Mimouni F, Khoury JC. Transplacental passage of insulin in pregnant women with insulin-dependent diabetes mellitus. Its role in fetal macrosomia. The New England Journal of Medicine. 1990;**323**(5):

309-315. DOI: 10.1056/NEJM199008023230505

[25] McCance DR, Casey C. Type 1 diabetes in pregnancy. Endocrinology and Metabolism Clinics of North America. 2019;**48**(3):495-509. DOI: 10.1016/j.ecl.2019.05.008

[26] Jaffar F, Laycock K, Huda MSB. Type 1 diabetes in pregnancy: A review of complications and management. Current Diabetes Reviews. 2022;**18**(7): e051121197761. DOI: d10.2174/1573399818666211105124829

[27] Satoh T. Molecular mechanisms for the regulation of insulin-stimulated glucose uptake by small guanosine triphosphatases in skeletal muscle and adipocytes. International Journal of Molecular Sciences. 2014;**15**(10): 18677-18692. DOI: 10.3390/ijms151018677

[28] Selen DJ, Thaweethai T, Schulte CCM, Hsu S, He W, James K, et al. Gestational Glucose Intolerance and Risk of Future Diabetes. Diabetes Care. 2023 Jan 1;**46**(1):83-91. DOI: 10.2337/dc22-1390

[29] Mores A. Probleme des Kinderdiabetes. Bratislavské lekárske listy. 1939;**19**(9):1-19

Section 2

Open Questions

Chapter 6

Molecular Challenges and Advances in Clinical Islet Transplantation

Nithyakalyani Mohan and Anusha Sunder

Abstract

The pathophysiology of diabetes is related to the levels of insulin within the body, and the body's ability to utilize insulin. Patients with diabetes persistently go through life-threatening hypoglycaemia. Consequently, their quality of life gets affected, progressively leading them to micro- and macro-vascular complications. This is an unmanageable happening despite the technology advancements in insulin formulations. Nevertheless, islet transplantation is emerging as an alternative therapeutic option. Our chapter will elaborate on the recent advancements in this field highlighting the present-day challenges of clinical islet cell transplantation. Additionally, details about the advancements in cutting-edge clinical research, bio-molecular signaling with special reference to the pre and post transplant, the need for beta-cell replacement therapies, including the application of induced pluripotent stem cells and mesenchymal stem cells are also mentioned in this chapter.

Keywords: diabetes, β cell, islet transplantation, human pluripotent stem cells (PSCs), PSC-derived islet cells, immunosuppressant

1. Introduction

1.1 Overview of diabetes: incidence, intensity and implication of innovative therapies

Diabetes is one of the fastest growing health challenges of the twenty-first century, with the number of adults living with diabetes having more than tripled over the past 20 years [1]. Most forms of diabetes witness hyperglycemia, which has its pathogenesis focally in the islet β cell. Known diabetics (diagnosis confirmed) as well as those who are at-risk of developing the disease exhibit impairment or loss of propeptide processing and secretory function. For the purpose of prediction, diagnosis or prognostics, biomarkers and genetics are used to understand the state of a biological process, severity of a pathological condition, and response to an intervention. This holds true for both research and clinical settings. The current chapter will focus on the potential utility of genetic markers, circulating molecules, and immune cell phenotyping as β cell's biomarkers of cellular function. How these biomarkers complement the assessment of β-cell secretory function is also interestingly explained. Having essayed the vitality of islet β cell, the chapter will also touch upon the possible implications of its loss. And henceforth, the β-cell secretory function could itself be considered as a biomarker. However, steadfast advances in the field have set the stage for stem cell-based approaches to take over in the near future. Generation of functional pancreatic islet cells using Human pluripotent stem cells (PSCs), including human embryonic stem cells and induced pluripotent stem cells, are promising cell sources in regenerating pancreatic islets, and this will become possible based on the substantial progress made over the past years. The forthcoming decade will probably witness research driven towards the molecular mechanisms of PSC-derived islet cells and their entailed use in experimental disease treatment. Therapeutic efficacy and safety considerations of patient PSC-derived islet cells and transplantation delivery systems should also be researched upon.

1.2 Diabetes- an understanding at the molecular level

Diabetes is a serious public health challenge, and its types, especially type 1 & 2 are caused by a combination of genetic and environmental risk factors. For instance, an increase in human islet BCL11A expression decreases islet insulin secretion. Thus *BCL11A* expression is elevated during T2D and chronic hyperglycemia [2]. Being **polygenic**, they are related to a change, or defect, in multiple genes. This includes variations in important genes which are vital for glucose metabolism (regulation of fasting & postprandial blood glucose levels), insulin function (mainly insulin resistance) & triglyceride metabolism. The following figure, **Figure 1** illustrates the pathogenesis of diabetes at a molecular level.

Diseases like diabetes are now being diagnosed, monitored and treated through an effective, individualized model of care rather than the 'one size fits all' approach. Owing to its efficiency in personalized care, precision medicine has gained focus worldwide, and its emerging application has diabetes in the forefront [3, 4]. For instance, the gastrointestinal side effects of the hypoglycaemic drug metformin has been linked to the interaction between the genes encoding the organic cation transporter 1 (OCT1) and the serotonin reuptake transporter (SERT). The number of low-expressing SERT S* alleles increased the odds of metformin intolerance. Likewise, the presence of two deficient OCT1 alleles was associated with over a nine-fold higher odds of metformin intolerance in patients carrying L*L* genotype [5].

Understanding relevant genes may not only help determine who is at high risk for developing the disease, but may also be useful in guiding treatment regimens. Beyond treating diabetes, we have set foot in a new era of curing the disease with pancreatic

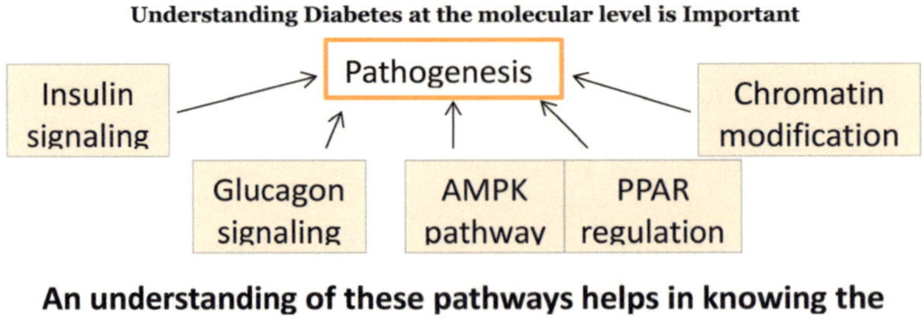

Figure 1.
Understanding diabetes at the molecular level is important.

islet cell transplantation. In islet transplantation, the requirement for immunosuppressive drug treatment to protect alloislets from alloimmune rejection and recurrent autoimmunity introduces additional risks that may be specific to the individual immunosuppressive drug agents as well as related more generally to immunosuppression. Thus recognition of inter-individual differences is gaining importance and is becoming possible through integration of pharmacogenetics, pharmacoproteomics, epigenetics, and noncoding RNAs data into clinical practice, thus emphasizing that *'Precision medicine is vital in transplantation'.* A panel of genetic variants for transplant recipients and donors can function as an additional tool at disposition of transplant physicians to provide individualized care.

2. Biological mechanisms that underlie Insulin dependence

Type 1 diabetes is a multifactorial autoimmune disease, which is characterized by T cell mediated damage to the insulin-secreting pancreatic β cells. The initial stages of the disease process feature insulitis, followed by the pancreatic islets' infiltration by mononuclear immune cells (including dendritic cells, macrophages, and T cells). This detrimental process leads to severe insulin depletion, and consequently

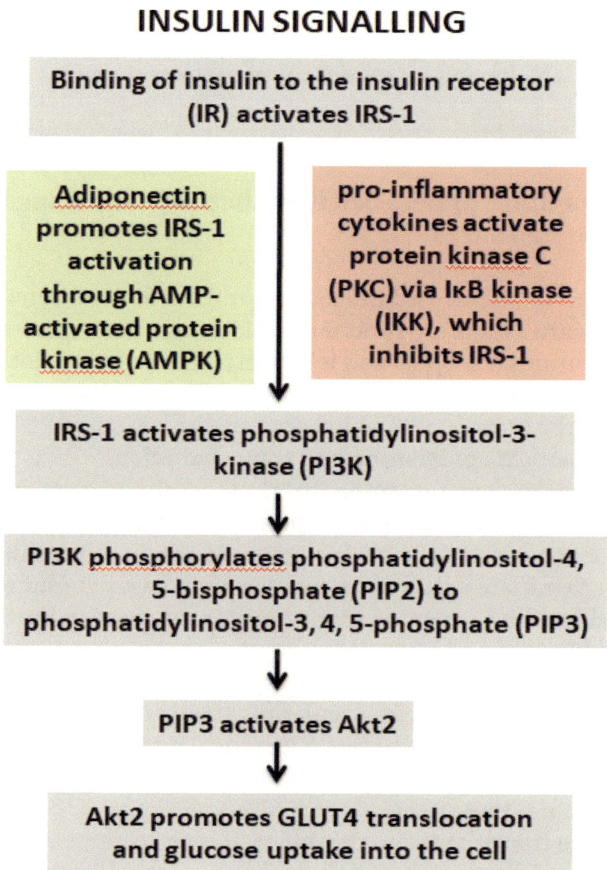

Figure 2.
Islet cells balance cellular glucose requirement with the glucose supply through blood.

hyperglycaemia. Underlying this hyperglycemia are reasons like hepatic overproduction of glucose by glycogenolysis and gluconeogenesis accompanied by a decrease in the cellular uptake of circulating glucose. Insulin's absence, increases fat breakdown and the consequence of fatty acid oxidation is excessive production of ketones. These metabolic disturbances are serious enough to progressively cause central nervous system depression, coma, and death, if left untreated. Therefore, type 1 diabetes necessitates lifetime treatment with exogenous insulin as a survival-essential. Pancreatic β cell destruction rate shows inter-individual differences, yet, tends to be more aggressive in infants and young children [6]. Type 1 diabetes represents approximately 10% of all cases with diabetes. Its incidence is increasing worldwide at a rate of about 3% per year. The latest edition of the International Diabetes Federation *(IDF), Diabetes Atlas* shows that 1.1 million children and adolescents under the age of 20 live with type 1 diabetes [1]. Islet cells balance cellular glucose requirement with the glucose supply through blood, and this is illustrated in the following figure, **Figure 2** through insulin signaling pathway.

For individuals with type 1 diabetes or insulin-deficient forms of pancreatogenic (type 3c) diabetes, isolation of islets from a deceased donor pancreas with intrahepatic transplantation of allogeneic islets can result in amelioration of hypoglycemia, on-target glycemic control, improved quality of life, and insulin independence. Recent progress in techniques for islet isolation, islet culture, and peritransplant management of the islet transplant recipient has resulted in substantial improvements in metabolic and safety outcomes for patients. The metabolic benefits of islet transplantation are dependent on the count of islets transplanted that survive engraftment [7].

3. Molecular semaphore of beta cell in diabetes: integrating biomarkers with functional measures

Circadian regulation of glucose homeostasis and insulin secretion is an important feature to assess whether islets are functional. Molecular clock mechanism is highly conserved among various cell types and is driven by a set of core clock genes that form interrelated transcriptional-translational complex. Thus understanding the molecular mechanism driving the inter relationship between disruption and islet functioning is crucial in context of disease prevention and transplantation.

The molecular mechanism governing this rhythmicity is based on complex program of gene expression. A number of interlocked transcriptional and posttranslational feedback loops are responsible for generation and maintenance of rhythms. It will be interesting to initiate a study to assess the basal levels of glut receptor; Ca2+, glucose kinase and Insulin expression immediately after the purification of islets are done. This will highlight the necessity to understand the molecular and physiological underpinnings responsible for the functionality of islets before the transplant. These basal levels of expression of all the molecular parameters will give the clinician an idea on functionality of islets even before it is transplanted. However after the transplant the levels should vary depending on the success of transplant surgery, circadian regulation and graft function [8–13].

Once the islets are transplanted to the donor, it is very important to assess the level of relevant molecular signatures in-vivo, which are involved in graft function or damage and these biomarkers decide the fate of the transplant. Optimizing engraftment and early survival after clinical islet transplantation is critical to long-term function.

Cell-free circulating DNA (cfDNA), is now recognized as a potential biomarker for a variety of diseases. In humans, the insulin promoter is predominantly unmethylated in islet β-cells and methylated in all other tissues. cfDNA-based estimation of beta cell death 24 hours after islet allotransplantation correlates with clinical outcome and could predict early engraftment [14].

To understand on the beta cell function and beta cell mass, high-quality pancreatic islets are essential as they correlate with better post transplantation endocrine function. Islet quality and yield get affected by stress during the isolation process. During isolation, islet-enriched microRNAs (miRNAs) -375 are released and they serve helpful in assessing the extent of islet damage by correlating with post transplantation endocrine function. Assessment of the absolute concentration of miR-375 C-peptide at various islet isolation steps, including digestion, dilution, recombination, purification, and bagging is possible. Measurement of the absolute quantity of miRNA-375 during islet isolation is a useful tool to assess islet damage. The quantity of released miRNA is indicative of post transplantation endocrine function in transplant patients [15–17].

Better engraftment and functioning of islets needs to be proved by the production of Insulin for the alleviating problematic hypoglycemia before and after islet transplant. This can be done by constantly monitoring the insulin level by various methods. CD30 levels are a predictor marker for acute rejection before and after the islet transplant. Elevated CD30 levels may reflect an immune state detrimental for islet allograft survival. In islet allograft recipients, post-transplant reduction in sCD30 levels can serve as a biomarker to monitor graft function. Furthermore, an insight on how various immunosuppression protocols impact the timing and extent of changes in post-transplant sCD30 levels may facilitate patient-specific tailoring of immunosuppression [18, 19].

HMGB1 is a mediator of immune system during islet transplant. HMGB1 is one of the best-characterized DAMP molecules associated with islet. HMGB1 seemed to be released by damaged islets before and after transplant. HMGB1 will be one of the useful bio signatures detecting islet damage in clinical situation. It is the need of the hour for more research and development of kits in these area to bring the islet product release criteria that screen preparations before and after clinical allogeneic islet cell transplantation that are currently unavailable to predict post-transplant success from failure. More sensitive and reliable islet viability, potency kits and assays that characterize cell composition and molecular profiles will be useful in further defining the islet product and may provide useful information on islet immunogenicity and pro-inflammatory potential to evaluate islet functionality in the clinical setting [20, 21]. The following figure, **Figure 3** is a pictorial representation of 'development of molecular Bio Signatures- pre and post- islet cell transplantation.

A transplantation outcome that curtails infection and rejection is desirable; still, the present day immunosuppression strategies using prophylactic antimicrobial medications do not guarantee this! Human leukocyte antigen matching is an important aspect of graft survival. However, other factors like extent of immunosuppression, infections and management of comorbidities is also crucial. Considering transplant patient's predisposing genetic modifiers for risk stratification and as a basis for applying precision pharmacotherapy may improve transplant outcomes [22].

The most important genes deciding the fate of a transplanted cell, tissue, or organ belong to what is termed the MHC (the major histocompatibility complex). The MHC antigens' primary function is to aid in distinguishing self from no-self through peptide presentation to the immune system. The MHC antigens are also termed as

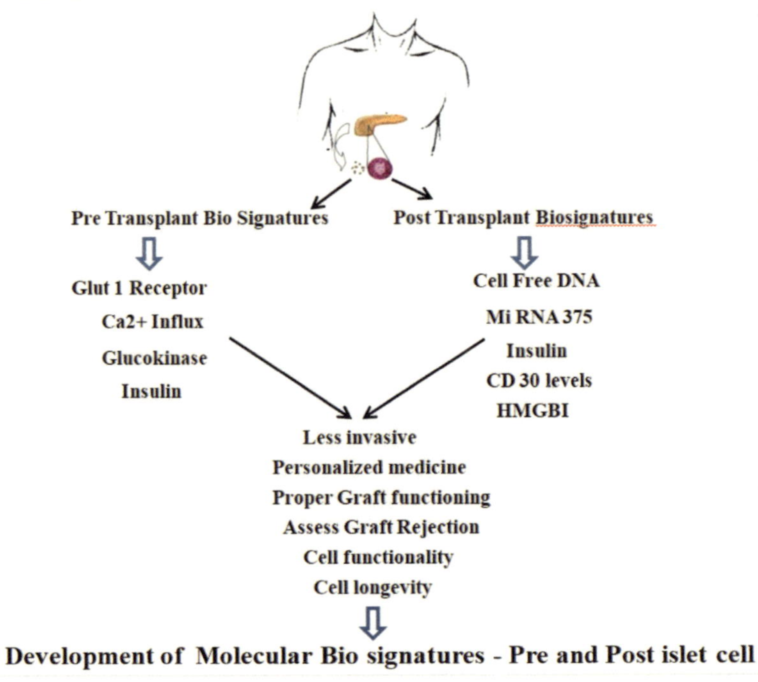

Figure 3.
Factors that govern the acceptance or rejection of an islet transplant.

HLA (human leukocyte antigens), and they comprise three regions, namely, class I (HLA-A, B, Cw), class II (HLA-DR, DQ, DP) and class III (no HLA genes). For acute rejection of an islet transplant, there is not any established treatment available. And hence transplantation of alloislets with HLAs reactive against even very low levels of preformed alloantibody in the recipient should be avoided even when T and B lymphocyte crossmatches are negative [23, 24].

Association of genetic assessment with demographic and clinical outcomes in a transplantation can potentially enable individualized risk stratification and immunosuppression through the identification of genetic variants relating to immune-mediated complications, post-transplant disease and also alterations in drug-metabolizing genes. Notably, immunosuppressive drug toxicity is of concern as the risk for impairment in kidney function relates with both calcineurin inhibitors and mTOR inhibitors. The drug Tacrolimus predominates immunosuppression in transplantation, and it is metabolized by the cytochrome P 450 3A (CYP3A) subfamily of enzymes in the liver and small intestine. In CYP3A5 gene, a polymorphism in intron 3 alters its expression affecting the enzyme activity and thereby tacrolimus drug metabolism. Tacrolimus drug level correlated well with presence or absence of CYP3A5 polymorphisms. Acute rejection episodes were more frequent in expressers, and they may require higher doses of tacrolimus. When alloislets are transplanted in patients with type 1 diabetes, the use of low-dose tacrolimus in combination with sirolimus is associated with decline in estimated GFR of ~5 mL/min/y/1.73 m^2. Therefore, CYP3A5 polymorphism analysis before transplant may help determine the optimal dose of tacrolimus in this population and prevent acute rejection episodes or tacrolimus toxicity [7, 25, 26].

3.1 Genes can impact the effectiveness of islet graft

The effectiveness of the islet graft depends both on beta cell function as well as the interaction between the graft and the host, and most importantly, these are governed by the expression of specific islet genes [27]. Components of specific cytokine pathways are upregulated in *bad* islet preparations (those which failed to reverse diabetes after transplantation). And these include tumor necrosis factor (TNF) machinery such as the TRAIL receptor TNFRSF10B that engage in β-cell death induced by T cells [28, 29]. The FAS and its ligand, FASL, can induce beta cell apoptosis [30, 31], and these are hiked in *bad* islets, suggesting that islet death-related pathways are already activated in these preparations even before transplantation. Adding on to apoptosis is the activation of NFκB and AP-1 transcription factors, which up-regulate expression of inflammatory cytokines [32]. A local proinflammatory environment is promoted by CCL2 (MCP1), which associates with islet death and diabetes [33, 34]. Also seen in b*ad* islets are higher expressions of the pattern recognition receptor TLR3, which relates with islet dysfunction and increased cytokine expression [35]. An elevated expression of tissue factor (F3) is pro-inflammatory and inhibits islet graft function [33, 36]. On the contrary, the TGFB2 and its receptor TGFBR1, and the IL13 receptor, OSMR, are other elevated chemokines which can initiate protective signals for islet cells [37–39]. Similarly, SERPINA3, also known as alpha-1-antichymotrypsin is upregulated and may promote wound healing [40, 41]. The SEPT9 gene is upregulated in bad islets and has recently been shown to be upregulated in islets of type 2 diabetics [42]. So it appears that the pathways leading to islet dysfunction are already triggered before transplantation, but that there is also the initiation of some counteractive measures.

A list of genes that were preferentially upregulated in *good* islet preparations (those which failed to reverse diabetes after transplantation) were relatable with the development and regeneration of pancreas. Hence a prior initiation of repair/regeneration pathways in damaged islets would prove effective after transplantation. Several such genes including ONECUT1 (HNF6) [43, 44], MNX1 (HB9) [45, 46], NKX2-2 [47, 48], INSM1 [49, 50], NKX6-1 [47, 51], FOXA2 [52–54], and PTCH1 [55, 56] interact in regulatory networks aiding embryonic pancreas development and regeneration following an injury. On the other hand, the NOTCH2 gene, is predominantly expressed in the *bad* islet preparations, possibly because of its significant role in expansion of the progenitor cell population through suppression of neurogenin3-dependent endocrine cell differentiation [57]. Gene encoding the rectifying potassium channel KCNMA1 which is upregulated in good islets has been shown to be important for repolarization of the membrane following insulin secretion. Loss of KCNMA1 suppresses insulin secretion and increases susceptibility to oxidative stress and apoptosis [58].

In the recipient inducing protective genes like heme oxygenase-1 (HO-1), A20/tumor necrosis factor alpha inducible protein3 (tnfaip3), biliverdin reductase (BVR), Bcl2, and others could synergistically improve islet graft survival and function. A similar effect is seen on administration of one or more of the products of HO-1 to the donor [59].

In heme degradation, HO-1 is the rate-limiting enzyme that produces equal molar amounts of carbon monoxide (CO), biliverdin, and iron. Biliverdin's rapid conversion by biliverdin reductase to bilirubin sequesters iron into ferritin. Being an ubiquitous stress protein, HO-1 gets induced in several cell types by various stimuli. Evidence piles up supporting HO-1 induction to offer cellular protection against transplant rejection. Induction of HO-1 pharmacologically or via gene transfer protects islets from stress-induced apoptosis in both the *in vitro* and the *in vivo* settings. HO-1 induction in β cell lines, or human islets protects against apoptosis induced by TNF-α and cyclohexamide (CHX), interleukin-1β (IL-1β), and Fas. In recepients, HO-1 induction with cobalt protoporphyrin (CoPP) pharmacologically improves islet function in a rodent model with marginal mass islet transplantation, wherein fewer islets are required to achieve normoglycemia when transplanted into a sygeneic recipient, whose been rendered diabetic by streptozotocin (STZ) treatment [60].

A20, also known as the TNF-α-induced protein 3 (TNFAIP3), is a zinc-ring finger protein. As a negative regulator of nuclear factor kappa B (NF-κB) activation, A20 is recognized as a central and ubiquitous regulator of inflammation and as a potent antiapoptotic gene in certain cell types, including β cells. Islets can be protected against apoptosis induced by IL-1β/INF-γ and Fas through adenovirus-mediated gene transfer causing overexpression of A20. A higher percentage of cure was seen after transplantation in recipients with suboptimal number of islets overexpressing A20 compared to control islets. Islets expressing A20 preserved functional β cell mass and are resistant to cell death. In β cells, expression of A20 renders a dual-protective effect through antiapoptosis and antiinflammation. The antiapototic effect of A20 attributes to its cytoprotective properties and is dependent on the abrogation of cytokine-induced NO (nitric oxide) production due to transcriptional blockade of iNOS induction [61–63].

Bilirubin administration reduced apoptosis and improved insulin secretion in an *in vitro* model in INS-1 cells when challenged with nonspecific inflammation induced by cytokines. Protective genes like HO-1 and bcl-2 were strongly expressed seen in in freshly isolated islets from bilirubin-treated donors. Also noticed was an evident suppression in the proinflammatory and proapoptotic genes including caspase-3, caspase-8, and MCP-1. Such a protective effect rendered by bilirubin reduces β-cell destruction post- transplantation, minimizes macrophage infiltration, and suppresses expression of MCP-1, BID, caspase-3, -8, and -9, TNF-α, iNOS, Fas, TRAIL-R, and CXCL10 in the graft after allogeneic transplantation [64, 65].

Exposing human islets to the nonpeptidyl low molecular weight radical scavenger IAC [bis(1-hydroxy-2,2,6,6-tetramethyl-4-piperidiny) decanedioate dihydrochloride] on isolated human islet cells protected them from isolation and culture-induced oxidative stress. Transduction of NOD islets with the antioxidative gene thioredoxin (TRX, reactive oxygen species scavenger and antiapoptotic) using a lentiviral vector before transplantation prolonged islet graft survival. Anthocyanins present in Chinese Bayberry have the potential to upregulate HO-1, and thus protect β cells against hydrogen-peroxide-induced necrosis and apoptosis. Islets' viability and function improved with adenoviral transfection as X-linked inhibitor of apoptosis provided protection from inflammatory cytokines [66].

4. Islet transplantation- practical difficulties and resolving approaches

1. Immunosuppressant regimen

Islet transplantation is emerging as a treatment for type 1 diabetes mellitus in selected patients with inadequate glucose control despite insulin therapy. However, considering the 267 allografts transplanted since 1990, insulin independence was observed in only 12.4 percent for periods of more than 1 week, and merely 8.2 percent could sustain the beneficial outcome for more than a year. Predominantly in these procedures the immunosuppression regimen comprised of antibody induction with an antilymphocyte globulin combined with cyclosporine, azathioprine, and glucocorticoids. Many of these immunosuppression regimens pose a threat of damaging beta cells or induce peripheral insulin resistance. Immunosuppressive drugs that concentrate in the liver can be toxic to the islets, yet must be taken for the lifetime of the graft. Currently, we are stepping into an era of accessing new and more potent immunosuppressive agents that will provide greater immunologic protection without diabetogenic side effects. Such an approach is glucocorticoid-free immunosuppressive protocol that includes sirolimus, low-dose tacrolimus, and a monoclonal antibody against the interleukin-2 receptor (daclizumab) for use in a trial of islet transplantation alone for patients with brittle type 1 diabetes. This has shown to result in insulin independence with excellent metabolic control when glucocorticoid-free immunosuppression is combined with the infusion of an adequate islet mass. Additionally, this immunosuppressive protocol has not clinically evidenced any episodes of graft rejection, and it appears to be effective in preventing autoimmune recurrence of diabetes [67].

Islet transplantation has emerged as a promising treatment option for type 1 diabetes. Still its progress is challenged by barriers like patient accessibility and long-term graft function. These can be overcome by amalgamating emerging technologies in biomaterials with drug delivery and immunomodulation. The hepatic microenvironment and traditional systemic immunosuppression can stress the vulnerable islets and limit the success rate of transplantation [68].

2. Other challenges like limitation in islet engraftment and function, low oxygen tension, insulin-induced hepatic steatosis, lipotoxicity and inflammation

Intrahepatic transplantation is a minimally invasive portal infusion that results in islet entrapment within hepatic sinusoids. The islet engraftment and function is restrained by hepatic portal vasculature. An instant blood-mediated inflammatory reaction (IBMIR) is a resultant of vascular delivery. Also noticed are activated complement and coagulation cascades, and leucocyte infiltration leading to the loss of nearly two-thirds of the islets within the first few days after transplantation. Islets that survive inside the hepatic portal environment experience high glucose levels, low oxygen tension, and first-pass exposure to metabolites and pharmaceuticals. Intrahepatically transplanted islets may also be lost as a result of localized, insulin-induced hepatic steatosis, lipotoxicity and inflammation. A transformative approach to islet transplantation may be achieved through the adaptation of technologies for locally controlling the transplant microenvironment to promote engraftment and long-term function while minimizing or eliminating systemic non-specific immunosuppression with local immunomodulation or operational tolerance induction [68].

Resolving approaches

- Natural or synthetic biomaterials can be employed to engineer an extrahepatic space to localize islets and control the microenvironment after transplantation. Transplantation at extrahepatic and extravascular site is enabled through the support of biomaterial scaffold, which proves beneficial by avoiding the unfavorable influences on the liver environment and the IBMIR. Interestingly, the extrahepatically implanted biomaterial scaffolds can be retrieved, facilitating the adoption of insulin-producing cells derived from stem cells.

- Porous scaffolds are emerging as a suitable vehicle for islet transplantation. The reason being the ease of seeding islets into the pores as well as the porosity supporting rapid cell infiltration for integration with the host tissue. The composition of microporous scaffolds include biocompatible, biodegradable copolymer of lactide and glycolide (PLG) which are approved by the US Food and Drug Administration. The PLG create and maintain a space for transplanted islets while exerting control on their density and distribution. Similar to this, rapid ingrowth and revascularization can also be supported through degradable hydrogels such as collagen, fibrin and clotted plasma.

- Isolation employing non-degradable natural or synthetic hydrogels such as alginate and polyethylene glycol is an alternate to engraftment. These hydrogels have manifold benefits, including prevention against cellular attack by the immune system, avoidance of cell ingrowth, vascularisation and re-innervation. The aforementioned benefits can potentially target glucose sensing, insulin secretion and long-term beta cell turnover

- The interaction between islet and Extracellular matrix modellling (ECM) crucially determines islet survival signals. During islet isolation, the enzymatic and mechanical processes disrupt the islet cell's specialized basement membrane of ECM proteins. Applying biomaterial technology to supply ECM proteins to islets may significantly enhance engraftment and function owing to the structural support provided, alongside the binding of cell-surface integrins which mediate adhesion and activate intracellular signaling pathways.

- During the early stages of post-transplantation, the islet cell death is relatable to a loss in integrin signaling, which may trigger apoptosis (also known as anoikis). To enhance engraftment and transplantation, biomaterial surfaces or hydrogels can be formed or modified with ECM molecules, adhesive peptides or other biochemical signals.

- Specific cellular processes stimulated by the trophic factor delivery may associate with islet survival and engraftment to maximize transplant success. The transplanted islet survival and function is enhanced by specific factors including, insulinotropic factors such as IGF-1, prolactin and exendin-4 or anti-apoptotic factors like BCL2-associated X protein (BAX)-inhibiting peptide. Regulation of beta cell mass, its proliferation and regeneration are determined by IGF-1. Exendin-4 is a long-acting glucagon-like peptide-1 agonist that stimulates beta cell proliferation, protects against apoptosis and improves outcomes in islet transplantation. Prolactin signaling during pregnancy is responsible for beta cell proliferation, and prolactin pre-incubation and injection have been shown to improve transplanted islet engraftment and revascularisation. Islet cell apoptosis is a major contributor to islet loss in the early post-transplant period. It is triggered by cues such as loss of ECM contacts, DNA damage, hypoxia and nutrient starvation. Pre-treatment with or induced production of BAX-inhibiting peptide in islet transplants can enhance engraftment by minimizing apoptosis. Delivery of angiogenic factors like vascular endothelial growth factor (VEGF) can enhance islet engraftment and glucose sensing by improving revascularization [68–72].

5. Promise and challenges of stem cell derived islet cell transplant- can it become a clinical reality?

People who are insulin dependent require multiple insulin injections, sometimes with an insulin pump, coupled with regular blood glucose monitoring. Diabetes management has improved with the availability of modified insulin's, each with peaks of activity at varying times and conditions. Transplantation of cadaveric islets coupled with immune suppression has been impressive results leading to insulin independence in patients with Type 1 Diabetes. But again there is not a perfect balance between the available donors populations compared to diabetic load. Continuous availability of beta cells to the patients at an appropriate timelines is the need of the hour in any country. This can be made a reality with the use of pluripotent stem cells, to produce a virtually unlimited and uniform supply of human islet-like clusters by directed differentiation can solve many issues.

Stem cells, being undifferentiated, are capable of self-renewal, and can virtually produce any tissue or organ [73–78]. Stem cells can be broadly classified on the basis of their origin as embryonic stem cells (ESCs), fetal stem cells (FSCs), adult stem cells (ASCs), and induced pluripotent stem cells (iPSCs). The iPSCs and ESCs are pluripotent stem cells (PSCs), while ASCs are unipotent or oligopotent [79–81].

Human-induced PSCs (iPSCs) and human embryonic stem cells (ESCs), serve as a reproducible source of human cells even at early developmental stages owing to their potential of forming any cell type in the adult body [82–84]. From a viewpoint of preservation of β-cells through islet protection and regeneration, the human-induced PSCs (iPSCs), hematopoietic stem cells (HSCs), human cord blood-derived multipotent stem cells (CB-SCs), and MSCs are being used. Additionally, stem cells are capable of re-establishing peripheral tolerance towards β-cells by remodeling of immune responses alongside inhibition of autoreactive T-cell function [85, 86]. Stem cells have the potential to increase islet mass owing to their capability of differentiation to β-cells-like organoids. They inhibit the immune responses of T cell and Th1 cells through TGF-β and inflammatory pathways, and thus reconstitute immunotolerance. Type 1 diabetes being an autoimmune disease is featured by activated immune cells which target and destroy pancreatic β-cells. Thus stem cell therapy for treating T1DM should take into account the stem cell's immunomodulatory properties of and also its capability of differentiation into insulin-producing cells.

Nevertheless, challenges demanding resolution are plenty, like the ethical problem in using autologous and allogeneic stem cells to preserve the β-cells' function. Even though research focused on stem cell-derived β-cell replacement is gaining momentum year by year, enormous effort on the interventions with stem cell transplantation is required in the future to aid in achieving remission of T1DM by β-cell replacement.

6. Conclusion and perspectives

A potentially promising therapeutic option for diabetes (especially T1DM) treatment can be stem cell treatment, as it cures the disease rather than treating or managing them. Major advances in research on the derivation of IPCs from hPSCs have improved our chance of reestablishing glucose-responsive insulin secretion in patients with T1DM. There are many questions and technical hurdles that still need to be solved.

The major problems include the following five aspects:

1. Can we generate more mature functional β-like cells in vitro from hPSCs.
2. Is there a possibility to improve the differentiation efficiency of IPCs from hPSCs.
3. How to protect implanted IPCs from autoimmune attack.
4. Need of the hour to generate sufficient numbers of desired cell types for clinical transplantation.
5. How to establish thorough insulin independence to make it a clinical reality.

Despite these obstacles, the application of stem cell-based therapy for T1DM represents the most advanced approach for curing type 1diabetes.

Acknowledgements

Indian Council for Medical Research (ICMR), New Delhi.
Apollo group of Hospitals, Chennai.
Apollo Hospital and Research Foundation, Chennai.
Dr. Viswanadham D, Vice President, IKP.
IKP Knowledge Park, Telangana.

Conflict of interest

We hereby declare that we have no conflict of interest of any form pertaining to our chapter titled, 'Molecular Challenges and Advances in Clinical Islet Transplantation'.

Author details

Nithyakalyani Mohan* and Anusha Sunder
Apollo Hospital and Research Foundation, Apollo Hospitals, Chennai, Tamilnadu, India

*Address all correspondence to: mmnithya@gmail.com

References

[1] de Lapertosa SG, de Moura AF, Decroux C, Duke L, Hammond L, Jacobs E, et al. International Diabetes Federation (IDF). Diabetes Atlas. 9th ed. Brussels, Belgium; 2019. Available from: https://www.diabetesatlas.org/en/. ISBN: 978-2-930229-87-4

[2] Peiris H, Park S, Louis S, et al. Discovering human diabetes-risk gene function with genetics and physiological assays. Nature Communications. 2018;**9**:3855. DOI: 10.1038/s41467-018-06249-3

[3] Mohan V, Unnikrishnan R. Precision diabetes: Where do we stand today? The Indian Journal of Medical Research. 2018;**148**(5):472-475. Available from: https://www.ncbi.nlm.nih.gov/pmc/articles/PMC6366260/

[4] Ragia G, Petridis I, Tavridou A, Christakidis D, Manolopoulos VG. Presence of CYP2C9*3 allele increases risk for hypoglycemia in Type 2 diabetic patients treated with sulfonylureas. Pharmacogenomics. 2009;**10**(11):1781-1787. Available from: https://www.ncbi.nlm.nih.gov/pubmed/19891554/

[5] Dujic T, Zhou K, Tavendale R, Palmer CN, Pearson ER. Effect of serotonin transporter 5-HTTLPR polymorphism on gastrointestinal intolerance to metformin: A GoDARTS study. Diabetes Care. 2016;**39**(11):1896-1901. DOI: 10.2337/dc16-0706

[6] Kelly MA, Rayner ML, Mijovic CH, Barnett AH. Molecular aspects of type 1 diabetes. Molecular Pathology. 2003;**56**(1):1-10. DOI: 10.1136/mp.56.1.1

[7] Rickels MR, Robertson RP. Pancreatic islet transplantation in humans: Recent progress and future directions. Endocrine Reviews. 2019;**40**(2):631-668. DOI: 10.1210/er.2018-00154

[8] Klec C, Ziomek G, Pichler M, Malli R, Graier WF. Calcium signaling in ß-cell physiology and pathology: A revisit. International Journal of Molecular Sciences. 2019;**20**(24):6110. DOI: 10.3390/ijms20246110

[9] Moccia F, Berra-Romani R, Tanzi F. Update on vascular endothelial Ca(2+) signalling: A tale of ion channels, pumps and transporters. World Journal of Biological Chemistry. 2012;**3**(7):127-158. DOI: 10.4331/wjbc.v3.i7.127

[10] Bouché C, Shanti Serdy C, Kahn R, Goldfine AB. The cellular fate of glucose and its relevance in Type 2 diabetes. Endocrine Reviews. 2004;**25**(5):807-830. DOI: 10.1210/er.2003-0026

[11] Kahn SE, Chen YC, Esser N, et al. The β cell in diabetes: Integrating biomarkers with functional measures. Endocrine Reviews. 2021;**42**(5):528-583. DOI: 10.1210/endrev/bnab021

[12] Meda P. The in vivo β-to-β-cell chat room: Connexin connections matter. Diabetes. 2012;**61**(7):1656-1658. DOI: 10.2337/db12-0336

[13] Weitz J, Menegaz D, Caicedo A. Deciphering the complex communication networks that orchestrate pancreatic islet function. Diabetes. 2021;**70**(1):17-26. DOI: 10.2337/dbi19-0033

[14] Gala-Lopez BL, Neiman D, Kin T, et al. Beta cell death by cell-free DNA and outcome after clinical islet transplantation. Transplantation. 2018;**102**(6):978-985. DOI: 10.1097/TP.0000000000002083

[15] Kanak MA, Takita M, Shahbazov R, et al. Evaluation of MicroRNA375 as

a novel biomarker for graft damage in clinical islet transplantation. Transplantation. 2015;**99**(8):1568-1573. DOI: 10.1097/TP.0000000000000625

[16] Erener S, Mojibian M, Fox JK, Denroche HC, Kieffer TJ. Circulating miR-375 as a biomarker of β-cell death and diabetes in mice. Endocrinology. 2013;**154**(2):603-608. DOI: 10.1210/en.2012-1744

[17] Poy MN, Hausser J, Trajkovski M, et al. miR-375 maintains normal pancreatic alpha- and beta-cell mass. Proceedings of the National Academy of Sciences of the United States of America. 2009;**106**(14):5813-5818. DOI: 10.1073/pnas.0810550106

[18] Saini D, Ramachandran S, Nataraju A, et al. Activated effector and memory T cells contribute to circulating sCD30: Potential marker for islet allograft rejection. American Journal of Transplantation. 2008;**8**(9):1798-1808. DOI: 10.1111/j.1600-6143.2008.02329.x

[19] Hire K, Hering B, Bansal-Pakala P. Relative reductions in soluble CD30 levels post-transplant predict acute graft function in islet allograft recipients receiving three different immunosuppression protocols. Transplant Immunology. 2010;**23**(4):209-214. DOI: 10.1016/j.trim.2010.06.007

[20] Papas KK, Suszynski TM, Colton CK. Islet assessment for transplantation. Current Opinion in Organ Transplantation. 2009;**14**(6):674-682. DOI: 10.1097/MOT.0b013e328332a489

[21] Itoh T, Takita M, SoRelle JA, et al. Correlation of released HMGB1 levels with the degree of islet damage in mice and humans and with the outcomes of islet transplantation in mice. Cell Transplantation. 2012;**21**(7):1371-1381. DOI: 10.3727/096368912X640592

[22] Yang JY, Sarwal MM. Transplant genetics and genomics. Nature Reviews. Genetics. 2017;**18**(5):309-326. DOI: 10.1038/nrg.2017.12

[23] Giannoukakis N, Thomson A, Robbins P. Gene therapy in transplantation. Gene Therapy. 1999;**6**:1499-1511. DOI: 10.1038/sj.gt.3300981

[24] Hernandez A, Evers BM. Functional genomics: Clinical effect and the evolving role of the surgeon. Archives of Surgery. 1999;**134**(11):1209-1215. DOI: 10.1001/archsurg.134.11.1209

[25] Nair SS, Sarasamma S, Gracious N, George J, Anish TS, Radhakrishnan R. Polymorphism of the CYP3A5 gene and its effect on tacrolimus blood level. Experimental and Clinical Transplantation. Apr 2015;**13**(Suppl. 1): 197-200. Available from: https://pubmed.ncbi.nlm.nih.gov/25894154/

[26] Nobakht E, Jagadeesan M, Paul R, Bromberg J, Dadgar S. Precision medicine in kidney transplantation: Just hype or a realistic hope? Transplantation Direct. 2021;**7**(2):e650. DOI: 10.1097/TXD.0000000000001102

[27] Kurian SM, Ferreri K, Wang CH, et al. Gene expression signature predicts human islet integrity and transplant functionality in diabetic mice. PLoS One. 2017;**12**(10):e0185331. DOI: 10.1371/journal.pone.0185331

[28] Cheung SS, Metzger DL, Wang X, et al. Tumor necrosis factor-related apoptosis-inducing ligand and CD56 expression in patients with type 1 diabetes mellitus. Pancreas. 2005;**30**(2):105-114. DOI: 10.1097/01.mpa.0000148515.77497.4b

[29] Ou D, Metzger DL, Wang X, Huang J, Pozzilli P, Tingle AJ.

TNF-related apoptosis-inducing ligand death pathway-mediated human beta-cell destruction. Diabetologia. 2002;**45**(12):1678-1688. DOI: 10.1007/s00125-002-0926-2

[30] Loweth AC, Williams GT, James RF, Scarpello JH, Morgan NG. Human islets of Langerhans express Fas ligand and undergo apoptosis in response to interleukin-1beta and Fas ligation. Diabetes. 1998;**47**(5):727-732. DOI: 10.2337/diabetes.47.5.727

[31] Maedler K, Spinas GA, Lehmann R, et al. Glucose induces beta-cell apoptosis via upregulation of the Fas receptor in human islets. Diabetes. 2001;**50**(8):1683-1690. DOI: 10.2337/diabetes.50.8.1683

[32] Firestein GS, Manning AM. Signal transduction and transcription factors in rheumatic disease. Arthritis and Rheumatism. 1999;**42**(4):609-621. DOI: 10.1002/1529-0131(199904)42:4<609::AID-ANR3>3.0.CO;2-I

[33] Bertuzzi F, Marzorati S, Maffi P, et al. Tissue factor and CCL2/monocyte chemoattractant protein-1 released by human islets affect islet engraftment in type 1 diabetic recipients. The Journal of Clinical Endocrinology and Metabolism. 2004;**89**(11):5724-5728. DOI: 10.1210/jc.2004-0659

[34] Melzi R, Piemonti L, Nano R, et al. Donor and isolation variables associated with human islet monocyte chemoattractant protein-1 release. Transplantation. 2004;**78**(10):1564-1567. DOI: 10.1097/01.tp.0000144184.20085.41

[35] Shibasaki S, Imagawa A, Tauriainen S, et al. Expression of toll-like receptors in the pancreas of recent-onset fulminant type 1 diabetes. Endocrine Journal. 2010;**57**(3):211-219. DOI: 10.1507/endocrj.k09e-291

[36] Johansson H, Lukinius A, Moberg L, et al. Tissue factor produced by the endocrine cells of the islets of Langerhans is associated with a negative outcome of clinical islet transplantation. Diabetes. 2005;**54**(6):1755-1762. DOI: 10.2337/diabetes.54.6.1755

[37] Russell MA, Cooper AC, Dhayal S, Morgan NG. Differential effects of interleukin-13 and interleukin-6 on Jak/STAT signaling and cell viability in pancreatic β-cells. Islets. 2013;**5**(2):95-105. DOI: 10.4161/isl.24249

[38] El-Gohary Y, Tulachan S, Guo P, et al. Smad signaling pathways regulate pancreatic endocrine development. Developmental Biology. 2013;**378**(2):83-93. DOI: 10.1016/j.ydbio.2013.04.003

[39] Xiao X, Wiersch J, El-Gohary Y, et al. TGFβ receptor signaling is essential for inflammation-induced but not β-cell workload-induced β-cell proliferation. Diabetes. 2013;**62**(4):1217-1226. DOI: 10.2337/db12-1428

[40] Hoffmann DC, Textoris C, Oehme F, et al. Pivotal role for alpha1-antichymotrypsin in skin repair. The Journal of Biological Chemistry. 2011;**286**(33):28889-28901. DOI: 10.1074/jbc.M111.249979

[41] Zhang B, Abreu JG, Zhou K, et al. Blocking the Wnt pathway, a unifying mechanism for an angiogenic inhibitor in the serine proteinase inhibitor family. Proceedings of the National Academy of Sciences of the United States of America. 2010;**107**(15):6900-6905. DOI: 10.1073/pnas.0906764107

[42] Dayeh T, Volkov P, Salö S, et al. Genome-wide DNA methylation analysis of human pancreatic islets from type 2 diabetic and non-diabetic donors identifies candidate genes that influence insulin secretion. PLoS Genetics.

2014;**10**(3):e1004160. DOI: 10.1371/journal.pgen.1004160

[43] Zhang H, Ables ET, Pope CF, et al. Multiple, temporal-specific roles for HNF6 in pancreatic endocrine and ductal differentiation. Mechanisms of Development. 2009;**126**(11-12):958-973. DOI: 10.1016/j.mod.2009.09.006

[44] Jacquemin P, Durviaux SM, Jensen J, et al. Transcription factor hepatocyte nuclear factor 6 regulates pancreatic endocrine cell differentiation and controls expression of the proendocrine gene ngn3. Molecular and Cellular Biology. 2000;**20**(12):4445-4454. DOI: 10.1128/MCB.20.12.4445-4454.2000

[45] Bonnefond A, Vaillant E, Philippe J, et al. Transcription factor gene MNX1 is a novel cause of permanent neonatal diabetes in a consanguineous family. Diabetes & Metabolism. 2013;**39**(3):276-280. DOI: 10.1016/j.diabet.2013.02.007

[46] Jeon J, Correa-Medina M, Ricordi C, Edlund H, Diez JA. Endocrine cell clustering during human pancreas development. The Journal of Histochemistry and Cytochemistry. 2009;**57**(9):811-824. DOI: 10.1369/jhc.2009.953307

[47] Lyttle BM, Li J, Krishnamurthy M, et al. Transcription factor expression in the developing human fetal endocrine pancreas. Diabetologia. 2008;**51**(7):1169-1180. DOI: 10.1007/s00125-008-1006-z

[48] Sussel L, Kalamaras J, Hartigan-O'Connor DJ, et al. Mice lacking the homeodomain transcription factor Nkx2.2 have diabetes due to arrested differentiation of pancreatic beta cells. Development. 1998;**125**(12):2213-2221. DOI: 10.1242/dev.125.12.2213

[49] Mellitzer G, Bonné S, Luco RF, et al. IA1 is NGN3-dependent and essential for differentiation of the endocrine pancreas. The EMBO Journal. 2006;**25**(6):1344-1352. DOI: 10.1038/sj.emboj.7601011

[50] Zhang T, Wang H, Saunee NA, Breslin MB, Lan MS. Insulinoma-associated antigen-1 zinc-finger transcription factor promotes pancreatic duct cell trans-differentiation. Endocrinology. 2010;**151**(5):2030-2039. DOI: 10.1210/en.2009-1224

[51] Schaffer AE, Taylor BL, Benthuysen JR, et al. Nkx6.1 controls a gene regulatory network required for establishing and maintaining pancreatic Beta cell identity. PLoS Genetics. 2013;**9**(1):e1003274. DOI: 10.1371/journal.pgen.1003274

[52] Ejarque M, Cervantes S, Pujadas G, Tutusaus A, Sanchez L, Gasa R. Neurogenin3 cooperates with Foxa2 to autoactivate its own expression. The Journal of Biological Chemistry. 2013;**288**(17):11705-11717. DOI: 10.1074/jbc.M112.388173

[53] Lantz KA, Vatamaniuk MZ, Brestelli JE, Friedman JR, Matschinsky FM, Kaestner KH. Foxa2 regulates multiple pathways of insulin secretion. The Journal of Clinical Investigation. 2004;**114**(4):512-520. DOI: 10.1172/JCI21149

[54] Gao N, LeLay J, Vatamaniuk MZ, Rieck S, Friedman JR, Kaestner KH. Dynamic regulation of Pdx1 enhancers by Foxa1 and Foxa2 is essential for pancreas development. Genes & Development. 2008;**22**(24):3435-3448. DOI: 10.1101/gad.1752608

[55] Nakayama S, Arakawa M, Uchida T, et al. Dose-dependent requirement of patched homologue 1 in mouse pancreatic beta cell mass. Diabetologia. 2008;**51**(10):1883-1892. DOI: 10.1007/s00125-008-1080-2

[56] Grieco FA, Moretti M, Sebastiani G, et al. Delta-cell-specific expression of hedgehog pathway Ptch1 receptor in murine and human endocrine pancreas. Diabetes/Metabolism Research and Reviews. 2011;**27**(8):755-760. DOI: 10.1002/dmrr.1247

[57] Cras-Méneur C, Li L, Kopan R, Permutt MA. Presenilins, Notch dose control the fate of pancreatic endocrine progenitors during a narrow developmental window. Genes & Development. 2009;**23**(17):2088-2101. DOI: 10.1101/gad.1800209

[58] Düfer M, Neye Y, Hörth K, et al. BK channels affect glucose homeostasis and cell viability of murine pancreatic beta cells. Diabetologia. 2011;**54**(2):423-432. DOI: 10.1007/s00125-010-1936-0

[59] Wang H, Ferran C, Attanasio C, Calise F, et al. Induction of protective genes leads to islet survival and function. Journal of Transplantation. 2011;**2011**(141898):10. DOI: 10.1155/2011/141898

[60] Gozzelino R, Jeney V, Soares MP. Mechanisms of cell protection by heme oxygenase-1. Annual Review of Pharmacology and Toxicology. 2010;**50**:323-354. DOI: 10.1146/annurev.pharmtox.010909.105600

[61] Grey ST, Arvelo MB, Hasenkamp W, Bach FH, Ferran C. A20 inhibits cytokine-induced apoptosis and nuclear factor kappaB-dependent gene activation in islets. The Journal of Experimental Medicine. 1999;**190**(8):1135-1146. DOI: 10.1084/jem.190.8.1135

[62] Grey ST, Longo C, Shukri T, et al. Genetic engineering of a suboptimal islet graft with A20 preserves beta cell mass and function. Journal of Immunology. 2003;**170**(12):6250-6256. DOI: 10.4049/jimmunol.170.12.6250

[63] Liuwantara D, Elliot M, Smith MW, et al. Nuclear factor-kappaB regulates beta-cell death: A critical role for A20 in beta-cell protection. Diabetes. 2006;**55**(9):2491-2501. DOI: 10.2337/db06-0142

[64] Wang H, Lee SS, Dell'Agnello C, et al. Bilirubin can induce tolerance to islet allografts [published correction appears in Endocrinology. 2006 Oct;147(10):4842. D'Avilla, Joanna [corrected to d'Avila, Joana Costa Pinto]]. Endocrinology. 2006;**147**(2):762-768. DOI: 10.1210/en.2005-0632

[65] Lee SS, Gao W, Mazzola S, et al. Heme oxygenase-1, carbon monoxide, and bilirubin induce tolerance in recipients toward islet allografts by modulating T regulatory cells. The FASEB Journal. 2007;**21**(13):3450-3457. DOI: 10.1096/fj.07-8472com

[66] Zhang B, Kang M, Xie Q, et al. Anthocyanins from Chinese bayberry extract protect β cells from oxidative stress-mediated injury via HO-1 upregulation. Journal of Agricultural and Food Chemistry. 2011;**59**(2):537-545. DOI: 10.1021/jf1035405

[67] Shapiro AM, Lakey JR, Ryan EA, et al. Islet transplantation in seven patients with type 1 diabetes mellitus using a glucocorticoid-free immunosuppressive regimen. The New England Journal of Medicine. 2000;**343**(4):230-238. DOI: 10.1056/NEJM200007273430401

[68] Gibly RF, Graham JG, Luo X, Lowe WL Jr, Hering BJ, Shea LD. Advancing islet transplantation: From engraftment to the immune response. Diabetologia. 2011;**54**(10):2494-2505. DOI: 10.1007/s00125-011-2243-0

[69] Ghofaili KA, Fung M, Ao Z, et al. Effect of exenatide on beta cell function after islet transplantation

in type 1 diabetes. Transplantation. 2007;**83**(1):24-28. DOI: 10.1097/01.tp.0000251379.46596.2d

[70] Giannoukakis N, Mi Z, Rudert WA, Gambotto A, Trucco M, Robbins P. Prevention of beta cell dysfunction and apoptosis activation in human islets by adenoviral gene transfer of the insulin-like growth factor I. Gene Therapy. 2000;**7**(23):2015-2022. DOI: 10.1038/sj.gt.3301333

[71] Johansson M, Olerud J, Jansson L, Carlsson PO. Prolactin treatment improves engraftment and function of transplanted pancreatic islets. Endocrinology. 2009;**150**(4):1646-1653. DOI: 10.1210/en.2008-1318

[72] Rivas-Carrillo JD, Soto-Gutierrez A, Navarro-Alvarez N, et al. Cell-permeable pentapeptide V5 inhibits apoptosis and enhances insulin secretion, allowing experimental single-donor islet transplantation in mice. Diabetes. 2007;**56**(5):1259-1267. DOI: 10.2337/db06-1679

[73] Wen SJ, Zheng XM, Liu LF, et al. Effects of primary microglia and astrocytes on neural stem cells in *in vitro* and *in vivo* models of ischemic stroke. Neural Regeneration Research. 2021;**16**(9):1677-1685. DOI: 10.4103/1673-5374.306093

[74] Sultan N, Amin LE, Zaher AR, Grawish ME, Scheven BA. Dental pulp stem cells stimulate neuronal differentiation of PC12 cells. Neural Regeneration Research. 2021;**16**(9):1821-1828. DOI: 10.4103/1673-5374.306089

[75] Hu XM, Li ZX, Zhang DY, et al. A systematic summary of survival and death signalling during the life of hair follicle stem cells. Stem Cell Research & Therapy. 2021;**12**(1):453. DOI: 10.1186/s13287-021-02527-y

[76] Francese R, Fiorina P. Immunological and regenerative properties of cord blood stem cells. Clinical Immunology. 2010;**136**(3):309-322. DOI: 10.1016/j.clim.2010.04.010

[77] Hu XM, Zhang Q, Zhou RX, et al. Programmed cell death in stem cell-based therapy: Mechanisms and clinical applications. World Journal of Stem Cells. 2021;**13**(5):386-415. DOI: 10.4252/wjsc.v13.i5.386

[78] Yang R, Liu F, Wang J, Chen X, Xie J, Xiong K. Epidermal stem cells in wound healing and their clinical applications [published correction appears in Stem Cell Res Ther. 22 Oct 2020;**11**(1):447]. Stem Cell Research & Therapy. 2019;**10**(1):229. DOI: 10.1186/s13287-019-1312-z

[79] Ilic D, Polak JM. Stem cells in regenerative medicine: Introduction. British Medical Bulletin. 2011;**98**:117-126. DOI: 10.1093/bmb/ldr012

[80] Bongso A, Richards M. History and perspective of stem cell research. Best Practice & Research. Clinical Obstetrics & Gynaecology. 2004;**18**(6):827-842. DOI: 10.1016/j.bpobgyn.2004.09.002

[81] Yang R, Yang S, Zhao J, et al. Progress in studies of epidermal stem cells and their application in skin tissue engineering [published correction appears in Stem Cell Res Ther. 2022 May 5;**13**(1):183]. Stem Cell Research & Therapy. 2020;**11**(1):303. DOI: 10.1186/s13287-020-01796-3

[82] Parmar M, Grealish S, Henchcliffe C. The future of stem cell therapies for Parkinson disease. Nature Reviews. Neuroscience. 2020;**21**(2):103-115. DOI: 10.1038/s41583-019-0257-7

[83] Thomson JA, Itskovitz-Eldor J, Shapiro SS, et al. Embryonic stem cell

lines derived from human blastocysts [published correction appears in Science 1998 Dec 4;282(5395):1827]. Science. 1998;**282**(5391):1145-1147. DOI: 10.1126/science.282.5391.1145

[84] Takahashi K, Tanabe K, Ohnuki M, et al. Induction of pluripotent stem cells from adult human fibroblasts by defined factors. Cell. 2007;**131**(5):861-872. DOI: 10.1016/j.cell.2007.11.019

[85] Tahbaz M, Yoshihara E. Immune protection of stem cell-derived islet cell therapy for treating diabetes. Frontiers in Endocrinology (Lausanne). 2021;**12**:716625. DOI: 10.3389/fendo.2021.716625

[86] Buron F, Reffet S, Badet L, Morelon E, Thaunat O. Immunological monitoring in beta cell replacement: Towards a pathophysiology-guided implementation of biomarkers. Current Diabetes Reports. 2021;**21**(6):19. DOI: 10.1007/s11892-021-01386-4

Chapter 7

Controversies in Platelet Functions in Diabetes Mellitus Type 1

Gordon Ogweno and Edwin Murungi

Abstract

Individuals with diabetes mellitus (DM) are at high risk of thrombosis in which hyperactive platelets are implicated. The platelet hyperactivity has been linked to hyperglycemia. This hypothesis is supported by studies in type II diabetes mellitus showing increased sensitivity of platelets to stimulating agonists in the context of tissue resistance to high-circulating insulin. However, controversy still exists regarding the altered platelet functions in type 1 diabetes mellitus (T1DM) and the link to modifying factors such as blood glucose, hyperlipidemia, metabolic acidosis and insulin treatment. Moreover, increased insulin dosage or treatment appears to have antagonistic actions: diminished functions at low doses and enhanced activation at high doses, the switch being attributable to insulin-like growth factor. The physiological role of insulin in suppressing platelet activation is lost in T1DM, a scenario that favors increased platelet sensitivity to stimulating agonists. Furthermore, the response to antiplatelet agents and statins is sub-optimal in diabetics presenting clinical and research knowledge gap regarding the ideal antiplatelet treatment in DM in general and T1DM in particular. This chapter reviews the unique characteristics of platelet functions in T1DM highlighting the controversial areas linking unique behavior of platelets and the abnormal response to therapeutic interventions.

Keywords: type 1 diabetes mellitus, platelets, hyperactivity, thrombosis, platelet functions

1. Introduction

Diabetes mellitus (DM) is a metabolic disorder characterized by high blood glucose levels. There are two major types: type 1DM (T1DM) or insulin-dependent DM (IDDM) due to insulin deficiency or absence; and type 2 DM (T2DM) or non-insulin-dependent DM (NIDDM) is due to insulin resistance.

Diabetes mellitus and impaired glucose tolerance are associated with cardiovascular risk [1, 2] and thrombosis [3] considered to be platelet in origin [4]. Data on platelet functions have largely been derived from T2DM, since it is the most prevalent. However, T1DM is unique in that platelets are exposed to hyperglycemia in the absence of insulin, while in T2DM they are exposed to both hyperglycemia and hyperinsulinemia. It is increasingly debatable the roles of these factors in alteration of platelet functions in T1DM owing to the acuteness and short duration of exposure. More so, the role of insulin on platelet functions is controversial [5] given the paucity of its receptors [6], and that the platelet glucose transporters are independent of it [6].

IntechOpen

2. Platelet Indices and Morphology in T1DM

2.1 Platelet indices

Platelet indices such as platelet count, mean platelet volume (MPV), platelet distribution width (PDW), and platelet large cell ratio (P-LCR) are elevated in patients with IDM type 1 than non-diabetic controls [7] and are associated with cardiovascular complications [8]. These strongly correlate with duration of blood sugar control as assessed by extent of HbA1c [9] suggesting link with metabolic impairment. Notably, MPV size positively correlated with fasting blood glucose and HbA1C [10]. However, as to whether these changes are due to glucose and attendant osmotic effects or part of disease process remains largely unexplored.

2.2 Bone Marrow and megakaryocytes in T1DM

Changes in platelet indices in DM correlate with mekaryocyte DNA content or ploidy [11] reflecting direct influence on bone marrow function even prior to systemic circulation observations. The thrombopoiesis associated with T1DM releases an enormous amount of hyperactive platelets from the bone marrow into circulation [12]. Moreover, the newly released large but immature platelets from bone marrow have increased synthetic capacity for thromboxane and thrombospondin, have enhanced membrane surface expression of receptors such as GPIIbIIIa, CD61, and CD63, [13, 14], and have enhanced aggregation [14, 15]. In DM, the hyperglycemia acts through neutrophils to stimulate thrombopoietin (TPO) production in the liver and enhance megakaryocyte thrombopoiesis [16]. In T1DM, increased circulating TPO has been shown to be linked to elevated blood sugar levels and HbA1c HbA1C [17] providing evidence linking bone marrow megakaryopoiesis and metabolic state.

2.3 Platelet morphology and ultrastructure in T1DM

Peripheral blood smears of patients with diabetic complications show occasional giant platelets [8]. Biochemical examination has revealed altered membrane lipid composition, as well as Na +-K+ ATPase and Ca++-ATPase, which are sensitive to glucose concentrations compared with control from non-diabetic subjects [18].

Ultra structural examinations show prominence of dense granules.

3. Platelet hemostatic functions in T1DM

Diabetes mellitus is a pro-thrombotic condition and platelets are implicated. This has been confirmed by number of laboratory methods such adhesion to immobilized surfaces, granule content secretion, aggregation, clot retraction, and membrane surface expression of activation biomarkers.

3.1 Platelet Adhesion in T1DM

In T1DM, there is evidence of increased platelets adherence to surfaces such as collagen and fibrinogen [19–21], and this corresponds to elevated plasma vWF Ag and activity [22] and low ADAMTS-13 Ag and activity [23]. These features are related to glycemic control [24] and only if vWF is present and elevated in plasma [25].

However, it is not yet established whether the increased adhesiveness are linked to aggregation and linked to or derived from ensuing endothelial injury.

3.2 Aggregation

In DM, platelets exhibit hyperactivity and increased sensitivity to agonists such as ADP, AA, collagen, and epinephrine [26], which augments successive increased secretion of and response to prostaglandins [21, 27]. Specifically, there is greater platelet reactivity in T1DM compared with T2DM and healthy controls as evaluated by light transmission aggregometry (LTA) and platelet function analyzer-100 (PFA-100) [28, 29]. Notably, aggregation curves are biphasic at low agonist concentrations showing greater augmentation of second wave [26] indicating increased secretion of and response to prostaglandins [27]. The mechanism for the biphasic wave response is due to altered ATP/ADP metabolism [30], nucleotide and thromboxane secretion [31], and calcium fluxes [32]. These are because, upon agonist stimulation, there is an initial phase characterized by glycogenolysis with minimal ATP synthesis causing translocation of alpha granule-containing glucose transporter 3 (Glut-3) to the surface, followed by a second phase of enhanced Glut-3 glucose entry, glycolysis, and ATP synthesis leading to both alpha and delta granule translocation and degranulation [33]. These processes are exaggerated in the presence of high vWF, cholesterol and poor glycemic control in T1DM [24].

In contrast, others have found no change in ADP-induced platelet aggregation in T1DM [34, 35]. The lack of consistency with other studies probably suggests loss of adhesive molecules into platelet microparticles [36] or modulation by factors extrinsic to the platelets such as magnesium ions [37], insulin [38], and acidosis [39].

3.3 Membrane surface receptor expression and platelet-leukocyte aggregates (PLA)

Evaluation of platelets from T1DM patients has shown increased membrane surface expression of activation markers such as P-selectin, platelet-leukocyte aggregates (PLA)(platelet-monocyte, platelet-granulocytes) [17, 40, 41]. Importantly, it has been demonstrated that first relatives of T1DM patients at risk of T1DM have increased expression of P-selectin, CD63, and thrombospondin compared with at-no-risk controls [42]. Given that these changes are also observed in megakayryocytes, and peripherally, there is ongoing debate whether the changes are predetermined and intrinsic to disease process or epigenetic secondary to the altered metabolic milieu, are yet to be resolved.

3.4 Secretion and other soluble markers of activation

Urinary excretion of thromboxane B2 (TXB2) was found higher in DM than in healthy controls [35]. This is in contrast to another study that found decreased levels of TXB2, β-Thromboglobulin (BTG) and platelet factor-4 (PF-4) in diabetic patients with uncontrolled blood sugar and high HbA1C [34].

3.5 Platelet microparticle

Platelet microparticles (PMPs) or membrane-covered vesicles that bleb or vesiculate off in response to oxidative stress are elevated in T1DM [43]. The elevated PMP in T1DM compared with T2DM [44] has not been explained. Nevertheless, the levels are predictive of vasculopathy [1].

4. Platelet: inflammation cross talk in T1DM

There is cross talk between inflammation and platelets in T1DM where leukocytes and platelets activate each other [45] and both leukocytes, especially monocytes, and platelets are hyperactivated [41, 46]. Whereas platelets release cytokines [47], and increased levels of these factors have been found in circulation in individuals with T1DM [40], a cause and effect relationship has been questioned [48]. What is known is that cytokines, especially IL-6 and IL-8, are platelet activators [49], but whether they are the cause of platelet hyperactivity in T1DM remains largely unknown.

5. Modifiers of platelet function

Although platelet hyperactivity are vital to the pathophysiology of diabetes mellitus [42, 50–52], there are other factors in systemic circulation that modify disease progression. These factors include hyperglycemia and its control, insulin deficiency and therapy, acute metabolic acidosis, inflammatory markers that precede and coexist during disease states, and body calcium-magnesium fluxes levels.

5.1 Acute metabolic acidosis

Unlike in type 2 DM, acute metabolic diabetes keto-acidosis (DKA) characterized by lactic acidosis and ketonemia occurs in T1DM with a rate between 20 and 70% depending on the intensity of glucose control [53]. Subjects in DKA have increased blood levels of β-Thromboglobulin (β-TG), platelet factor-4 (PF-4), but their platelets are paradoxically less sensitive to aggregation agonists such as ADP and prostacyclin. The agonist sensitivity improves with glycemic control [54]. The initial depressed platelet function that improves with treatment is similar to previous findings by Janka [55] and Ileri et al [56].

Although ketones contribute to acidosis in DKA, only effects of lactic acid on platelets are well studied. Lactic acid dose dependently reduces platelet secondary wave aggregation *in vitro* [57–60]. The effect of pH changes is on impairing intracellular Ca++ store release [61, 62], thus interfering with cytoskeletal changes [63], facilitating platelet reactions [64]. In addition, the changes affect membrane surface expression of GP1b and P-selectin under anaerobic conditions [65] indicating metabolic effects. However, addition of lactic acid together with known platelet inhibitors such as aspirin is not additive but instead attenuates the effects [66, 67]. The paradoxical behavior can probably be accounted for by lactate being metabolized to produce ATP for platelet activation processes leaving protons to be buffered by other means.

5.2 Blood glucose and platelet functions in T1DM

Although platelet hyperactivity in T1DM has partly been ascribed to hyperglycemia, however, empirical evidence has been conflicting. Study results have ranged from no effects, decreased to increased platelet functions. The ambiguity may be attributed to confounders, depending on study designs, dose, and duration of exposure. Specifically, non-diabetic or healthy controls do not have the coexisting inflammatory biomarker seen in diabetics (T1DM from T2DM) who additionally have hyperlipidemia. Thus, in diabetics, duration of disease determines the level of non-enzymatic glycation. The route of glucose administration also matters. Oral intake is accompanied by post-prandial secretion of gut and counter regulatory hormones while direct or parenteral administration bypasses the gut, with *in vitro* mixing with platelet-rich plasma excluding the leukocytes contribution.

Bridges and coworkers [19] first demonstrated the link between blood glucose and platelet function. They showed that either a postprandial oral glucose load or intravenous infusion increased platelet stickiness in both diabetics and nob-diabetics. The observation has since been confirmed by others mostly in T2DM [68–71]. Surprisingly, in one study of hyperglycemia platelet p-selectin expression was decreased during hyperglycemia compared with levels before oral intake [72]. These results are confounded other factors concurrently activating platelets such as post-prandial hyperglycemia on counter regulatory hormones [73], procoagulant platelet microparticles [74], combined effect with insulin [75, 76], neutrophil-megakaryocyte thrombopoiesis [16], and hyperlipidemia [25, 77, 78].

In order to avoid the many confounders inherent in *in vivo* hyperglycaemia, *in vitro* studies designed to define the particular role of glucose have yielded mixed results. It has been shown that *in vitro* incubation of healthy PRP platelets with glucose upto 50 mmol has no effect on agonist-induced aggregation to ADP, AA or collagen, secretion of MDA or TXB2 [79] indicating no direct effects on platelets. Many *in vitro* studies involving short incubation periods with varying concentrations of glucose have shown no effects [80, 81]. However, studies have shown that glucose paradoxically increases platelet aggregation or surface P-selectin expression depending on the type of agonist [82–85].

The discordance in effects of glucose on platelets can be explained by the duration of exposure. While acute or short duration of exposure is associated with no or minimal effects, longer duration or chronic exposure stimulates thrombopoiesis in which reticulocytes increase adhesive receptors and are hyperactive to agonists [16]. The duration of glucose exposure correlates with HbA1c levels [86]. Contrary to popular belief, hyperactive platelets are evident even before observable metabolic features in individuals predisposed to T1DM with normal blood [41]. Early evidence of the influence of glucose on platelet functions via metabolic reactions was provided by Murer et al. [87] and Chaudhry et al. [88]. The two groups reported the presence of aggregation in media containing glucose or substitute substrates, the extent of which was related to glucose consumption and carbon dioxide production due to metabolism. In these experiments, addition of metabolic inhibitors inhibited aggregation. Moreover, alterations of membrane properties and energy requiring processes have been noted upon incubation of platelets with varying glucose concentrations [18] suggesting other mechanisms are at play.

Several preclinical animal studies have confirmed the dependency of platelet functions on glucose uptake and subsequent metabolism [33, 89]. Under resting conditions, the plasma membrane localized GLUT-1 glucose transporter facilitates glucose entry into platelets, activation glycolysis, and ATP production [90]. Upon stimulation with agonists such as thrombin, alpha granules containing both P-selectin and GLUT-3 translocate and fuse with plasma membrane to increase glucose uptake [91]. The resulting alpha granules degranulation, glucose influx, and increased ATP synthesis lead to P-selectin expression and aggregation [33, 92].

It appears that hyperglycemia in itself has little bearing on platelet activation unless accompanied by other changes. In a study of T1DM and T2DM, despite postprandial elevation of blood glucose in both types, however, markers of platelet activation were only increased in T2DM. Interestingly, insulin levels did not change in T1DM unlike in T2DM. Administration of insulin pre-meal was accompanied by increase of postprandial platelet activation markers [74, 76, 93]. However, platelet-activating effects of insulin in T1DM are evident only when there is concurrent hypoglycemia [94]. At low extracellular glucose, insulin potentiates action of thrombin to increase glucose entry via Glut-3 with concomitant increase in surface expression of P-selectin and aggregation. Conversely, at high glucose concentrations, insulin becomes inhibitory through its action on protein kinase B (PKB) and hampers thrombin activation mechanisms leading to decreased platelet activation and aggregation [92].

5.3 Hypertriglyceridemia/hyperlipidemia

In T1DM, the frequency of occurrence of hyperlipidemia is variable [95–97], but when it occurs is associated with platelet hyper-activation [46] and aggregation [98]. The link between post-prandial lipids and platelet secretions [99] and aggregations has been known for a long time [100]. The case was made stronger by observations that treatments lowering the plasma lipids led to normalization of platelet aggregation [101] and glycoprotein expression [102]. Hyper lipidemia associated with uncontrolled T1DM thus becomes an added dimension in platelet hyperactivity together with roles of glucose and insulin.

5.4 Pharmacological treatments

5.4.1 Insulin treatment

Platelet hyperactivity, which largely occurs together with hyperglycemia and hyperinsulinemia, is well known in T2DM [103]. Notably, despite the absolute or relative deficiency of insulin in T1DM, platelet hyperactivity also occurs in T1DM. This phenomenon has elicited debate on the role of insulin in platelet functions. The data available on platelet functions in T1DM are usually at the beginning of insulin treatment or follow-up, which have reported mixed results: no change [86, 104, 105], reduced functions [38], or enhanced activity [24]. These discrepancies in study results can be accounted for by the differences in insulin dosages that produce hypoglycemia, duration of disease, individual peculiarities such as obesity, hyperlipidemia, and plasma calcium and magnesium balances.

Low dose or physiological levels of insulin inhibit platelet aggregation through several mechanisms [38, 106]. These include: decreasing intracellular cAMP levels [38], decreasing calcium mobilization [107] but increasing magnesium influx [108], nitric-oxide-mediated increase in cGMP [38], stimulation of prostacyclin synthesis [109]. Low-dose Insulin prevents second wave aggregation in diabetics, an effect augmented by calcium channel blockers [110]. It is therefore apparent that physiological levels of insulin suppress platelet function, effects that are reversed in its absence during diabetes mellitus type1.

The studies that showed increased platelet hyperactivity concurrent with hyperinsulinemia induced hypoglycemia [94], with attendant increase in counter-regulatory hormones such as adrenaline [111, 112] and increase in vWF-platelet adhesiveness [24], results which were similar to findings in T2DM [113].

Experimental *in vitro*, insulin has antagonistic effects on PRP activation in healthy humans. While at low levels, it decreases platelet aggregation to ADP, at supraphysiological levels, aggregation to ADP is increased [114]. *In vitro,* in healthy controls, supraphysiological insulin enhances ADP-induced whole blood platelet expression of

P-selectin as well as fibrinogen binding, in addition to PRP aggregation. These effects are independent of extracellular calcium and glucose [115]. Insulin, both at physiological and supranormal levels, enhances platelet P-selectin, fibrinogen binding, and platelet-leukocyte aggregates in whole blood [115, 116]. Insulin at low doses decreases platelet aggregation, while at high doses enhances platelet aggregation due to the paradoxical changes in intraplatelet cGMP levels [114].

Whereas low-dose insulin decreases platelet aggregation, high dose increases platelet aggregation in vitro [115, 117]. These effects are mediated by paradoxical changes in intraplatelet cGMP levels [116] and co-operativity with insulin-like growth factor on platelets [118]. Indeed platelets pose few insulin receptors and responses are weak but potentiated by IGF-1 [118] in the presence of extracellular calcium [119]. This is because insulin and IGF-1 circulate together and share a lot of similarities in both structure and receptors [120, 121]. Thus, at high insulin concentrations, the effects of IGF-1 predominate, thus explaining the increased platelet aggregation and response to agonists in patients on hyperinsulinemia.

In healthy, non-diabetic non-obese subjects, insulin decreases platelet adherence to collagen surfaces, decreases agonist-induced (ADP, collagen, AA, and TRAP) platelet aggregation but increases intracellular cGMP. These responses are abolished or blunted in obese individuals [122].

5.4.2 Anti-platelet treatments

Aspirin suppressed platelet functions TXA secretion, LTA, and PFA although there are no observable differences between healthy and DM individuals [35]. In case of stable (>1 month) dual 100 mg aspirin and 75 mg clopidogrel, insulin-treated DM has elevated platelet reactivity as assessed by LTA and PFA compared with NIDM and non-diabetic controls [29]. The refractory effect of antiplatelets in the presence of insulin has been reported [123]. Aspirin has been shown to attenuate maximum aggregation in newly diagnosed T1DM via its effects on ADP, epinephrine, and thrombin. The effects are most marked in reducing the secondary [26] indicating propensity for secretory phase. The refractory state to anti-platelets responses of platelets to agonists in the presence of high glucose is dependent on the signaling pathways tested. For example, hyperglycemia blocks the NO-cGMP-protein kinase pathway but spares the thromboxane secretion [124].

5.4.3 Statins

In patients with hyperlipidemia type II, statins reduced ADP-induced platelet aggregation regardless of the type of drug. However, there was no change with collagen or ristocetin agonist. In addition, the changes were not observed in fibrinogen levels, spontaneous aggregation, and adhesion [125]. The effect of lipid lowering agents in attenuating platelet functions appears to be related to changes in fibrinogen levels [126], suggesting modulation through inflammatory mediators.

5.5 Inflammation

Inflammation is common to both T1DM and T2DM. However, in T1DM inflammation is upstream involving cellular interactions that release cytokines and fibrinogen [127]. The cytokines and fibrinogen have been found to influence platelet activation independent of hyperglycemia [123, 128]. Since fibrinogen is an acute phase protein associated with acute inflammatory conditions, its correlation with platelet functions points to the role of inflammation in the modulation platelet response after stimulation.

6. Mechanisms of altered platelet functions in T1DM

6.1 Oxidative stress

Owing to the absence or deficiency of insulin in T1DM glucose undergoes auto-oxidation with accumulation of reactive oxygen species [129]. The consequence is peroxidation of membrane lipids and proteins [130] promoting platelet aggregation [131].

However, it is still controversial whether oxidative stress is a consequence of metabolic complications in T1DM or the cause of the disease [47].

6.2 Hyperglycemia

Persistent hyperglycemia leads to formation of non-enzymatic glycation of proteins, so-called advanced glycation end products (AGEs). Accumulation of these products facilitates cytoskeletal reorganization causing externalization of membrane phosphatidyleserine (PS) [132], altered membrane fluidity [133], and increased expression of glycoproteins GPIb, IIbIIIa [134], P-selectin, and PLA [135].

Hyperglycemia induces secretion of TPO that potentiates agonist-induced activation of mature platelets. Levels positively correlate with blood glucose and level of control HbA1C [17].

6.3 Signal transduction mechanisms

Collagen at low dose selectively promotes granule secretions through GPVI receptors, a finding not found with high doses or thrombin [136].

DM platelets have upregulated protein C Kinase promoting aggregation [137], downregulation of cAMP, and subsequent increased expression of P2y12

6.4 Ca++signaling

Calcium fluxes are essential for platelet functions, and abnormalities in regulation contributed by prolonged exposure (24 hours) to high glucose are associated with platelet hyperactivity [138].

In T1DM, there is coexistence of insulin deficiency/absence and hypomagnesaemia [139]. Hypomagnesaemia is associated with oxidative stress [140] and increases in platelet baseline intracellular Ca++. The consequence of un-opposed intracellular calcium leads to signal transduction sequences that eventually promote membrane glycoprotein expression, adhesion, secretion, and aggregation [141, 142].

6.5 Lipids

DM subjects have hypertriglyceridaemia, apo E, and HDL receptors that modify cation transporters and nitric oxide synthase involved in platelet aggregation and activation [143–145].

6.6 Prostacyclin

Endothelium of individuals with diabetes mellitus is deficient in prostacyclin thought to contribute to enhanced platelet hyperactivity. However, in vitro testing found platelets from DM were less sensitive to PGI2 than normal controls [146].

6.7 Immune mechanisms

Inflammatory markers such as TNFα, cytokines, and immune complexes are abundant in diabetes, and these are thought to play a role in platelet activation. Cytokines contribute to platelet activation [147–149], and these are amplified by the presence of glucose and ADP [150].

6.8 Platelet-Neutrophil interaction

Animal studies have provided evidence for indirect platelet activation in DM that in the presence of hyperglycemia, neutrophils are stimulated to release S-100 calcium-binding proteins A8/A9 that lead to production of TPO from the liver. The released TPO consequently acts on bone marrow megakaryocytes to release reticulocytes [16]. Reticulocytes have high surface expression of GPIIbIIIa, P-selectin, and release cytokines [16]. The expressed P-selectin interacts with SGL-P on neutrophils to release neutrophil extracellular traps (NETs).

6.9 Thrombopiesis

DM and hyperglycemia are associated with release of large, immature platelets [12]. This indicates that the platelet hyperactivity in diabetic subjects is partly central from bone marrow, thus explaining lack of sensitivity to antiplatelet agents [151].

7. Clinical significance of platelet functions

Microangiopathy is common in T1DM and is associated with hyperactive platelets expressing agonist stimulated P-selectina and platelet-leucocyte aggregates [41]. A number of clinical trials have reported decreased efficacy of anti-platelets in DM subjects [152]. The reasons are multifactorial, but can be summarized as lack of effect in leukocyte-platelet interactions, chronic effects of hyperglycemia especially oxidative stress, insulin resistance, and inability of megakaryocytes to respond.

8. Conclusion

T1DM is associated with platelet hypersensitivity to stimulating agonists. Hyperglycemia, in a dose and duration-dependent manner, provides the substrates for energy generation that powers alpha granule translocation to the membrane surface. Enhanced expression of P-selectin and GPIIbIIIa contributes to increased platelet aggregation evident in T1DM. Platelet hyperactivity in T1DM represents a reversal of the attenuating effects of low dose or physiological insulin. This is augmented by the attendant hyperlipidemia. However, the paradoxical hyperactivity in the presence of hyperinsulinemia is due to counter-regulatory hormones and potentiation by insulin-like growth factor. Overall, platelet activation in T1DM occurs through multiple signal transduction pathways not targeted by currently available antiplatelet agents. These pathways offer avenues for the development of novel antiplatelet remedies with improved therapeutic efficacy.

Author details

Gordon Ogweno[1*] and Edwin Murungi[2]

1 Department of Medical Physiology, Kenyatta University, Kenya

2 Department of Medical Biochemistry, Kisii University, Kenya

*Address all correspondence to: ogweno.gordon@ku.ac.ke

References

[1] Salem MAEK, Adly AAM, Ismail EAR, Darwish YW, Kamel HA. Platelets microparticles as a link between micro- and macro-angiopathy in young patients with type 1 diabetes. Platelets. 2015;**26**(7):682-688

[2] Tominaga M, Eguchi H, Manaka H, Igarashi K, Kato T, Sekikawa A. I m p a i red glucose tolerance is a risk factor for cardiovascular disease, but not impaired fasting glucose. The Funagata Diabetes Study. Diabetes Care. 1999;**22**(6):920-924

[3] Vazzana N, Ranalli P, Cuccurullo C, Davì G. Diabetes mellitus and thrombosis. Thrombosis Research. 2012;**129**(3):371-377

[4] Shechter M, Bairey Merz CN, Paul-Labrador MJ, Kaul S. Blood glucose and platelet-dependent thrombosis in patients with coronary artery disease. Journal of the American College of Cardiology. 2000;**35**(2):300-307

[5] Nusca A et al. Platelet effects of anti-diabetic therapies : New perspectives in the management of patients with diabetes and cardiovascular disease. Frontiers in Pharmacology. 2021;**12**:670155

[6] Ebeling P, Koistinen HA, Koivisto VA. Insulin-independent glucose transport regulates insulin sensitivity. FEBS Letters. 1998;**436**(3):301-303

[7] Malachowska B et al. Altered Platelets' morphological parameters in children with type 1 diabetes – a case-control study. BMC Endocrinology Disorders. 1998;**15**(1):17

[8] Jindal S et al. Platelet indices in diabetes mellitus : Indicators of diabetic microvascular complications Platelet indices in diabetes mellitus : Indicators of diabetic microvascular complications. Hematology. 2011;**16**(2):86-89

[9] Findikli HA, Kirac CO. Evaluation of the relationship between blood glucose regulation and hematological indices in patients with diabetes mellitus. EJMI. 2022;**6**(2):240-244

[10] Manoj S, Swami YK, Meena SR. Study of impact of glycemic status (HbA1c) on platelet activity measured by mean platelet volume & vascular complications in. The Journal of the Association of Physicians of India. 2019;**67**:26-29

[11] Brown AS et al. Megakaryocyte ploidy and platelet changes in human diabetes and atherosclerosis. Arteriosclerosis, Thrombosis, and Vascular Biology. 1997;**17**(4):802-807

[12] Tschoepe D et al. Large platelets circulate in an activated state in diabetes mellitus. Seminars in Thrombosis and Hemostasis. 1991;**17**(4):433-438

[13] Wisinski JA, Kimple ME. Platelet dysfunction in type 1 diabetes: Stressing the thromboxanes. Diabetes. 2016;**65**(2):349-351

[14] Fraser JK, Leahy MF, Berridge MV. Expression of antigens of the platelet glycoprotein IIb/IIIa complex on human hematopoietic stem cells. Blood. 1986;**68**(3):762-769

[15] Berridge MV, Ralph SJ, Tan AS. Cell-lineage antigens of the stem cell-megakaryocyte-platelet lineage are associated with the platelet IIb-IIIa glycoprotein complex. Blood. 1985;**66**(1):76-85

[16] Kraakman MJ et al. Neutrophil-derived S100 calcium-binding proteins A8/A9 promote reticulated thrombocytosis and atherogenesis in diabetes. The Journal of Clinical Investigation. 2017;**127**(6):2133-2147

[17] Bosco O et al. Thrombopoietin contributes to enhanced platelet activation in patients with type 1 diabetes mellitus. International Journal of Molecular Sciences. 2021;**22**(13):1-12

[18] Mazzanti L et al. Altered platelet membrane dynamic properties in type 1 diabetes. Diabetes. 1997;**46**(12):2069-2074

[19] Bridges JM, Dalby AM, Millar JHD, Weaver JA. An effect of D-glucose on platelet stickiness. Lancet. 1965;**285**(7376):75-77

[20] Heath H, Gridgen WD, Canever JV, Pollock J, Kelsey J, Bloom A. Platelet adhesiveness and aggregation in relation to diabetic retinopathy. Diabetologia. 1971;7:308-315

[21] Colwell JA, Nair RMG, Halushka PV, Rogers C, Whetsell A, Sage J. Platelet adhesion and aggregation in diabetes mellitus. Metabolism. 2003;**28**(74):394-400

[22] Chan NN, Fuller JH, Rubens M, Colhoun HM. Von Willebrand factor in type 1 diabetes: Its relationship with endothelial nitric oxide production and coronary artery calcification. Medical Science Monitor. 2003;**9**(7):297-304

[23] Skeppholm M, Kallner A, Kalani M, Jörneskog G, Blombäck M, Wallén HN. ADAMTS13 and von willebrand factor concentrations in patients with diabetes mellitus. Blood Coagulation & Fibrinolysis. 2009;**20**(8):619-626

[24] Mohamed SM, El-kinany HA, Abdel-fattah MA. Platelet aggregation and von Willebrand factor in children with insulin dependent diabetes mellitus and their relation to glycemic control abstract : Introduction: Subjects and methods : Results and discussion. Alexander Journal of Pdiatrics. 1998;**12**(2):329-338

[25] Dittmar S, Polanowska-Grabowska R, Gear ARL. Platelet adhesion to collagen under flow conditions in diabetes mellitus. Thrombosis Research. 1994;**74**(3):273-283

[26] Sagel J, Ch B, Colwell JA, Ph D, Crook L, Ph D. Increased platelet aggregation in early diabetus mellitus. Annals of Internal Medicine. 1975;**82**(6):733-738

[27] Colwell JA, Halushka PV, Sarji KE, Sagel J. Platelet function and diabetes mellitus. The Medical Clinics of North America. 1978;**62**(4):753-766

[28] Angiolillo DJ et al. Platelet dunction profiles in patients With type 2 diabetes and coronary artery disease on combined aspirin and clopidogrel treatment. Diabetes. 1978;**54**:2430-2435

[29] Angiolillo DJ et al. Insulin therapy is associated with platelet dysfunction in patients with type 2 diabetes mellitus on dual oral antiplatelet treatment. Journal of American College Cardiology. 1978;**48**(2):298-304

[30] Michno A, Bielarczyk H, Pawełczyk T, Jankowska-Kulawy A, Klimaszewska J, Szutowicz A. Alterations of adenine nucleotide metabolism and function of blood platelets in patients with diabetes. Diabetes. 2007;**56**(2):462-467

[31] Li Z, Zhang G, Le Breton GC, Gao X, Malik AB, Du X. Two waves of platelet secretion induced by thromboxane A2 receptor and a critical

role for phosphoinositide 3-kinases. The Journal of Biological Chemistry. 2003;**278**(33):30725-30731

[32] Emery M, O'Dell BL. Biphasic platelet aggregation in rat plasma and the effect of calcium flux modulators. Thrombosis Research. 1987;**46**:617-623

[33] Fidler TP et al. Glucose transporter 3 potentiates degranulation and is required for platelet activation. Arteriosclerosis, Thrombosis, and Vascular Biology. 2017;**37**(9):1628-1639

[34] Kutti J, Wadenvik H, Henestam B. Evaluation of platelet reactivity in diabetes mellitus. Acta Medica Scandinavica. 1986;**219**:195-199

[35] Al-sofiani ME et al. Diabetes and platelet response to low-dose aspirin. The Journal of Clinical Endocrinology and Metabolism. 2018;**103**:4599-4608

[36] Omoto S et al. Significance of platelet-derived microparticles and activated platelets in diabetic nephropathy. Nephron. 1999;**81**(3):271-277

[37] Sobczak AIS, Phoenix FA, Pitt SJ, Ajjan RA, Stewart AJ. Reduced plasma magnesium levels in type-1 diabetes associate with prothrombotic changes in fibrin clotting and fibrinolysis. Thrombosis and Haemostasis. 2020;**120**(2):243-252

[38] Trovati M, Anfossi G, Cavalot F, Massucco P, Mularoni E, Emanuelli G. Insulin directly reduces platelet sensitivity to aggregating agents. Studies in vitro and in vivo. Diabetes. 1988;**37**(6):780-786

[39] Etulain J et al. Acidosis downregulates platelet haemostatic functions and promotes neutrophil proinflammatory responses mediated by platelets. Thrombosis and Haemostasis. 2012;**107**:99-110

[40] Yngen M, Östenson CG, Hu H, Li N, Hjemdahl P, Wallén NH. Enhanced P-selectin expression and increased soluble CD40 Ligand in patients with Type 1 diabetes mellitus and microangiopathy: Evidence for platelet hyperactivity and chronic inflammation. Diabetologia. 2004;**47**(3):537-540

[41] Hu H, Li N, Yngen M. Enhanced leukocyte – platelet cross-talk in Type 1 diabetes mellitus: Relationship to microangiopathy. Journal of Thrombosis and Haemostasis. 2004;**2**:58-64

[42] Tschoepe D, Driesch E, Schwippert B, Lampeter EF. Activated platelets in subjects at increased risk of IDDM. Diabetologia. 1997;**40**(5):573-577

[43] Bergen K, Mobarrez F, Jörneskog G, Wallén H, Tehrani S. High levels of endothelial and platelet microvesicles in patients with type 1 diabetes irrespective of microvascular complications. Thrombosis Research. 1997;**196**:78-86

[44] Sabatier F et al. Type 1 and type 2 diabetic patients display different patterns of cellular microparticles. Diabetes. 2002;**51**(9):2840-2845

[45] Popp SK, Vecchio F, Brown DJ, Fukuda R, Suzuki Y, Takeda Y, et al. Circulating platelet-neutrophil aggregates characterize the development of type 1 diabetes in humans and NOD mice. JCI insight. 2022;**7**(2):e153993. DOI: 10.1172/jci.insight.153993

[46] Zahran AM, El-Badawy O, Mohamad IL, Tamer DM, Abdel-Aziz SM, Elsayh KI. Platelet activation and platelet–leukocyte aggregates in type I diabetes mellitus. Clinical Application in Thrombosis. 2002;**24**(9):230-239

[47] Chen Y, Zhong H, Zhao Y, Luo X, Gao W. Role of platelet biomarkers in inflammatory response. Biomark Research. 2020;**8**(1):28

[48] Haller MJ, Schatz DA. Cytokines and type 1 diabetes complications : Casual or causal association ? Pedriatric Diabetes. 2008;**9**(11):1-2

[49] Lumadue JA, Lanzkron SM, Kennedy SD, Kuhl DT, Mt BS, Kickler TS. Cytokine induction of platelet activation. American Journal of Clinical Pathology. 1996;**106**:795-798

[50] Bern MM. Platelet functions in diabetes mellitus. Diabetes. 1978;**2**(3):342-350

[51] BETTERIDGE DJ, TAHIR KEHE, RECKLESS JPD, WILLIAMS KI. Platelets from diabetic subjects show diminished sensitivity to prostacyclin. European Journal of Clinical Investigation. 1982;**12**(5):395-398

[52] Kim JH, Bae HY, Kim SY. Clinical marker of platelet hyperreactivity in diabetes mellitus. Diabetes and Metabolism Journal. 2013;**37**(6):423-428

[53] Cesur M, Sayin I. Diabetic Ketoacidosis, In: Type 1 Diabetes. London, United Kingdom: IntechOpen; 2013. DOI: 10.5772/53199 Available from: https://www.intechopen.com/chapters 10/pp 251-291/43299

[54] Campbell RR, Foster KJ, Stirling C, Mundy D, Reckless JPD. Paradoxical platelet behaviour in diabetic ketoacidosis. Diabetic Medicine. 1986;**3**(2):161-164

[55] Janka HU, Mehmet H. No rationale for antiplatelet drug treatment in diabetic ketoacidosis. Diabetologia. 1982;**23**:1982

[56] Ileri NŞ et al. Evaluation of the haemostatic system during ketoacidotic deterioration of diabetes mellitus. Haemostasis. 1999;**29**(6):318-325

[57] Goldschmidt B. Effect of lactic acid on the aggregation of human platelets induced by ADP, adrenaline and collagen. Specialia. 1973;**15**(11):1399-1401

[58] Foley ME, Mcnicol GP. An in-vitro study of acidosis, platelet function, and perinatal cerebral intraventricular haemorrhage. Lancet. 1977;**11**:1230-1232

[59] Lanier CJ, Taintor JS, Christopherson PW, Spangler EA. Effect of lactic acid addition to equine whole blood on platelet aggregation measured by impedance aggregometry. Veterinary Clinical Pathology. 2022;**51**(1):65-69

[60] Lawson CA, Spangler EA. The effect of adding lactic acid to canine whole blood on platelet aggregation as measured by impedance aggregometry. Veterinary Clinical Pathology. 2020;**49**(2):217-221

[61] Marumo M, Suehiro A, Kakishita E, Groschner K, Wakabayashi I. Extracellular pH affects platelet aggregation associated with modulation of store-operated Ca2+ entry. Thrombosis Research. 2001;**104**(5):353-360

[62] Laskay G, Kálmán K, Van Kerkhove E, Steels P, Ameloot M. Store-operated Ca2+-channels are sensitive to changes in extracellular pH. Biochemical and Biophysical Research Communications. 2005;**337**(2):571-579

[63] Nachmias VT, Yoshida K, Glennon MC. Lowering pH in blood platelets dissociates myosin phosphorylation from shape change and myosin association with the

cytoskeleton. The Journal of Cell Biology. 1987;**105**(4):1761-1769

[64] Djaldetti M, Fishman P, Bessler H, Chaimoff C. Platelet ultrastructural alterations. A possible mechanism for impaired platelet aggregation. Archives of Surgery. 1979;**114**:707-710

[65] Bertolini F, Porretti L, Lauri E, Rebulla P, Sirchia G. Role of lactate in platelet storage lesion. Vox Sanguinis. 1993;**65**(3):194-198

[66] Kobzar G, Mardla V, Samel N. Short-term exposure of platelets to glucose impairs inhibition of platelet aggregation by cyclooxygenase inhibitors. Platelets. 2011;**22**(5):338-344

[67] Kobzar G, Mardla V, Samel N. Lactate is a possible mediator of the glucose effect on platelet inhibition. Platelets. 2014;**25**(4):239-245

[68] Przygodzki T, Luzak B, Kassassir H, Mnich E, Boncler M, Siewiera K, et al. Diabetes and Hyperglycemia Affect Platelet GPIIIa Expression. Effects on Adhesion Potential of Blood Platelets from Diabetic Patients under In Vitro Flow Conditions. International journal of molecular sciences. 2020;**21**(9):3222. DOI: 10.3390/ijms21093222

[69] Gresele P et al. Hyperglycemia-induced platelet activation in type 2 diabetes is resistant to aspirin but not to a nitric oxide – donating agent. Diabetes Care. 2010;**33**(6):1262-1268

[70] Worthley MI et al. The deleterious effects of hyperglycemia on platelet function in diabetic patients with acute coronary syndromes. Mediation by superoxide production, resolution with intensive insulin administration. Journal of the American College of Cardiology. 2007;**49**(3):304-310

[71] Li N, Sudic D, Forslund M, Razmara M. Acute hyperglycaemia enhances platelet activation: Involvement of multiple mechanisms. Blood. 2004;**104**(11):3884-3884

[72] Yngen M, Ostenson C-G, Li N, Hjemdahl P, Wallen NH. Acute hyperglycemia increases soluble P- selectin in male patients with mild diabetes mellitus. Blood Coagulation & Fibrinolysis. 2001;**12**(2):109-116

[73] Santilli F et al. Postprandial hyperglycemia is a determinant of platelet activation in early type 2 diabetes mellitus. Journal of Thrombosis and Haemostasis. 2010;**8**(4):828-837

[74] Spectre G et al. Meal intake increases circulating procoagulant microparticles in patients with type 1 and type 2 diabetes mellitus. Platelets. 2019;**30**(3):348-355

[75] Vaidyula VR, Rao AK, Mozzoli M, Homko C, Cheung P, Boden G. Effects of hyperglycemia and hyperinsulinemia on circulating tissue factor procoagulant activity and platelet CD40 ligand. Diabetes. 2006;**55**(1):202-208

[76] Spectre G, Stålesen R, Östenson C, Hjemdahl P. Meal-induced platelet activation in diabetes mellitus type 1 or type 2 is related to postprandial insulin rather than glucose levels ☆. Thrombosis Research. 2016;**141**:93-97

[77] Knobler H, Savion N, Shenkman B, Kotev-Emeth S, Varon D. Shear-induced platelet adhesion and aggregation on subendothelium are increased in diabetic patients. Thrombosis Research. 1998;**90**(4):181-190

[78] Pawelczyk M, Kaczorowska B, Baj Z. The impact of hyperglycemia and hyperlipidemia on plasma P-selectin

and platelet markers after ischemic stroke. Archives of Medical Science. 2017;**13**(5):1049-1056

[79] Best L, Jones PBB, Preston FE. Effect of glucose on platelet thromboxane biosynthesis. Lancet. 1979;**314**(8146):790

[80] Ogweno GO. The Effects of Crystalloid Solutions on the Human Blood Coagulation System. Kenyatta University; 2016. dc.identifier.uri. Available from: http://ir-library.ku.ac.ke/handle/123456789/14948

[81] Wilder DM, Reid T, Bakaltcheva IB. Hypertonic resuscitation and blood coagulation: In vitro comparison of several hypertonic solutions for their action on platelets and plasma coagulation. Thrombosis Research. 2002;**107**(5):255-261

[82] Tang WH et al. Glucose and collagen regulate human platelet activity through aldose reductase induction of thromboxane. The Journal of Clinical Investigation. 2011;**121**(11):4462-4476

[83] De La Cruz JP et al. Influence of glucose concentration on the effects of aspirin, ticlopidine and clopidogrel on platelet function and platelet-subendothelium interaction. European Journal of Pharmacology. 2004;**484**(1):19-27

[84] Sudic D, Razmara M, Forslund M, Ji Q, Hjemdahl P, Li N. High glucose levels enhance platelet activation: Involvement of multiple mechanisms. British Journal of Haematology. 2006;**133**(3):315-322

[85] Keating FK, Sobel BE, Schneider DJ. Effects of increased concentrations of glucose on platelet reactivity in healthy subjects and in patients with and without diabetes mellitus. The American Journal of Cardiology. 2003;**92**(11):1362-1365

[86] Jones DB, Davis TME, Bown E, Carter RD, Infirmary R, Unit S. Determinants of ADP-induced platelet aggregation in diabetes mellitus. Diabetologia. 1986;**29**:291-294

[87] Mürer EH, Hellem AJ, Rozenberg MC. Energy metabolism and platelet function. Scandinavian Journal of Clinical and Laboratory Investigation. 1967;**19**(3):280-282

[88] Chaudhry AA, Sagone AL, Metz EN, Balcerzak SP. Relationship of glucose oxidation to aggregation of human platelets. Blood. 1973;**41**(2):249-258

[89] Fidler TP et al. Glucose metabolism is required for platelet hyperactivation in a murine model of type 1 diabetes. Diabetes. 2019;**68**(5):932-938

[90] Whiteheart SW. Fueling platelets: Where does the glucose come from? Arteriosclerosis, Thrombosis, and Vascular Biology. 2017;**37**(9):1592-1594

[91] Heijnen HFG, Oorschot V, Sixma JJ, Slot JW, James DE. Thrombin stimulates glucose transport in human platelets via the translocation of the glucose transporter GLUT-3 from α-granules to the cell surface. The Journal of Cell Biology. 1997;**138**(2):323-330

[92] Ferreira IA, Mocking AIM, Urbanus RT, Varlack S, Wnuk M, Akkerman JWN. Glucose uptake via glucose transporter 3 by human platelets is regulated by protein kinase B. The Journal of Biological Chemistry. 2005;**280**(38):32625-32633

[93] Spectre G, Östenson CG, Li N, Hjemdahl P. Postprandial platelet activation is related to postprandial plasma insulin rather than glucose in patients with type 2 diabetes. Diabetes. 2012;**61**(9):2380-2384

[94] Jarek-Martynowa IR et al. Influence of hyperinsulinemic - hypoglycemic clamp on induced platelet aggregation, activity of physiological anticoagulants and von willebrand factor in patients with type I diabetes. Diabetes Mellitus. 2018;**21**(2):84-91

[95] Bulut T, Demirel F, Metin A. The prevalence of dyslipidemia and associated factors in children and adolescents with type 1 diabetes. Journal of Pediatric Endocrinology & Metabolism. 2017;**30**(2):181-187

[96] Mona HM, Sahar SA, Hend SM, Nanees A-WA. Dyslipidemia in type 1 diabetes mellitus: Relation to diabetes duration, glycemic control, body habitus, dietary intake and other epidemiological risk factors. Egyptian Pediatric Associated Gazette. 2015;**63**(2):63-68

[97] Alrasheed AA. Dyslipidemia among patients with type 1 diabetes and its associated factors in Saudi Arabia: An analytical cross-sectional study. Cureus Journal of Medical Science. 2022;**14**(2):e1923

[98] Ewald U, Kobbah M, Vessby B, Tevemo T. Increased platelet aggregability in diabetic children: Relation to serum lipid and fatty acid composition. Diabetologia. 1983;**25**:382-385

[99] Betteridge DJ, Zahavi J, Jones NAG, Shine B, Kakkar VV, Galton DJ. Platelet function in diabetes mellitus in relationship to complications, glycosylated haemoglobin and serum lipoproteins. European Journal of Clinical Investigation. 1981;**11**(4):273-277

[100] Fuhrman B, Brook JG, Aviram M. Increased platelet aggregation during alimentary hyperlipemia in normal and hypertriglyceridemic subjects. Annals of Nutrition & Metabolism. 1986;**30**(4):250-260

[101] Kobbah AM, Ewald U, Tuvemo T, Hospital A. Platelet aggregability during the first two years of type 1 (insulin-deependent) diabetes mellitus in children. Diabetologia. 1989;**32**:729-735

[102] Hiramatsu K, Nozaki H, Arimori S. Reduction of platelet aggregation induced by euglycaemic insulin clamp. Diabetologia. 1987;**30**(5):310-313

[103] Ferroni P, Basili S, Falco A, Davì G. Platelet activation in type 2 diabetes mellitus. Journal of Thrombosis and Haemostasis. 2004;**2**(8):1282-1291

[104] Roshan B et al. Improved glycemic control and platelet function abnormalities in diabetic patients with microvascular disease. Metabolism. 2000;**49**(1):88-91

[105] Singer J, Weissler Snir A, Leshem-Lev D, Rigler M, Kornowski R, Lev EI. Effect of intensive glycemic control on platelet reactivity in patients with long-standing uncontrolled diabetes. Thrombosis Research. 2014;**134**(1):121-124

[106] Westerbacka J, Turpeinen A, Rissanen A, Vehkavaara S, Lassila R. Inhibition of platelet-collagen interaction. An in vivo action of insulin abolished by insulin resistance in obesity. An in vivo action of insulin abolished by insulin resistance in obesity. Arteriosclerosis, Thrombosis, and Vascular Biology. 2002;**22**:167-172

[107] Ferreira IA, Eybrechts KL, Mocking AIM, Kroner C, Akkerman JWN. IRS-1 mediates inhibition of Ca2+ mobilization by insulin via the inhibitory G-protein Gi. The Journal of Biological Chemistry. 2004;**279**(5):3254-3264

[108] Hwang DL, Yen CF, Nadler JL. Insulin increases intracellular magnesium transport in human platelets. The Journal of Clinical Endocrinology and Metabolism. 1993;**76**(3):549-553

[109] Kahn NN, Bauman WA, Hatcher VB, Sinha AK. Inhibition of platelet aggregation and the stimulation of prostacyclin synthesis by insulin in humans. American Journal of Physiology. 1993;**265**:H2160

[110] Lee YS, Hahm K-S, Lee SY. Effects of calcium channel blockers and insulin on the platelet function in patients with diabetes mellitus. Yonsei Medical Journal. 1993;**27**(2):132

[111] Hutton RA, Mikhailidis D, Dormandy KM, Ginsburg J. Platelet aggregation studies during transient hypoglycaemia. A potential method for evaluating platelet function. Journal of Clinical Pathology. 1979;**32**(5):434-438

[112] Trovati M et al. Studies on mechanisms involved in hypoglycemia-lnduced platelet activation. Diabetes. 1986;**35**:818-825

[113] Kahal H et al. Platelet function following induced hypoglycaemia in type 2 diabetes. Diabetes & Metabolism. 2018;**44**(5):431-436

[114] Anfossi G et al. Insulin exerts opposite effects on platelet function at physiological and supraphysiological concentrations. Thrombosis Research. 1996;**82**(1):57-68

[115] Yngen M, Li N, Hjemdahl P, HWallen NH. Insulin enhances platelet activation in vitro. Thrombosis Research. 2001;**104**:85-91

[116] Hu H, Hjemdahl P, Li N. Effects of insulin on platelet and leukocyte activity in whole blood. Thrombosis Research. 2002;**107**(5):209-215

[117] Murer EH, Gyda MA, Martinez NJ. Insulin increases the aggregation response of human platelets to ADP. Thrombosis Research. 1994;**73**:69-74

[118] Hunter RW, Hers I. Insulin/IGF-1 hybrid receptor expression on human platelets: Consequences for the effect of insulin on platelet function. Journal of Thrombosis and Haemostasis. 2009;**7**(12):2123-2130

[119] Motani AS, Angard EE, Ferns GAA. Recombinant Insulin-like growth factor-1 modulates aggregation in human platelets via extracellular calcium. Life Sciences. 1996;**58**(15):269-274

[120] Hers I. Insulin-like growth factor-1 potentiates platelet activation via the IRS/PI3Kα pathway. Blood. 2007;**110**(13):4243-4252

[121] Stolla MC, Li D, Lu L, Woulfe DS. Enhanced platelet activity and thrombosis in a murine model of type I diabetes are partially insulin-like growth factor 1-dependent and phosphoinositide 3-kinase-dependent. Journal of Thrombosis and Haemostasis. 2013;**11**(5):919-929

[122] Westerbacka J, Turpeinen A, Rissanen A, Vehkavaara S, Lassila R. An in vivo action of insulin abolished by insulin resistance in obesity. Arteriosclerosis, Thrombosis, and Vascular Biology. 2002;**22**:167-172

[123] Gaborit B, FrèRe C, Cuisset T, Alessi MC, Dutour A. Enhanced post-clopidogrel platelet reactivity in diabetic patients is independently related to plasma fibrinogen level but not to

glycemic control. Journal of Thrombosis and Haemostasis. 2009;7(11):1939-1941

[124] Russo I et al. High glucose inhibits the aspirin-induced activation of the nitric oxide/cGMP/cGMP-dependent protein kinase pathway and does not affect the aspirin-induced inhibition of thromboxane synthesis in human platelets. Diabetes. 2012;**61**(11):2913-2921

[125] Sikora J, Kostka B, Marczyk I, Krajewska U, Chałubiński M, Broncel M. Effect of statins on platelet function in patients with hyperlipidemia. Archives of Medical Science. 2013;**9**(4):622-628

[126] De Man FH et al. Activated platelets in patients with severe hypertriglyceridemia: Effects of triglyceride-lowering therapy. Atherosclerosis. 2000;**152**(2):407-414

[127] Bending D, Zaccone P, Cooke A. Inflammation and type one diabetes. International Immunology. 2012;**24**(6):339-346

[128] Triolo G et al. Circulating immune complexes and platelet thromboxane synthesis in patients with insulin-dependent (type I) diabetes mellitus. Diabetes. 1984;**33**(8):728-731

[129] Dominguez C, Ruiz E, Gussinye M, Carrascosa A. Oxidative stress at onset and in early stages of type 1 diabetes in children and adolescents. Diabetes Care. 1998;**21**:1736-1742

[130] Chen J, Stimpson SE, Fernandez-bueno GA, Mathews CE, Al CET. Mitochondrial reactive oxygen species and type 1 diabetes. Antioxidants & Redox Signaling. 2018;**29**(14):1361-1372

[131] Malladi N et al. Understanding the activation of platelets in diabetes and its modulation by allyl methyl sulfide, an active metabolite of garlic. Hindawi. 2021;**2021**:12

[132] Wang Y et al. Advanced glycation end products elicit externalization of phosphatidylserine in a subpopulation of platelets via 5-HT 2A / 2C receptors. American Journal of Physiology. Cell Physiology. 2007;**293**:C328-C336

[133] Winocour PD, Watala C, Perry DW, Kinlough-rathbone RL. Decreased platelet membrane fluidity due to glycation or acetylatîon of membrane proteins. Thrombosis and Haemostasis. 1992;**68**(5):577-582

[134] Gawlowski T et al. Advanced glycation end products strongly activate platelets. European Journal of Nutrition. 2009;**48**(8):475-481

[135] Gawlowski T, Stratmann B, Stirban AO, Negrean M, Tschoepe D. AGEs and methylglyoxal induce apoptosis and expression of Mac-1 on neutrophils resulting in platelet-neutrophil aggregation. Thrombosis Research. 2007;**121**(1):117-126

[136] Ollivier V et al. Collagen can selectively trigger a platelet secretory phenotype via glycoprotein VI. PLoS One. 2007;**9**(8):e104712

[137] Assert R, Scherk G, Bumbure A, Pirags V, Schatz H, Pfeiffer AFH. Regulation of protein kinase C by short term hyperglycaemia in human platelets in vivo and in vitro. Diabetologia. 2001;**44**:188-195

[138] Li Y, Woo V, Bose R. Platelet hyperactivity and abnormal CA2+ homeostasis in diabetes mellitus. American Journaal of Physiology. 2001;**280**(4):1480-1489

[139] Andac B, Bulbul BY, Durak DM. Relationship of magnesium level with glycemic control and lipid profile in adult patients with TYPE 1 diabetes mellitus. Journal of Elementology. 2021;**26**(2):307-317

[140] Van Dijk PR, Waanders F, Qiu J, De Boer HHR, Van Goor H, Bilo HJG. Hypomagnesemia in persons with type 1 diabetes : Associations with clinical parameters and oxidative stress. Therapeutic Advances in Endocrinology and Metabolism. 2020;**11**:1-9

[141] Hwang DL, Yen CF, Nadler JL. Effect of extracellular magnesium on platelet activation and intracellular calcium mobilization. American Journal of Hypertension. 1992;**5**:700-706

[142] Sheu J, Hsiao G, Shen M, Fong T, Chen Y. Mechanisms involved in the antiplatelet activity of magnesium in human platelets. British Journal of Haematology. 2002;**119**:1033-1041

[143] Rabini RA et al. Influence of low density lipoprotein from insulin-dependent diabetic patients on platelet functions. The Journal of Clinical Endocrinology and Metabolism. 1999;**84**(10):3770-3774

[144] Ferretti G et al. Glycated low density lipoproteins modify platelt properties : A compositional and functional study. The Journal of Clinical Endocrinology and Metabolism. 2002;**87**(5):2180-2184

[145] Pedren J, Hurt-camejo E, Wiklund O, Badimo L. Platelet function in patients with familial hypertriglyceridemia: Evidence that platelet reactivity is modulated by apolipoprotein E content of very–low-density lipoprotein particles. Metabolism. 2000;**49**(7):942-949

[146] Akai T, Naka K, Okuda K, Takemura T, Fujii S. Decreased sensistivity of platelets to prostacyclin in patients with diabetes mellitus. Hormone and Metabolic Research. 1983;**15**:523-526

[147] Lumadue JA, Lanzkron SM, Kennedy SD, Kuhl DT, Mt BS, Kickler TS. Cytokine-induced alteration of platelet and hemostatic function. American Journal of Clinical Pathology. 1996;**106**:795-798

[148] Kim SW, Lim YA. Effects of cytokines on platelet activation. Journal of Korean Society. 2002;**1**(13):1-9

[149] Maione F, Cicala C, Liverani E, Mascolo N, Perretti M, D'Acquisto F. IL-17A Increases ADP-induced platelet aggregation. Biochemical and Biophysical Research Communication. 2011;**408**(4):658-662. DOI: 10.1016/j.bbrc.2011.04.080. Epub 2011 Apr 22. PMID: 21530487; PMCID: PMC3182527

[150] Davizon-Castillo P et al. TNF-a–driven inflammation and mitochondrial dysfunction define the platelet hyperreactivity of aging. Blood. 2019;**134**(9):727-740

[151] Guthikonda S et al. Reticulated platelets and uninhibited COX-1 and COX-2 decrease the antiplatelet effects of aspirin. Journal of Thrombosis and Haemostasis. 2007;**5**:490-496

[152] Kakouros N, Rade JJ, Kourliouros A, Resar JR. Platelet function in patients with diabetes mellitus: From a theoretical to a practical perspective. International Journal of Endocrinology. 2007;**2011**:74219

Chapter 8

The Role of Apoptosis in Autoimmune Destruction of Pancreatic b-Cells

Anna Vladimirovna Lugovaya, Vladimir Phylippovich Mitreikin and Natalia Mikhailovna Kalinina

Abstract

The purpose of this section of the monograph is to familiarize readers with the role of programmed cell death type 1—apoptosis in autoimmune destruction of the pancreas in type 1 diabetes mellitus (T1DM-1). The task of focusing the reader's attention on the mechanisms of pancreatic b-cells apoptosis is explained by the fact that the interest of scientists in this problem continues to grow. Sections of the chapter are devoted to the modern concept of T1DM-1 immunopathogenesis, the role of insufficient apoptosis of circulating effector T cells, on the one hand, and enhanced apoptosis of b-cells, on the other hand. Special attention is paid to the prospects for the treatment and prevention of T1DM. The chapter presents the results of experimental studies on the role of apoptosis in the immunopathogenesis of T1DM. Separately, the results of the authors' own studies are considered. The chapter was based on sources from international data bases: Scopus, Springer, PubMed. The authors express the hope that the chapter will contribute not only to a deeper understanding of the pathogenesis of T1DM, but also to arouse interest in the prospects for the treatment and prevention of this disease. The chapter is intended for students of medical universities and a wide range of readers with higher medical and biological education.

Keywords: apoptosis, autoimmune mechanisms of pancreatic destruction, efferocytosis, autoreactive T cells, proinflammatory cytokines, perforin, granzyme, T helpers, cytotoxic T cells, type 1 diabetes mellitus, C-peptide, b-cells

1. Introduction

The authors of this chapter have been dealing with programmed cell death in T1DM for many years. The area of scientific interests is the assessment of apoptosis of peripheral blood lymphocytes in the closest relatives of DM1 patients with a high risk of developing DM1. The risk group for DM1 was included by the first author of this chapter in her thesis on "Apoptosis of peripheral blood mononuclear cells in patients with type 1 diabetes mellitus."

The study of the mechanisms and significance of genetically programmed cell death began in the 1960s. The authorship of the term "apoptosis" belongs to the

English scientists—J. Kerr, E. Wylie and A. Kerry, who first put forward and substantiated the concept of a fundamental difference between physiological cell death (apoptosis) and their pathological death (necrosis). To date, tens of thousands of scientific papers have been devoted to the theory of apoptosis, revealing the main mechanisms of its development at the physiological, genetic, and biochemical levels. There is an active search for its regulators. Of particular interest are studies that allow the practical use of apoptosis regulation in the treatment of oncological, autoimmune, and neurodystrophic diseases.

Apoptosis (from the Greek ἀπόπτωσις—fall), the process of self-destruction or "leaf fall". However, not everything is so clear. Recent studies convincingly show that the processes of apoptosis and regeneration can be strongly interrelated. The removal of non-functioning cells by apoptosis can simultaneously serve as a signal for regenerative processes through the transmission of information through apoptotic bodies. The need for a clear coordination of tissue regeneration processes raises the question of the coordinators of this regulation and the signaling pathways through which different types of cells perform their functions in this process.

And since there is only one step from cell death to regeneration, the authors of the chapter are working hard to unravel the mystery: what molecules and what mechanisms can coordinate these processes? The issues of pancreatic cell regeneration in T1DM are the subject of research that we are currently doing in our laboratory.

2. Modern ideas about the immunopathogenesis of type 1 diabetes mellitus

Type 1 diabetes mellitus (T1DM) is an organ-specific autoimmune disease that develops as a result of the selective destruction of b-cells of the pancreatic islet apparatus by cytotoxic T lymphocytes (CTL), T helper type 1 (Th1) and autoantibodies [1, 2]. Together with interleukin 1b (IL-1b) and tumor necrosis factor α (TNF-α), interferon-g (IFN-g) is able to increase the expression of molecules of the major histocompatibility complex of the second class on pancreatic b-cells. This leads to recognizing them as alien [3, 4]. As a result of the gradual destruction of b-cells, insulin deficiency occurs, leading to a breakdown in glucose homeostasis and the manifestation T1DM. Clinically classic symptoms of T1DM—hyperglycemia and ketosis, appear only when 80–90% of the islets of Langerhans are destroyed [5].

Despite the active study of the immunopathogenesis of T1DM, many key points in the development and progression of this disease remain unclear. The problems of early diagnosis of T1DM, ensuring a stable course of the disease and combating its secondary complications are still relevant [6]. The manifestation of T1DM is preceded by a long asymptomatic period—the prediabetic stage. It should be emphasized that during the asymptomatic stage T1DM there is an active production of autoantibodies to pancreatic b-cells and the formation of inflammatory infiltrates, the so-called "insulitis" [2]. In connection with the trend towards "rejuvenation" of the age of patients with T1DM, leading to early disability, an increase in the incidence rate, clarification of the mechanisms of immunopathogenesis and the development of new methods for the timely diagnosis of T1DM are relevant.

The key point in the initiation of T1DM is the resistance of autoreactive T lymphocytes to apoptosis. Escape of autoreactive cells from immunological surveillance leads to active destruction of b-cells and subsequent manifestation of the disease [7, 8]. It has been established that in mice of the NOD (nonobese diabetic) line, which are a model of spontaneous autoimmune diabetes similar to human T1DM, Th1-cells and cytotoxic T lymphocytes, even when the influence of IL-2, a factor that promotes the proliferation of T lymphocytes, is blocked on them exhibit increased resistance to apoptosis. At the same time, T-helpers are more resistant to apoptosis than cytotoxic T lymphocytes, which disrupts the normal balance of Th1-cells/cytotoxic T cells and contributes to the maintenance of autoimmune Th1-inflammation. Resistance of T lymphocytes of NOD mice to apoptosis is explained by increased expression of the apoptosis inhibitor Bcl-xL protein by T cells [9], as well as disturbances in the Fas/FasL system, which provides the receptor-mediated pathway for apoptosis [10].

Autoreactive lymphocytes resistant to apoptosis migrate from the bloodstream to the target organ—the pancreas and form insulitis, consisting of T and B cells, as well as macrophages, dendritic cells (DC), natural killer cells (NK cells) and natural killer T cells (T-NK cells) [2]. Immunocompetent cells infiltrating the islet tissue produce pro-inflammatory cytokines TNF-α, IFN-g, and IL-1b, nitric oxide, cytotoxic enzymes (perforin and granzyme B), excess free radicals, and other compounds that cause b-cell death by apoptosis [4, 5]. IL-1b alone or in combination with TNF-α and IFN-g enhances Fas-receptor expression on b-cells, which leads to their apoptosis as a result of interaction with autoreactive lymphocytes expressing Fas-ligand [1]. Some authors consider Fas-mediated apoptosis as the leading mechanism of b-cell destruction [11, 12].

In the pathogenesis of T1DM, disturbances in Fas-mediated apoptosis of lymphocytes, which play a major role in maintaining peripheral autotolerance, are important. The Fas/FasL system is involved in the clonal deletion of autoreactive T cells in peripheral lymphatic organs, in the elimination of activated T cells, and thus is central to the regulation of the peripheral immune respons. In the immune system, Fas receptor (FasR) and Fas ligand (FasL) are involved in the regulation of immune responses and in T-lymphocyte-mediated cytotoxicity. FasL is mainly expressed by activated CD4+ and CD8+ T cells [13]. FasR is constitutively expressed by mature T lymphocytes, but its expression is increased after antigen activation, making T cells more susceptible to apoptosis. If there is a defect in the Fas/FasL system, activated lymphocytes can accumulate [14–16]. Thus, if these cells are not eliminated by Fas-mediated apoptosis, the probability of developing an autoimmune disease increases [17].

Thus, from the modern point of view, T1DM is considered as a polygenic, multifactorial disease, in which a genetic predisposition in combination with environmental triggers triggers the activation of specific autoimmune processes leading to the death of b-cells. The leading links in the pathogenesis of autoimmune damage to pancreatic b-cells are immune dysregulation and programmed cell death. Disturbances in the processes of initiation and implementation of apoptosis become fundamental in the development of the disease [18]. Meanwhile, pathogenetic factors and markers of programmed cell death in autoimmune lesions have not yet been sufficiently studied, which is of interest for further research.

3. Role of apoptosis in immune-mediated death of pancreatic b-cells in type 1 diabetes mellitus

3.1 The role of Fas-mediated apoptosis in the pathogenesis of T1DM

It is known that the Fas/FasL system plays a central role in maintaining peripheral autotolerance and tissue homeostasis of the organism [19, 20]. Fas-mediated apoptosis is induced by binding of the Fas(CD95/APO-1/TNFRSF6) receptor to the

Fas(CD95L/CD178/TNFSF6) ligand on the corresponding cells [21]. Triggering the expression of cell surface Fas receptors (Fas) regulates the elimination of autoreactive T- and B-lymphocytes by apoptosis.

Fas-mediated apoptosis is the initiating phase of apoptotic signal transduction and refers to an extrinsic (receptor) pathway for triggering cell death.

Depending on the triggering mechanism of the apoptotic cascade, there are two main signaling pathways leading to the induction of apoptosis in mammalian cells: extrinsic (receptor) and intrinsic (mitochondrial or Bcl-2-regulated) [19, 22]. The extrinsic pathway is mediated by DR (Death Receptor) cell receptors, which include the Fas receptor (Fas). Fas contains the domain DD (Death Domain), the central physiological regulator of apoptosis, in its cytoplasmic part. Binding of Fas to the Fas ligand (FasL) activates the Fas-associated death domain adapter protein FADD (Fas-Associated Death Domain protein), which leads to the formation of the DISC effector complex (Death Initiating Signaling Complex) [23–25]. DISC activates procaspase-8, which undergoes autocatalytic cleavage and transforms into its active form, caspase-8, which initiates apoptosis of the target cell [26, 27].

The Fas (CD95/APO-1/TNFRSF6) receptor is a membrane protein that is a member of the tumor necrosis factor receptor superfamily (TNFRSF-Tumor Necrosis Factor Receptor Super Family) and belongs to the DR (Death Receptor) group of receptors [20]. The latest literature reports that Fas is normally ubiquitously expressed in human tissues at the basal level, and its activation threshold must be strictly regulated to avoid excessive cell death [18, 20]. There is a functionally active soluble form of Fas, which is the result of proteolytic cleavage of membrane-bound receptors or is formed during alternative splicing [28, 29].

Fas/APO-l-ligand (FasL/CD178/TNFSF6) is a membrane protein and is a member of the tumor necrosis factor (TNF) superfamily of ligands, which belong to cytokines [20, 28]. Like the TNF ligand, FasL can be released from the cell surface and be physiologically active in a soluble form [29–31].

Fas-mediated apoptosis ensures the elimination of cells of the immune system that are undesirable for the organism, and is also involved in the regulatory suppression of immune responses and cytotoxicity of T-lymphocytes [20].

According to literature, the role of death receptors in the destruction of b-cells in type 1 diabetes mellitus (T1DM) is widely discussed [1, 5, 20]. Studies using isolated human pancreatic islets have shown that exposure to stress factors (hyperglycemia, excess free radicals, reactive oxygen species, production of IL-1b by microenvironment cells) enhances Fas expression on b-cells, which leads to their death by mechanism of the Fas-mediated apoptosis [17]. Immunocompetent cells infiltrating pancreatic islet tissue produce pro-inflammatory cytokines: IL-1b, TNF-a, and IFN-g, which are known for their pro-apoptogenic properties [20, 32, 33]. IL-1b induces an increase in Fas expression on b-cells, which increases their readiness for Fas-mediated apoptosis, which is realized by autoreactive T cells expressing FasL. Activated cytotoxic T lymphocytes (CD8 + CTL), which are part of the inflammatory infiltrates of the pancreas (insulitis), can also destroy b-cells in a Fas-dependent receptor way [18, 30].

There are conflicting data in the literature on the surface expression of the Fas receptor on peripheral blood T lymphocytes in T1DM. In experimental studies in NOD mice, a decrease in the expression of the proapoptotic Fas antigen on the surface of T lymphocytes was revealed [8, 9]. The results of our own studies revealed a statistically significant increase in Fas receptor expression in certain subpopulations of peripheral blood T lymphocytes in T1DM patients, regardless of the duration and state of disease compensation, compared with the control group [34].

We examined 63 patients with a reliably established diagnosis of T1DM and 15 individuals with a high risk of developing T1DM. The control group (Group I) consisted of 30 healthy individuals, comparable in sex and age to patients with T1DM. The distribution of patients into groups was carried out depending on the phase of compensation and the duration of the course of the disease. Group II (decompensated T1DM) consisted of 17 patients with newly diagnosed T1DM (group IIa) and 19 patients with an average duration of T1DM of 15.3 ± 5.1 years (group IIb). Group III (the state of compensation for T1DM) included 13 patients with a disease duration of up to 1 year (group IIIa) and 14 patients with an average duration of T1DM of 15.1 ± 5.4 years (group IIIb). Group IV consisted of 15 persons with a high risk of developing T1DM, who are immediate family members of the examined patients with T1DM. Additional selection criteria for the risk group were an increased titer (>1/20) of autoantibodies to cytoplasmic antigens of islet cells (Islet Cell Autoantibodies) in serum and impaired glucose tolerance.

Immunophenotyping of peripheral blood mononuclear cells was performed by flow cytometry using the following monoclonal antibodies manufactured by "Immunotech" (Beckman Coulter Corporation, USA): anti-CD3 conjugated with FITC (Fluorescein Isothiocyanate), anti-CD4-FITC, anti-CD8-FITC, anti- CD16-FITC, anti-CD20-FITC, anti-CD25-FITC, anti-HLA-DR-FITC, anti-CD95-FITC and their isotype controls.

To assess apoptotic processes in individual subpopulations of T lymphocytes, the level of surface expression of the Fas receptor was determined using a double fluorescent label—FITC (Fluorescein Isothiocyanate) and PE (Phycoerythrin). The study was performed using the following combinations of antibodies: anti-CD3-FITC/anti-CD95-PE, anti-CD4-FITC/anti-CD95-PE and anti-CD8-FITC/anti-CD95-PE. Cytometric analysis of lymphocytes was performed on an EPICS XL flow cytometer (Beckman Coulter Corporation, USA).

Determination of soluble forms of the Fas receptor (sFas) and Fas ligand (sFasL) in blood serum was carried out by indirect enzyme-linked immunosorbent assay (ELISA) using the "Human sFas Ligand ELISA" test systems (Bender MedSystems, Austria) and "Human Fas ELISA" test systems (BD Biosciences, USA).

The data we obtained are presented in **Table 1**. The maximum increase in the relative and absolute content of T-lymphocytes expressing the Fas receptor was found during decompensation of T1DM, which is explained by the influence of hyperglycemia, a secondary immune response to the so-called "late apoptotic" b-cells due to their inefficient phagocytic clearance and is consistent with the data literature [2]. It has been established that hyperglycemia increases the sensitivity of T cells to Fas-mediated apoptosis due to increased expression of the Fas receptor on their surface, and also induces p53-mediated apoptosis of target cells with the participation of effector caspase-3 [35, 36].

The maximum increase in the relative and absolute amount of CD95+ cells and the number of T-lymphocytes expressing the Fas receptor (Fas) was found in T1DM decompensation, regardless of the duration of the disease (groups IIa and IIb). These data indicate that in T1DM, an increase in the readiness of immunocompetent cells for apoptosis does not depend on the duration of the disease, but is clearly associated with the decompensation of carbohydrate metabolism and the level of glycemia.

Figure 1 shows a comparative assessment of the level of surface expression of the Fas receptor (CD95+) in individual subpopulations of T-lymphocytes in T1DM patients in a state of carbohydrate metabolism decompensation and in the control group.

Groups	CD95+- cells		CD3+CD95+ lymphocytes	CD4+CD95+ lymphocytes	CD8+CD95+ lymphocytes
	The relative amount,%	The absolute amount, mm3	The relative amount, %		
I	4.2	80	3.0	2.3	0.9
Ia	12.4**	260**	10.8**	7.3**	6.0***
IIb	13.2**	222**	11.1**	8.1**	6.7***
IIIa	8.6*	212*	7.3*	5.1*	3.9**
IIIb	8.2*	152*	6.9*	4.8*	3.7**
IV	4.9	90	3.5	3.0	2.1*

*Notes: (1) I—control group (healthy persons); Ia group—the state of decompensation, newly diagnosed T1DM; IIb group—he state of decompensation, the average duration of the T1DM is 15.3 ± 5.1 years; IIIa group—the state of compensation, the average duration of the T1DM is 0.6 ± 0.2 years; IIIb group—the state of compensation, the average duration of the T1DM is 15.1 ± 5.4 years; IV group—persons with a high risk of developing T1DM. (2) *Differences in the studied indicator with the control group (I) are statistically significant (p < 0.05); (2) **differences in the studied indicator with the control group (I) are statistically significant (p < 0.01); (3) *** differences in the studied indicator with the control group (I) are statistically significant (p < 0,001).*

Table 1.
The relative and absolute amount of CD95+-cells and T-lymphocytes expressing the Fas receptor in the peripheral blood of patients with T1DM and persons with a high risk of developing T1DM.

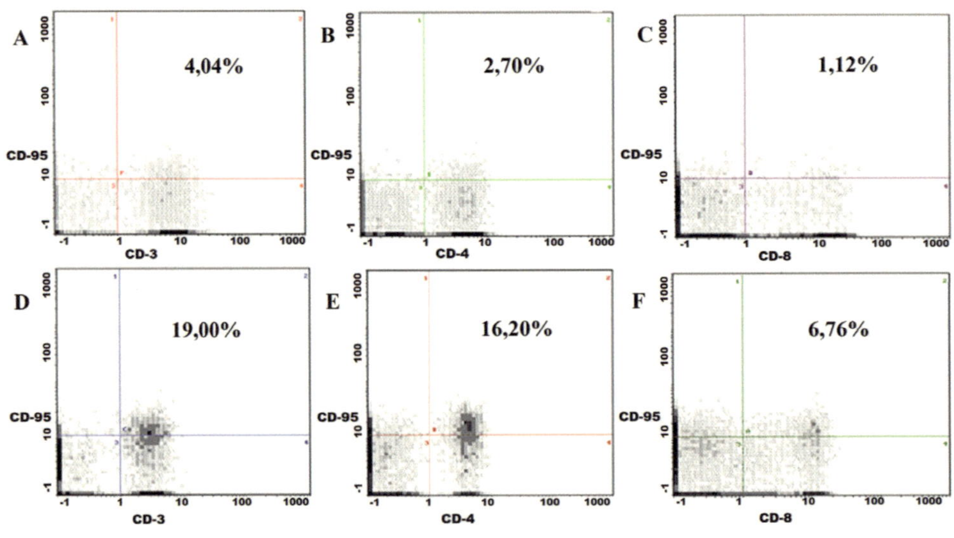

Figure 1.
The histogram shows the number of CD3+CD95+-, CD4+CD95+- and CD8+CD95+ -lymphocytes in the control group (A–C) and in the group of T1DM patients in the state of carbohydrate metabolism decompensation (D–F).

Among the subpopulations of T-lymphocytes, a significant increase in the percentage of CD8+CD95+-cells from the total amount of cytotoxic T-lymphocytes (CD8+CTLs) in all groups of examined patients should be noted compared to the control group (**Figure 2**). The increase in the relative amount of Fas-expressing CD8+CTLs is most pronounced with disease decompensation (groups IIa and IIb). An increase in the number of cells with the CD8+CD95+ phenotype in T1DM is probably

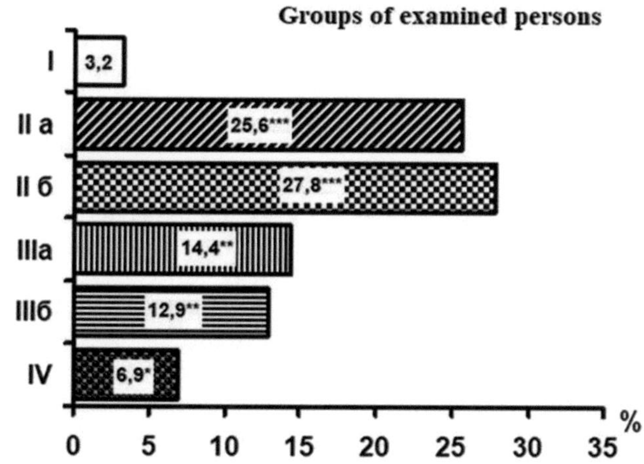

Figure 2.
*Percentage of CD8+CD95+ cells from the total number of cytotoxic T-lymphocytes. Notes: (1) *Differences in the studied indicator with the control group (I) are statistically significant ($p < 0.05$); (2) **differences in the studied indicator with the control group (I) are statistically significant ($p < 0.01$); (3) *** differences in the studied indicator with the control group (I) are statistically significant ($p < 0.001$).*

a compensatory mechanism aimed at the elimination of autoreactive cytotoxic T-lymphocytes by apoptosis. According to the literature, it is the effector CD8+CTLs that play the dominant role in the destruction of pancreatic β-cells [2, 20].

At the same time, a significant increase in the number of cells with the CD8+CD95+ phenotype in the blood of individuals with a high risk of developing T1DM (group IV) compared with the control group (group I) is an unfavorable prognostic factor. These data indicate that already in the latent stage of T1DM there is an expansion of autoreactive clones of cytotoxic T-lymphocytes in peripheral blood, followed by their migration to the target organ (pancreas), which leads to the progression of the autoimmune process.

In addition to assessing the surface expression of the Fas receptor and Fas ligand, it is necessary to consider the pathogenetic significance of soluble forms of Fas and FasL in the development of autoimmunity in T1DM, since the diagnostic and prognostic significance of these indicators of Fas-mediated apoptosis is actively studied in systemic and organ-specific autoimmune diseases, in sepsis, acute renal failure, oncological diseases [29, 32, 37]. A comprehensive assessment of the effectiveness of Fas-mediated apoptosis with the determination of all biomarkers (surface and soluble) involved in this variant of the receptor pathway for triggering the apoptotic program can provide a more accurate understanding of the mechanisms and significance of Fas/FasL system dysregulation in the pathogenesis of T1DM.

We found that the content of soluble forms of Fas (sFas – soluble Fas) and FasL (sFasL – soluble FasL) in the blood serum of T1DM patients did not depend on the duration of the disease, but changed depending on the state of carbohydrate metabolism compensation. In patients with T1DM in the phase of decompensation of the disease, a significant increase in the content of sFas was observed compared with the control group and other examined groups of patients (patients in the phase of T1DM compensation, persons with a high risk of developing T1DM) [34]. Our results are consistent with literature data on the relationship between an increase in the concentration of sFas in the serum of patients and worsening of the course of the disease. It has been reported that a high level of serum sFas correlates with the severity of the septic process [28]. It has been shown that the content of sFas in the blood increased with increasing renal dysfunction in patients with acute kidney injury [29, 31].

According to the literature data, the soluble form of Fas competes with the membrane Fas receptor for the binding of the Fas ligand, which prevents the "physiological" apoptosis of the cells to be eliminated. With an increase in the sFas content in the circulation, not all "defective" cells can implement their apoptotic program. As a result, they accumulate in the peripheral blood, which leads to an aggravation of the pathological process.

We also studied the content of the soluble form of Fas-ligand in the serum of T1DM patients and those at risk for developing T1DM.

The content of sFasL with compensation for T1DM was significantly higher than in the decompensation group and significantly lower than in the risk group (**Table 2**). It should be noted a significant increase in the content of sFasL in the risk group, which is consistent with the literature data. According to the authors, an increase in sFasL in the latent stage of T1DM has a protective value and is aimed at eliminating autoaggressive lymphocyte clones by Fas-mediated apoptosis [8].

Thus, our results indicate a pronounced dysregulation in the Fas/FasL system, which is observed at all stages of the development of T1DM.

Disturbances in the functioning of the Fas receptor (Fas) and Fas ligand (FasL), as key inducers of receptor-dependent apoptosis, are actively studied in the pathogenesis of diseases associated with both inhibition and enhancement of apoptosis in cells of shock organs [30]. It has recently been found that Fas-mediated caspase-8 activation plays an important role in the regulation of pathogenic mechanisms in bacterial infections [26]. It has been shown that an increase in the soluble form of FasL in the blood is one of the early markers of heart failure progression [29].

In the pathogenesis of T1DM, disturbances in Fas-mediated apoptosis are of a bivalent nature. So, if in relation to b-cells the development of apoptosis is associated with the progression of the disease, then from the point of view of the elimination of activated autoreactive lymphocytes, apoptosis is desirable and can slow down the destruction of pancreatic b-cells. The dual role of the receptor (external) pathway for triggering apoptosis in the pathogenesis of T1DM is due to the expression of its mediating molecules (Fas and FasL) by both effector cells (autoreactive T cells) and target cells (pancreatic b-cells) [20].

Indicator	Control group (n = 28)	Patients with T1DM		Persons with a high risk of developing T1DM (n = 15)
		The state of decompensation (n = 26)	The state of compensation (n = 24)	
	I	II	III	IV
sFas (ng/ml)	778	1501*	789	864
sFasL (pg/ml)	0.102	0.118	0.243*	0.403**

*Notes: (1) n—the number of examined persons; (2) *differences in the studied indicator with the control group (I) are statistically significant (p < 0.05); (2) **differences in the studied indicator with the control group (I) are statistically significant (p < 0.01).*

Table 2.
The concentration of the soluble form of the Fas receptor and Fas ligand in the blood serum of patients with T1DM and in persons with a high risk of developing T1DM.

Efficient elimination of autoreactive T lymphocytes from the peripheral blood requires maintaining a balance between cells expressing Fas and FasL. It is important to consider the possible role of the soluble Fas receptor (sFas) in the inhibition of apoptosis via the Fas pathway [30].

Our results on an increase in serum sFas in the state of decompensation of T1DM are consistent with the results of a number of authors who reported an increase in the content of the soluble form of Fas in some systemic and organ-specific autoimmune diseases [31, 37].

The concentration of sFasL in the T1DM compensation group was significantly higher than in the decompensation group and significantly lower than in the risk group (**Table 2**). It should be noted a significant increase in the level of sFasL in the risk group, which is consistent with the literature data [8].

Several experimental studies have shown that both membrane and soluble forms of the Fas ligand (sFasL) are involved in the removal of autoreactive human cells [20, 21]. According to the literature, in an experimental study, preliminary cultivation of diabetogenic T lymphocyte clones with sFasL completely inhibited the development of autoimmune diabetes in mice, which were then transplanted with diabetogenic T cells [20]. This means that the increase in sFasL in T1DM has a protective value and is aimed at establishing peripheral tolerance, which is necessary for protection against autoimmune aggression against b-cells. An increase in sFasL was reported in individuals at high risk of developing T1DM against the background of a decrease in the number of autoreactive CD4+CD95+- and CD8+CD95+-lymphocytes in the blood, in connection with which the authors suggest the involvement of sFasL in the removal of pathogenic T cells at the preclinical stage of the disease [8]. According to the literature, an increase in the soluble form of the Fas ligand (sFasL) is a compensatory mechanism aimed at the elimination of activated autoreactive peripheral blood lymphocytes and plays a protective role.

3.2 Apoptosis in the regulation of immune mechanisms involved in the pathogenesis of T1DM

Both humoral and cellular immunity factors are involved in the development of T1DM. Islet cell autoantigens are recognized by autoantibodies and autoreactive effector T lymphocytes resistant to apoptosis, which are involved in the destruction of b-cells through the release of a triad of pro-inflammatory cytokines TNF-α, IL-1b, IFN-g, cytotoxic enzymes (perforin, granzyme B) and other compounds, including free radicals [7]. Experimental studies on mice of the NOD (nonobese diabetic) line on the creation of autoimmune diabetes, close to human T1DM, showed that the central role in the pathogenesis of this disease belongs to autoreactive T-lymphocytes, specific for pancreatic islet b-cells [1, 5].

Autoreactive clones of T cells that react with the islets of Langerhans have been described both in animals and in humans [5, 7]. From the peripheral blood of children with newly diagnosed T1DM, a clone of T-lymphocytes (CD4Th1 + cells) was isolated, which recognizes glutamate decarboxylase, an epitope of the B-chain of the insulin molecule, and other autoantigens of the islets of Langerhans. It has been shown that by transplanting autoreactive T lymphocytes of a sick animal, it is possible to induce T1DM in a healthy syngeneic animal. Strong evidence for the involvement of T cells in the immunopathogenic mechanisms of T1DM is that monoclonal antibodies to the

CD3 antigen can interrupt early T1DM in NOD mice and restore their tolerance to b-cell autoantigens [38, 39]. Most often, diabetogenic clones of T-lymphocytes consist of CD4+ cells, but there are clones formed by CD8+ cells. Some authors believe that CD8+-lymphocytes without the presence of CD4+ cells are not able to lead to the destruction of b-cells [38–40].

In recent years, the cellular mechanisms of death of b-cells of the islets of Langerhans are considered leading [5, 7]. The direct effect of immunocompetent cells on target cells (including b-cells), leading to the destruction of the latter, is referred to as cellular cytotoxicity. Two main pathways for the realization of cellular cytotoxicity have been described, involving perforin- and Fas-dependent mechanisms. It has recently been established that in some cases such destruction is accompanied by the development of apoptosis [1, 7]. A specific feature of the development of apoptosis in this case is the primary damage to the membrane of target cells, which is atypical for this process, with the penetration of granzyme proteins into them. It is believed that it is the latter that include the mechanism of programmed cell death [7]. If CD8+CTLs realize their cytotoxicity by activating both mechanisms, then natural killer cells use exclusively the perforin-dependent pathway, while CD4+ lymphocytes activate Fas-dependent mechanisms and are restricted by the major histocompatibility complex of the second class [1, 2]. Here it is necessary to mention the role of cytokines in the immune-mediated destruction of b-cells. Together with IL-1 and TNF-a, IFN-g is able to increase the expression of molecules of the major histocompatibility complex of the second class on the cells of the pancreatic islets. This leads to recognizing them as alien. The death of pancreatic islet cells occurs as a result of apoptosis, direct cytotoxic action of TNF-a and cytotoxic T lymphocytes (CD8+CTL), as well as by antibody-dependent cytotoxicity [6]. According to a number of researchers [41, 42], the initial step in the development of T1DM is the presentation by macrophages or dendritic cells of specific autoantigens of b-cells to T helpers, which is carried out in association with molecules of the major histocompatibility complex of the second class.

In accordance with modern concepts, type 1 diabetes mellitus is considered as an autoimmune insulitis, in the pathogenesis of which, in addition to autoantibodies, the role of cellular immunity reactions is undeniable [2]. Autoreactive lymphocytes migrate from the bloodstream to the target organ (pancreas) and penetrate into the islets of Langerhans, forming inflammatory infiltrates—insulitis. This is evidenced by the results of histological studies that reveal lymphocytic infiltration of pancreatic islets, formed mainly by CD8+ and CD4+ T cells [1, 5, 7].

Activated macrophages secrete IL-12, which stimulates CD4+ cells that secrete IFN-g and IL-2. IFN-g activates "resting" macrophages, which in turn produce IL-1b and TN-Fa, which is accompanied by a sharp rise in the level of free radicals in b-cells [7]. IL-2 causes the migration of peripheral CD8+ lymphocytes to the islets of Langerhans, probably due to the induction of the expression of specific homing receptors. Naive cytotoxic T cells that carry specific receptors for b-cell autoantigens differentiate into effector cytotoxic CD8+ lymphocytes after recognizing a specific b-cell peptide associated with molecules of the major histocompatibility complex of the first class, which occurs in the presence of CD4+ lymphocytes. Then CD8+ lymphocytes start the process of destruction of b-cells due to the secretion of perforin and granzyme B. CD4+ lymphocytes expressing the Fas-ligand destroy b-cells by the mechanism of Fas-mediated apoptosis, as well as indirectly—due to the secretion of cytokines IFN-g and TNF-a. In this way, macrophages, CD4+ and CD8+ cells are thought to act synergistically to destroy b-cells, leading to the onset of autoimmune diabetes [41, 42].

3.3 Apoptosis as the final mechanism of immune-mediated destruction of pancreatic b-cells

The most important stage in the pathogenesis of T1DM is the dysregulation of apoptosis processes associated with the preservation of autoreactive clones of lymphocytes that are tropic for b-cells and are able to "escape" from apoptosis [11].

To date, most studies in the field of studying the role of apoptosis of immune-mediated destruction of pancreatic b-cells in T1DM have been performed on experimental models of type 1 diabetes mellitus in vivo and in vitro. However, it should be emphasized that the induction and regulation of apoptosis in animal models of T1DM may differ significantly in T1DM in humans [2]. In particular, nicotinamide, which effectively protects rat b-cells from apoptosis [43], can protect human b-cells from necrosis caused by free radicals, but not from cytokine-induced apoptosis [44]. Data obtained in experiments in vitro show that the sensitivity of human b-cells is definitely lower than that of animal b-cells [45, 46], which must be considered when approximating the results from model systems to the human body.

The detection of apoptosis in vivo and the study of its role in the destruction of b-cells in T1DM encounters significant methodological difficulties. However, in some models of T1DM in experimental animals, it is possible to detect apoptosis in pancreatic b-cells and show a correlation between the degree of insulitis and apoptosis of b-cells. In particular, it has been shown that apoptosis is the predominant mechanism of b-cell death in NOD mice [11].

3.3.1 Signal proteins involved in the implementation of apoptosis of pancreatic b-cells

When apoptosis is induced by cytokines produced by T-helpers and macrophages, the death of b-cells can be mediated by signaling systems associated with ceramides or with mitogen-activated protein kinases (MAPK). The combination of the cytokines TNF-a, IL-1b, and IFN-γ has been shown to induce beta cell death in vitro [5]. Cell death is induced by activation of the transcription factors JNK (c-Jun N-terminal kinase), NF-κB (nuclear factor kappa-light-chain-enhancer of activated B cells), and STAT-1 (Signal Transducers and Activators of Transcription), which induce iNOS transcription. and subsequent production of the free radical NO. Inactivation of the JNK pathway makes b-cells less susceptible to IL-1-mediated death through a NO-independent process [47, 48]. Other components of the MAPK signaling pathway, p38 and ERK1/2 (extracellular signal-regulated kinase1/2), also play a possible role in cytokine-induced b-cell death [49, 50].

3.3.2 Bcl-2 family members in b-cell apoptosis

In addition to the signaling proteins listed above, members of the Bcl-2 family play a significant role in the regulation of b-cell apoptosis in humans. The Bcl-2 family is known to include both the anti-apoptotic Bcl-2 and Bcl-xL proteins and the pro-apoptotic Bax, Bim, Bik, and Bak proteins. These proteins are regulators of the mitochondrial apoptosis triggering pathway [51], which plays an important role in b-cell death in T1DM [5, 52]. The Bax/Bcl-2 ratio regulates the balance between the processes of induction and inhibition of apoptosis [34, 53]. It has been established that overexpression of antiapoptotic proteins of the Bcl-2 family protects b-cells from apoptosis in T1DM [53–55]. Bcl-2 inhibits apoptosis by blocking the transport of cytochrome C protein from mitochondria, which plays an important role in the realization of the death signal.

It is believed that therapeutic methods aimed at enhancing the expression of anti-apoptotic members of the Bcl-2 family can protect b-cells from apoptosis and reduce the area and degree of damage in T1DM. To date, convincing results in this area have been obtained only in experimental models using NOD mice [56]. Nevertheless, research into the therapeutic potential of Bcl-2 is ongoing.

3.3.3 The role of nitric oxide and inducible NO-synthase in the destruction of b-cells

The study of the biological significance of nitric oxide (NO) was a significant breakthrough in understanding the mechanisms of destruction of pancreatic b-cells. Nitric oxide is a relatively unstable free radical with a half-life of several seconds [57]. Takamura et al. found that in b-cells of transgenic mice that develop type 1 diabetes mellitus, an increased expression of induced NO synthase is determined, which confirms the role of excessive nitric oxide formation and the development of T1DM in these animals without signs of insulitis [46]. Nitric oxide produced by activated macrophages functions as a specific effector molecule, but can also be involved in the destruction of b-cells [5]. Corbett and Daniel showed that the expression of inducible NO-synthase in macrophages and the formation of nitric oxide by them practically does not affect the function of the pancreatic islets. At the same time, the expression of inducible NO synthase directly in b-cells and the formation of NO here completely inhibit insulin secretion [58]. Thus, the main damaging value is attached to nitric oxide, which is formed directly in the b-cell. Eizirik and Mandrup-Poulsen showed that b-cells of human pancreatic islets are more resistant to the damaging action of various alkylating compounds (alloxan, streptozotocin), cytokines, oxygen free radicals and nitric oxide compared to rat pancreatic islets [59]. Induction of NO synthase in human pancreatic islets is observed several days after simultaneous exposure to IL-1b, TNF-a and IFN-g. Darville and Eizirik showed that in human pancreatic islets the expression of induced NO synthase occurs with the obligatory participation of IL-1b and IFN-g [60]. The transcription factors c-fos (protooncogene), JNK, and the nuclear factor NF-kB are involved in the regulation of induced NO-synthase mRNA expression. In vitro experiments have shown that the expression of NO synthase, which is activated by cytokines and various endotoxins, is inhibited by dexamethasone and insulin, which may be important in the prevention of type 1 diabetes [57].

The synthesis of nitric oxide in b-cells induced by pro-inflammatory cytokines can lead to their death by apoptosis, which is preceded by the appearance of many biological signs of the apoptotic process, including internucleosomal DNA fragmentation [11].

3.3.4 Role of pro-inflammatory cytokines in apoptosis-mediated b-cell death

It should be emphasized that TNF-α is a pleiotropic cytokine that plays a key role in many physiological and pathological cellular processes, including the role of an inducer of activation apoptosis of target cells [61]. It was believed that TNF-α could directly destroy b-cells, since it contains a death domain in its receptor. However, experimental studies using b-cell culture have shown that this is not the case. It turned out that in the presence of TNF-α, NF-kB (Nuclear Factor of κ-chain B-lymphocytes) which is known for its antiapoptotic properties, is activated [56, 62]. This is supported by in vivo experimental studies using NOD mice indicating that inhibition of NF-kB in b-cells increases their susceptibility to TNF-α-mediated apoptosis [62, 63].

Recent studies show that the priority of the latest therapeutic developments in the field of type 1 diabetes is the suppression of inflammation in the target organ. Resolvin D1 has been shown to reduce the severity of streptozotocin-induced T1DM by reducing oxidative stress and suppressing inflammation. The action of the drug is largely aimed at suppressing the production of pro-inflammatory cytokines TNF-α and IL-6. As a result of the action of Resolvin D1 in the peripheral blood of experimental animals, a statistically significant decrease in the concentration of TNF-α and IL-6 was recorded compared to the initial values ($p < 0.001$) [5]. In another study, the use of immunomodulatory therapy in individuals with a high risk of developing type 1 diabetes contributed to the suppression of the production of TNF-α and IFN-g, in combination with an increase in the concentration of C-peptide compared to pre-treatment levels. Teplizumab treatment improved b-cell function, as evidenced by a quantitative and qualitative improvement in insulin secretion [64]. Thus, monitoring of the cytokine profile and timely therapy aimed at suppressing anti-inflammatory cytokines is of critical importance in the pre-diabetic stage. New approaches to preventing the progression of clinical T1DM. to irreversible destruction of b-cells and insulin deficiency are a promising direction in modern diabetology.

IL-1b, produced by macrophages, also plays a significant role in the destruction of b-cells. It has been established that after stimulation of pancreatic b-cells in vitro with IL-1b, the expression of Fas receptors increases on their surface, as a result of which b-cells become targets for T-lymphocytes carrying FasL [1]. Expression of Fas receptors by b-cells has been confirmed not only by in vitro studies, but also in vivo in experiments using laboratory animals [1, 6]. Thus, IL-1b is involved in the destruction of b-cells by stimulating the expression of the Fas receptor on the membranes of b-cells. In b-cells after their interaction with IL-1b, characteristic signs of apoptosis are revealed: DNA fragmentation, nuclear condensation and the formation of apoptotic bodies [65].

IFN-g usually acts in combination with other pro-inflammatory cytokines, such as TNF-a or IL-1b, and sometimes both. IFN-g stimulates the production of IL-1b APC [66]. When IFN-g and TNF-a bind to cognate receptors on b-cells, either caspase-dependent b-cell apoptosis is triggered or b-cell apoptotic death is activated by inducible NO synthase (iNOS) [62]. The triad of pro-inflammatory cytokines TNF-a, IFN-g, and IL-1b is detrimental to b-cells, since it promotes the triggering of various mechanisms of apoptotic death of the islets of Langerhans. Maintaining high concentrations of all three cytokines in the microenvironment of b-cells enhances their apoptotic death [67].

Thus, many signaling proteins are involved in the apoptotic death of b-cells in T1DM, each of which can become a potential therapeutic target in the development of new methods of therapy for this disease.

A general scheme of the mechanisms of apoptotic death of b-cells in T1DM is shown in **Figure 3**.

The B-cell antigen is captured by antigen-presenting cells (APCs). Antigen processing results in the formation of antigenic fragments that form a complex with MHC II. The antigen-MHC II complex is recognized by T cell receptors (TCRs). T-cell activation occurs due to antigen recognition and co-stimulation by secondary signals of co-stimulatory molecules—CD28-B7. An activated cytotoxic T lymphocyte (CD8+CTL) produces IFN-g, which subsequently stimulates APC to produce additional cytokines IL-1b and TNF-a. In addition, CD8+CTL produces proteins: granzyme B and perforin.

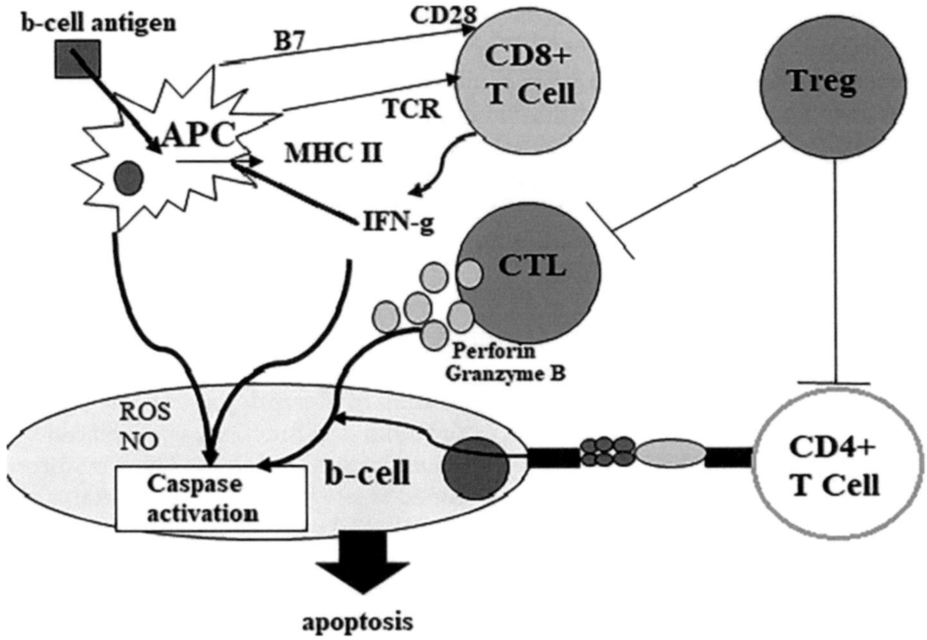

Figure 3.
The main mechanisms of pancreatic b-cells apoptosis in T1DM.

IL-1b increases expression of the Fas receptor on b-cells, which increases their sensitivity to Fas-mediated apoptosis mediated by CD8+ and CD4+ T cells. Conversely, regulatory T cells (T-regs) suppress CD8+ and CD4+ T cells [1].

4. Perspectives for the treatment and prevention of T1DM

It is clear from the above data that the process of apoptosis as the central mechanism of b-cell death in T1DM deserves further study. The field of research into the process of apoptosis is one of the most promising areas in cell biology. In the future, therapeutic intervention could be implemented at the level of immune cells and/or target cells.

The accumulation of knowledge about b-cell apoptosis is likely to progress rapidly in the near future. If apoptosis is the general mechanism by which b-cells die in T1DM in response to immune attacks by cytokines and/or T lymphocytes (cellular cytotoxicity), then new strategies may be developed to prevent the process of b-cell death, and hence the manifestation of the disease itself.

It has been established that protection against apoptosis can be implemented at four different levels: (1) “interception” of stimuli that induce apoptosis; (2) functional antagonism of apoptosis triggers; (3) intervention in the signal cascade; (4) blockade of catabolic enzymes involved in cell self-destruction. The study of all levels of intervention can serve as the basis for the development of a new strategy to prevent the death of b-cells [2, 7].

Treatment aimed at suppressing the initiation of the apoptosis process is promising. For example, some methods may include blockade of death ligand binding (TNF, FasL). In addition, the goals of therapy may be aimed at increasing resistance to apoptotic stimuli by increasing the expression of anti-apoptotic members of the bcl-2 family.

Insulin may have a potential positive effect in preventing disease at the preclinical stage, due to its potential immunomodulatory effect and its ability to induce b-cell "rest" [5].

Considering the numerous mechanisms by which apoptosis affects individual stages of the pathogenesis of T1DM, it is advisable to consider possible ways of its modulation in order to influence certain targets of the pathological process for therapeutic purposes.

5. Conclusion

Over the past 10 years, a real breakthrough has been made in immunology, both in the field of basic research and in clinical medicine. The rapid development of immunotherapy, the discovery and introduction into practice of new biomarkers, the improvement of immunological methods of laboratory diagnostics indicate that we live in an era of "every second" innovations. Using the example of T1DM, which is an autoimmune disease, we are seeing new advances in therapy and a significant improvement in the quality of life of patients. It should be emphasized that we owe all these achievements to experimental medicine, which is the first rung of the ladder leading to the success of clinical medicine.

The authors express the hope that this chapter will help readers to better understand the molecular mechanisms of T1DM immunopathogenesis, as well as to appreciate the significance of experimental studies in science and practical medicine. Perhaps the material presented in this section will inspire someone to their own scientific research.

Acknowledgements

Authors are grateful to Ivanov Andrei Mikhailovich, Head of the Department of Clinical Biochemistry and Laboratory Diagnostics of the S.M. Kirov Military Medical Academy for providing a base for research. We would also like to express our gratitude to the entire staff of the Department.

Conflict of interest

Authors declare no conflict of interest.

Author details

Anna Vladimirovna Lugovaya[1*], Vladimir Phylippovich Mitreikin[2] and Natalia Mikhailovna Kalinina[3,4]

1 First Pavlov State Medical University of Saint Petersburg, Russian Federation

2 Department of Pathological Physiology, First Pavlov State Medical University of Saint Petersburg, Russian Federation

3 Department of Immunology, First Pavlov State Medical University of Saint Petersburg, Russian Federation

4 Nikiforov Russian Center of Emergency and Radiation Medicine, Saint Petersburg, Russian Federation

*Address all correspondence to: g89213159748@gmail.com

References

[1] Ryan A, Murphy M, Godson C, et al. Diabetes mellitus and apoptosis: Inflammatory cells. Apoptosis. 2009;**14**:1435-1450. DOI: 10.1007/s10495-009-0340-z

[2] Vives-Pi M, Rodríguez-Fernández S, Pujol-Autonell I. How apoptotic β-cells direct immune response to tolerance or to autoimmune diabetes: A review. Apoptosis. 2015;**20**:263-272. DOI: 10.1007/s10495-015-1090-8

[3] Brozzi F, Nardelli TR, Lopes M, et al. Cytokines induce endoplasmic reticulum stress in human, rat and mouse beta cells via different mechanisms. Diabetologia. 2015;**58**:2307-2316. DOI: 10.1007/s00125-015-3669-6

[4] Bathina S, Das UN. Resolvin D1 decreases severity of streptozotocin-induced type 1 diabetes mellitus by enhancing BDNF levels, reducing oxidative stress, and suppressing inflammation. International Journal of Molecular Sciences. 2021;**22**:1-14. DOI: 10.3390/ijms22041516

[5] Thomas HE, McKenzie MD, Angstetra E, Campbell PD, Kay TW. Beta cell apoptosis in diabetes. Apoptosis. 2009;**14**:1389-1404. DOI: 10.1007/s10495-009-0339-5

[6] Fu D, Yu JY, Yang S, Wu M, Hammad SM, Connel AR, et al. Survival or death: A dual role for autophagy in stress-induce pericyte loss in diabetic retinopathy. Diabetologia. 2016;**59**:2251-2261. DOI: 10.1007/s00125-016-4058-5

[7] Thomas HE, Trapani JA, Kay TWH. The role of perforin and granzymes in diabetes. Cell Death and Differentiation. 2010;**17**:577-585. DOI: 10.1038/cdd.2009.165

[8] Tchorzewski H, Glowacka M, Banasik P, Lewkowicz M, Szalapska-Zawodniak M. Activated T lymphocytes from patients with high risk of type I diabetes mellitus have different ability to produce interferon-g, interleukin-6 and interleukin-10 and undergo anti-CD95 induced apoptosis after insulin stimulation. Immunology Letters. 2001;**75**:225-234

[9] Lamhamedi-Cherradi SE, Luan JJ, Eloy L, et al. Resistance of T-cells to apoptosis in autoimmune diabetes NOD mice is increased early in life and is associated with dysregulation of Bcl-xL. Diabetologia. 1998;**41**:178-184. DOI: 10.1007/s001250050887

[10] Walczak H, Krammer PH. The CD95 (APO-1/Fas) and the TRAIL (APO-2L) apoptosis system. Experimental Cell Research. 2000;**256**:58-66. DOI: 10.1006/excr.2000.4840

[11] Mauricio D, Mandrup-Poulsen T. Apoptosis and the pathogenesis of IDDM: A question of life and death. Diabetes. 1998;**47**:1537-1543. DOI: 10.2337/diabetes.47.10.1537

[12] Giordano C, Stassi G, Todaro M, et al. Low bcl-2 expression and increased spontaneous apoptosis in T-lymphocytes from newly-diagnosed IDDM patients. Diabetologia. 1995;**38**:953-958. DOI: 10.1007/BF00400585

[13] Nagata S. Apoptosis by death factor. Cell. 1997;**88**:355-365. DOI: 10.1016/s0092-8674(00)81874-7

[14] Cohen JJ, Duke RC, Fadok VA, et al. Apoptosis: Physiologic cell death. Journal of Clinical and Laboratory Medicine. 1994;**124**:761-765

[15] Cnop M, Welsh N, Jonas JC, et al. Mechanisms of pancreatic beta-cell death in type 1 and type 2 diabetes: Many differences, few similarities. Diabetes. 2005;**54**:97-107. DOI: 10.2337/diabetes.54.suppl_2.S97

[16] Eguchi K. Apoptosis in autoimmune diseases. Internal Medicine. 2001;**40**:275-284. DOI: 10.1007/s001250050887

[17] Takahashi T, Tanaka M, Brannan CI, et al. Generalized lymphoproliferative disease in mice, caused by a point mutation in the Fas ligand. Cell. 1994;**76**:969-976. DOI: 10.1016/0092-8674(94)90375-1

[18] De Franco S, Chiocchetti A, Ferretti M, et al. Defective function of the Fas apoptotic pathway in type 1 diabetes mellitus correlates with age at onset. International Journal of Immunopathology and Pharmacology. 2007;**20**:567-576. DOI: 10.1177/039463200702000314

[19] Esposti MD, Matarrese P, Tinari A, et al. Changes in membrane lipids drive increased endocytosis following Fas ligation. Apoptosis. 2017;**22**:681-695. DOI: 10.1007/s10495-017-1362-6

[20] Joglekar MV, Trivedi PM, Kay TW, et al. Human islet cells are killed by BID-independent mechanisms in response to FAS ligand. Apoptosis. 2016;**21**:379-389. DOI: doi.org/10.1007/s10495-016-1212-y

[21] Rossin A, Lounnas N, Jérôme DJ, et al. The Btk-dependent PIP5K1γ lipid kinase activation by Fas counteracts FasL-induced cell death. Apoptosis. 2017;**22**:1344-1352. DOI: 10.1007/s10495-017-1415-x

[22] Green DR. Cell death and the immune system: Getting to how and why. Immunological Reviews. 2017;**277**(1):4-8. DOI: 10.1111/imr.12553

[23] Garg AD, Romano E, Rufo N, Agostinis P. Immunogenic versus tolerogenic phagocytosis during anticancer therapy mechanisms and clinical translation. Cell Death and Differentiation. 2016;**23**:938-951. DOI: 10.1038/cdd.2016.5

[24] Green DR, Oguin TH, Martinez J. The clearance of dying cells: Table for two. Cell Death and Differentiation. 2016;**23**:915-926. DOI: 10.1038/cdd.2015.172

[25] Sachet M, Liang YY, Oehler R. The immune response to secondary necrotic cells. Apoptosis. 2017;**22**:1189-1204. DOI: 10.1007/s10495-017-1413-z

[26] Milisav I, Poljšak B, Ribarič S. Reduced risk of apoptosis: Mechanisms of stress responses. Apoptosis. 2017;**22**:265-283. DOI: 10.1007/s10495-016-1317-3

[27] Shukla V, Shakya AK, Perez-Pinzon MA, et al. Cerebral ischemic damage in diabetes: An inflammatory perspective. Journal of Neuroinflammation. 2017;**14**(21):1-22. DOI: 10.1186/s12974-016-0774-5

[28] Uchiyama R, Tsutsui H. Caspases as the key effectors of inflammatory responses against bacterial infection. Archivum Immunologiae et Therapiae Experimentalis. 2015;**63**:1-13. DOI: 10.1007/s00005-014-0301-2

[29] Bhatraju PK, Robinson-Cohen C, Mikacenic C, et al. Circulating levels of soluble Fas (sCD95) are associated with risk for development of a nonresolving acute kidney injury subphenotype. Critical Care. 2017;**21**(217):1-9. DOI: 10.1186/s13054-017-1807-x

[30] Khaitov RM. Immunology: Textbook. Moscow: GEOTAR-Media; 2018. p. 496 (In Russian)

[31] Liphaus BL, Kiss MHB, Carrasco S, et al. Increased serum sFas, sTRAIL, and reduced sFasL in juvenile-onset systemic lupus erythematosus. Clinical Rheumatology. 2017;**36**:2847-2852. DOI: 10.1007/s10067-017-3615-8

[32] Rieux-Laucat F, Magérus-Chatinet A, Neven B. The autoimmune lymphoproliferative syndrome with defective FAS or FAS-ligand functions. Journal of Clinical Immunology. 2018;**38**:558-568. DOI: 10.1007/s10875-018-0523-x

[33] Liang L, Ge K, Zhang F, et al. The suppressive effect of co-inhibiting PD-1 and CTLA-4 expression on H22 hepatomas in mice. Cellular & Molecular Biology Letters. 2018;**23**:58. DOI: 10.1186/s11658-018-0122-0

[34] Lugovaya AV, Kalinina NM, Mitreikin VP, Emanuel YV, Kovaltchuk YP, Artyomova AV, et al. Evaluation of efficiency of Fas-mediated apoptosis of peripheral blood lymphocytes in patients with type 1 diabetes mellitus. Medical Alphabet. Series «Modern Laboratory». 2019;**3**:26-31. DOI: 10.33667/2078-5631-2019-3-22(397)-26-32

[35] Baidwan S, Chekuri A, Hynds DL, Kowluru A. Glucotoxicity promotes aberrant activation and mislocalization of Ras-related C3 botulinum toxin substrate 1 [Rac1] and metabolic dysfunction in pancreatic islet β-cells: Reversal of such metabolic defects by metformin. Apoptosis. 2017;**22**:1380-1393. DOI: 10.1007/s10495-017-1409-8

[36] Sidarala V, Kowluru A. Exposure to chronic hyperglycemic conditions results in Ras-related C3 botulinum toxin substrate 1 (Rac1)-mediated activation of p53 and ATM kinase in pancreatic β-cells. Apoptosis. 2017;**22**:597-607. DOI: 10.1007/s10495-017-1354-6

[37] Nabipour I, Kalantarhormozi M, Assadi M, et al. Influence of levothyroxine treatment on serum levels of soluble Fas (CD95) and Fas ligand (CD95L) in chronic autoimmune hypothyroidism. Endocrine. 2010;**2010**(38):406-411. DOI: 10.1007/s12020-010-9401-x

[38] Schloot NC, Willemen S, Duinkerken G, et al. Cloned T-cells from a resent onset IDDM patient reactive with insulin B-chain. Journal of Autoimmunity. 1998;**2**:169-175. DOI: 10.1006/jaut.1997.0183

[39] Chatenoud L. Restoration of self-tolerance is feasible approach to control ongoing beta-cell specific autoreactivity: Its relevance for triatment in established diabetes and islet transplantation. Diabetologia. 2001;**44**:521-536. DOI: 10.1007/s001250051658

[40] Gearson CL, Hussain MJ, Vergani D, Peakman M. Lymphocyte vaccination protects prediabetic non-obese diabetic mice from developing diabetes mellitus. Diabetologia. 1997;**40**:1388-1395. DOI: 10.1007/s001250050840

[41] Yoon JW, Jun HS, Santamaria P. Cellular and molecular mechanisms for the initiation and progression of beta cell destruction resulting from the collaboration between macrophages and T cells. Autoimmunity. 1998;**27**:109-122. DOI: 10.3109/08916939809008041

[42] Yoon JW, Jun HS. Cellular and molecular roles of beta cell autoantigens, macrophages and T cells in the pathogenesis of autoimmune diabetes. Archives of Pharmacal Research. 1999;**22**:437-447. DOI: 10.1007/BF02979150

[43] Mandrup-Poulsen T. The role of interleukin-l in the pathogenesis of IDDM. Diabetologia. 1996;**39**:1005-1029. DOI: 10.1007/BF00400649

[44] Horens A, Pipeleers D. Nicotinamide protects human beta cells against chemically-induced necrosis, but not against cytokine-induced apoptosis. Diabetologia. 1999;**42**:55-59. DOI: 10.1007/s001250051113

[45] Signore A, Pozzilli P, Gale EAM, Andreani D, Beverly PCL. The natural history of lymphocyte subsets infiltrating the pancreas of NOD mice. Diabetologia. 1989;**32**:282-289. DOI: 10.1007/BF00265543

[46] Takamura T, Kato I, Kimura M, et al. Transgenic mice overexpressing type 2 nitric-oxide synthase in pancreatic b-cells develop insulin-dependent diabetes without insulitis. The Journal of Biological Chemistry. 1998;**273**:2493-2496. DOI: 10.1074/jbc.273.5.2493

[47] Ammendrup A, Maillard A, Nielsen K, et al. The c-Jun amino-terminal kinase pathway is preferentially activated by interleukin-1 and controls apoptosis in differentiating pancreatic beta-cells. Diabetes. 2000;**49**:1468-1476. DOI: 10.2337/diabetes.49.9.1468

[48] Bonny C, Oberson A, Negri S, et al. Cell-permeable peptide inhibitors of JNK: Novel blockers of beta-cell death. Diabetes. 2001;**50**:77-82. DOI: 10.2337/diabetes.50.1.77

[49] Chong MM, Thomas HE, Kay TW. Suppressor of cytokine signaling-1 regulates the sensitivity of pancreatic beta cells to tumor necrosis factor. The Journal of Biological Chemistry. 2002;**277**:27945-27952. DOI: 10.1074/jbc.M110214200

[50] Saldeen J, Lee JC, Welsh N. Role of p38 mitogen-activated protein kinase (p38 MAPK) in cytokine-induced rat islet cell apoptosis. Biochemical Pharmacology. 2001;**61**:1561-1569. DOI: 10.1016/S0006-2952(01)00605-0

[51] Li X, Shang B, Li Y, et al. IFNγ and TNFα synergistically induce apoptosis of mesenchymal stem/stromal cells via the induction of nitric oxide. Stem Cell Research & Therapy. 2019;**10**:18. DOI: 10.1186/s13287-018-1102-z

[52] Muhammad AR, Zaib Un N, Muhammad SA, et al. Assessment of metals induced histopathological and gene expression changes in different organs of non-diabetic and diabetic rats. Scientific Reports. 2020;**10**:1-11. DOI: 10.1038/s41598-020-62807-0

[53] Hyeon JY, Min JS, Dae WK, et al. Tat-CIAPIN1 protein prevents against cytokine-induced cytotoxicity in pancreatic RINm5F β-cells. BMB Reports. 2021;**54**(9):458-463. DOI: 10.5483/BMBRep.2021.54.9.040

[54] Yuan Z, Jie Y, Fan P, et al. Insulin and liraglutide attenuate brain pathology in diabetic mice by enhancing the Wnt/β-catenin signaling pathway. Experimental and Therapeutic Medicine. 2022;**24**(1):439. DOI: 10.3892/etm.2022.11366

[55] Bingzheng D, Zhenduo S, Yang D, et al. Quercetin ameliorates oxidative stress-induced cell apoptosis of seminal vesicles via activating Nrf2 in type 1 diabetic rats. Biomedicine & Pharmacotherapy. 2022;**151**:113108. DOI: 10.1016/j.biopha.2022.113108

[56] Kim S, Millet I, Kim HS, et al. NF-kappa B prevents beta cell death and autoimmune diabetes in NOD mice. Proceedings of the National Academy of Sciences of the United States of America. 2007;**104**:1913-1918. DOI: 10.1073/pnas.0610690104

[57] Bedard S, Marcotte B, Marette A. Insulin inhibits inducible nitric oxide synthase in skeletal muscle cells. Diabetologia. 1998;**41**:1523-1527. DOI: 10.1007/s001250051100

[58] Corbett JA, Daniel ML. Intraislet release of interleukine-1 inhibits beta-cell function by inducing beta-cell expression of inducible nitric oxide synthase. Journal of Experimental Medicine. 1995;**181**:559-568. DOI: 10.1084/jem.181.2.559

[59] Eizirik DL, Mandrup-Poulsen T. A choice of death—The signal-transduction of immune-mediated beta-cell apoptosis. Diabetologia. 2001;**44**:2115-2133. DOI: 10.1007/s001250100021

[60] Darville ML, Eizirik DL. Regulation by cytokines of the inducible nitric oxide synthase promoter in insulin-producing cells. Diabetologia. 1998;**41**:1101-1108. DOI: 10.1007/s001250051036

[61] Green EA, Eynon EE, Flavell RA. Local expression of TNF alpha in neonatal NOD mice promotes diabetes by enhancing presentation of islet antigens. Immunity. 1998;**9**:733-743. DOI: 10.1016/S1074-7613(00)80670-6

[62] Thomas HE, Angstetra E, Fernandes RV, et al. Perturbations in nuclear factor-kappaB or c-Jun N-terminal kinase pathways in pancreatic beta cells confer susceptibility to cytokine-induced cell death. Immunology and Cell Biology. 2006;**84**:20-27. DOI: 10.1111/j.1440-1711.2005.01397.x

[63] Eldor R, Yeffet A, Baum K, et al. Conditional and specific NF-kappaB blockade protects pancreatic beta cells from diabetogenic agents. Proceedings of the National Academy of Sciences of the United States of America. 2006;**103**:5072-5077. DOI: 10.1073/pnas.0508166103

[64] Emily KS, Brian NB, Kenneth S, et al. Teplizumab improves and stabilizes beta cell function in antibody-positive high-risk individuals. Science Translational Medicine. 2021;**13**(583):eabc8980. DOI: 10.1126/scitranslmed.abc8980

[65] Benoist C, Mathis D, Wilson AJ. Cell death mediators in autoimmune diabetes. No shortage of suspects. Cell. 1997;**89**:1-3. DOI: 10.1016/s0092-8674(00)80174-9

[66] Papaccio G, Graziano A, D'Aquino R, Valiante S, Naro F. A biphasic role of nuclear transcription factor (NF)-kappaB in the islet beta-cell apoptosis induced by interleukin (IL)-1beta. Journal of Cellular Physiology. 2005;**204**:124-130. DOI: 10.1002/jcp.20276

[67] McKenzie MD, Dudek NL, Mariana L, et al. Perforin and Fas induced by IFNgamma and TNFalpha mediate beta cell death by OT-I CTL. International Immunology. 2006;**18**:837-846. DOI: 10.1093/intimm/dxl020

Chapter 9

The Role of the Receptor for Advanced Glycation Endproducts (RAGE) in Type 1 Diabetes: An Immune Cell Perspective

Irina Buckle and Josephine M. Forbes

Abstract

Type 1 diabetes (T1DM) is an autoimmune disorder resulting in destruction of the insulin producing pancreatic β-cells that reside in the Islets of Langerhans. Despite significant progress in the understanding of T1DM pathogenesis, some fundamental contributing mechanisms remain to be fully elucidated. The receptor for advanced glycation end products (RAGE) and its ligands are increasingly believed to play a role in the development of T1DM, but this is not well understood. The location of RAGE gene is shared with major T1DM genetic susceptibility loci on chromosome 6 and polymorphism of this region confers risk for T1DM. Furthermore, changes in RAGE expression on and ligand binding by immune cells, in particular T cells, are associated with pro-inflammatory and autoimmune profiles key for T1DM development. Indeed, in murine models for T1DM, targeting of RAGE or its ligands decreased onset and severity of disease including favorable immune cell profiles and infiltration and improved beta cell insulin secretory function. Further understanding of RAGE expression and signaling in immune cells in T1DM will provide valuable insights into disease pathogenesis and therapy development. This chapter will discuss what is currently known about RAGE in the immune cells integral for the pathogenesis of T1DM.

Keywords: type 1 diabetes, RAGE, RAGE ligands, advanced glycation Endproducts, T cells, APCs, NK cells, neutrophils

1. Introduction

Type 1 diabetes (T1DM) is a complex autoimmune disorder resulting from the destruction of pancreatic insulin producing β-cells due to the loss of self-tolerance. There has been a rapid increase in disease incidence worldwide and T1DM is increasingly being diagnosed in even younger individuals and in those from diverse cultural backgrounds. Insulin replacement therapy remains the only viable option for individuals with T1DM. Ensuring any new therapies are meeting a very high safety bar and are superior to insulin replacement therapy remains a challenge. Indeed, treatment with global immunosuppression, while somewhat effective, has significant side

IntechOpen

effects and is not a practical solution to prevent T1DM which commonly develops in early life. Also, despite insulin's excellent safety profile, management of insulin replacement therapy involves multiple daily injections, pumps and continuous blood glucose monitoring or closed loop systems which are costly and complex to maintain, particularly in younger children. These therapies also bring increased risk for life-threatening high (hyperglycemia) or low (hypoglycemia) blood glucose concentrations as well as increased risk for chronic complications and shortened lifespan. Despite significant progress made in the development of therapeutics for T1DM and some remarkable results in the pre-clinical models, a successful translation into clinic is yet to occur. Due to the T1DM's multifactorial nature, the necessity to find links between genetic predisposition, immune system abnormalities and environmental triggers is becoming increasingly apparent. Therefore, exploring relationships between these contributing factors is necessary for better understanding of the disease progression and for design of the best therapeutic approaches. More recently, multiple studies have focused on the complex biology and involvement of the receptor for advanced glycation end products (RAGE) and its ligands in inflammation, autoimmunity, diabetes complications, apoptosis, and endoplasmic reticulum stress including the exploration of various ways to alleviate these. This presents an exciting new avenue for the development of targeted RAGE-related therapeutics and their translational potential from pre-clinical models to humans.

2. Preclinical murine models of T1DM

The non-obese diabetic (NOD) mouse model has been a useful tool to examine pathological mechanisms which contribute to and may be targeted in T1DM. Although there are several fundamental differences between murine and human disease [1, 2], the late timing of human disease manifestation, pancreas inaccessibility and lack of biomarkers in the peripheral blood continue to pose a significant challenge. Therefore, NOD mouse models remain instrumental in studying the disease pathophysiology and aids efforts to improve clinical translational potential of identified pathways and a first-line screening for effective therapies. Humanized mouse models, which are mice with a "human-like" immune system have proven to be an excellent platform to bridge the gap between preclinical mouse models and clinical studies by enabling researchers to assess the efficacy of treatments on human immune cells in a more physiological context than provided by cell culture [3]. In the T1DM field several excellent preclinical experimental approaches have also been proposed [4–6], although spontaneous T1DM disease development and sufficient similarity to human disease are still challenges.

3. RAGE in T1DM

RAGE is a member of the immunoglobulin superfamily It is postulated to play a role in host-pathogen defense and its expression increases during inflammation and in chronic inflammatory conditions including T1DM. The location of the RAGE gene (*AGER*) in humans is within the major histocompatibility complex on chromosome 6p21.3, a region implicated in various autoimmune disorders such as T1DM [7–9]. Similarly in mice, the *AGER* gene is located on chromosome 17 where several quantitative trait loci for T1DM have been reported [10]. RAGE is a multifunctional and promiscuous-ligand receptor, binding a wide array of ligands such as such as

DOI: http://dx.doi.org/10.5772/intechopen.108528

advanced glycation endproducts (AGEs), high mobility group box-1 (HMGB1), S100 proteins, β-amyloid fibrils, and others [11]. Upon binding to its ligands, the cytoplasmic domain associates with adaptor proteins including TIRAP and MyD88 followed by activation of downstream signaling of various pathways including NF-κB and STAT3 (**Figure 1**) [12].

Advanced Glycation Endproducts (AGEs) are canonical RAGE ligands but are low affinity and likely only bind RAGE when increased in concentration [13]. AGEs are formed as the result of non-enzymatic modifications to amino groups on lipids, proteins, peptides, and nucleic acids. Modern industrialization of food, flavor, and color enhancement as well as increased emulsification contribute significantly to formation of AGEs [9, 14, 15]. Prolonged exposure to AGEs has detrimental effects on β-cell function, insulin secretion and sensitivity and disease development in healthy humans and rodents [16]. Moreover, accumulation of AGEs and RAGE is associated with macro and micro vascular complications in diabetic patients [14, 17–19]. In the islet autoantibody positive individuals, the levels of circulating AGEs served as independent predictor for T1DM progression [20]. Chronic exposure of rodents to AGEs led to defects in insulin secretion and beta- cell death as well as defects in mitochondrial function supported by studies in isolated islets and beta cell lines such as MIN6N8. Following the treatment with AGE-lowering agent, the incidence of autoimmune diabetes was reduced in NOD mice [21].

HMGB1 is a non-histone chromosome protein present in all cells and may serve as a transcription factor in proinflammatory conditions [22]. Both RAGE and toll-like receptor 4 (TLR4) have been reported to serve as HMGB1 receptors, although SPR binding studies suggest that HMGB1 only binds to RAGE if associated with DNA fragments. Therapeutic potential of HMGB1 blockade has been shown in NOD mice, reducing T1DM incidence and autoimmunity [23, 24]. In newly diagnosed children

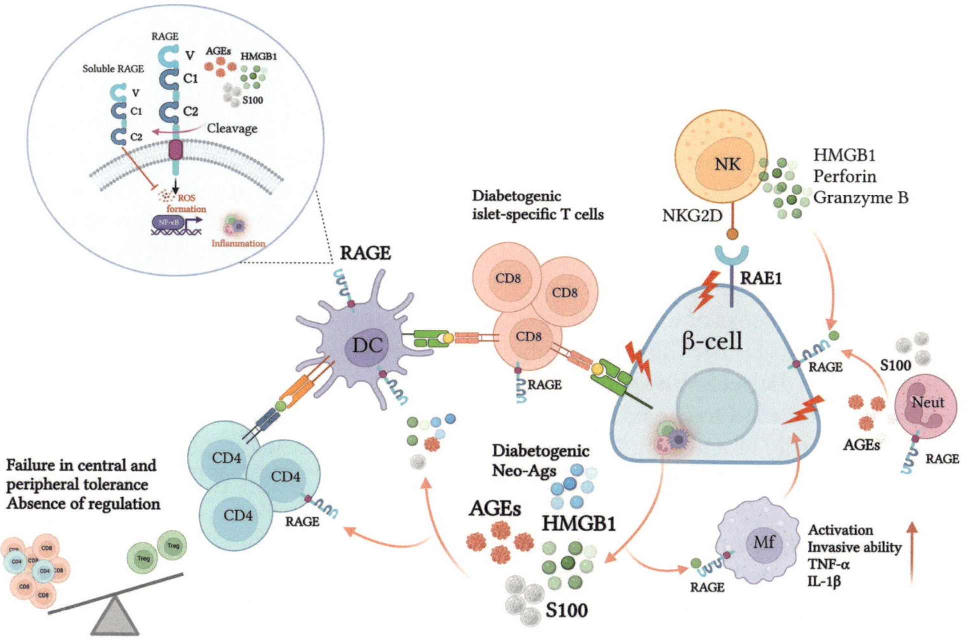

Figure 1.
RAGE cellular expression in immune cells important in T1DM development.

with T1DM, HMGB1 serum concentrations were significantly higher compared to controls suggesting its potential use as an inflammatory biomarker in the disease progression [25]. More recently, it was proposed that increases in HMGB1 impairs the stability of regulatory T cells (Tregs) in NOD mice and increases production of interferon-γ (IFN-γ). In individuals with T1DM increased levels of serum HMGB1 were directly correlated with increases in IFN-γ production by Tregs. Neutralizing HMGB1 antibody rescued Treg function and suppressed autoimmunity [23]. Furthermore, hyperglycemia may contribute to the release of HMGB1 by antigen presenting, natural killer and endothelial cells as well as necrotic and apoptotic cells leading to augmented autoimmunity [26].

Another set of proteins identified as RAGE ligands is S100 calgranulin family containing over 20 members with S100A8/9 and S100B binding RAGE [27]. Although their major site of manufacture is believed to be endothelial cells, they are known to be expressed by myeloid cells such as neutrophils, but expression by lymphocytes has not been reported. This proinflammatory heterodimer is implicated in several conditions including inflammatory bowel disease and rheumatoid arthritis. Furthermore, S100A8/A9 expression is associated with tumorigenesis, suppression of DC function and accumulation of myeloid-derived suppressor cells (MDSCs) [28].

RAGE can exist as both transmembrane protein and a truncated soluble form (sRAGE). The latter is present in serum and is postulated to act as a decoy receptor by competitively binding RAGE ligands and preventing downstream signaling [11, 12]. RAGE expression tends to be low in most tissues except for the skin and alveolar epithelial cells in the lung [29]. RAGE is expressed on a number of immune cells such as T lymphocytes, neutrophils, antigen presenting cells (APCs) including macrophages, dendritic cells (DCs) and B cells as well as endothelial cells [30]. The precise role of RAGE in these cell populations as well its ability to influence cell-cell interactions and behavior still eludes us. However, RAGE continues to serve as one of the major players in inflammatory and autoimmune conditions creating a perfect opportunity to investigate these links.

3.1 RAGE and T cells

Immune tolerance involves a diverse range of processes that prevent potentially harmful immune responses against self-antigens. Given that T1DM is a T cell mediated autoimmune disease, a key event in its development is the failure in the mechanisms of central tolerance, which allows for self-reactive T lymphocytes to escape deletion by the immune system. Once in the periphery, these effector T lymphocytes can exert deleterious effects with $CD4^+$ T lymphocytes believed to be important initiators and progressors of autoimmunity. Upon encounter of islet-antigen presented by dendritic cells (DCs), $CD4^+$ T lymphocytes become activated which promotes and perpetuates the diabetogenic process. The reasons as to why islet autoantigens are specifically presented to the immune system by DCs to amplify immune responses remains to be fully elucidated. Migration of DCs to pancreatic lymph nodes and islet-antigen presentation there amplifies recruitment and activation of $CD4^+$ and $CD8^+$ T lymphocytes.

An extensive pancreatic β- cell loss or loss of function is hallmark of T1DM. It is now well appreciated that autoreactive T cell are amongst key players in this process. $CD4^+$ T cells are thought to be initiators of the disease providing help for B cells in "auto"antibody production as well as enhancing effector activity of $CD8^+$ T cells and islet-resident macrophages. $CD8^+$ effector T cells are considered to cause pancreatic islet destruction and commonly dominate islet infiltrates [31–33].

Tregs are crucial for the maintenance of the peripheral tolerance where they dampen the effects of any self-reactive cells which have escaped deletion by central tolerance. In T1DM, there is impairment in function of and/or the numbers of Tregs present. This imbalance contributes to greater pathogenic activity of effector T lymphocytes and leads to a loss of peripheral tolerance. Peripheral tolerance is the local backstop to prevent self-antigen production and delete T cells with antigen specificity for self-antigens. Thymic derived Tregs (tTregs) defined as $CD4^+CD25^+Foxp3^+$ Tregs are responsible for suppression of effector T lymphocytes through secretion of anti-inflammatory cytokines and competition for IL-2. Both function and frequencies of this subset of Tregs is impaired in both humans and NOD mice [34]. Therefore, restoring their functionality and numbers appears to be an attractive option for preventing T1DM development and is certainly widely under investigation. Currently, there are a number of T cell-centered therapeutic approaches for treatment and prevention of T1DM under development. These include Treg enhancement and antigen-specific strategies, as well as strategies that dampen activation of T cells using CTLA-4-Ig (Abatacept) or anti-CD3 monoclonal antibody (Teplizumab) (reviewed here [35]). The latter has produced promising results in at risk antibody positive individuals significantly improving β-cell function [36, 37]. If this therapy progresses to clinic in the near future, it will make an excellent candidate for combination therapies.

RAGE expression is elevated on T cells from "at-risk" islet autoantibody positive (IAb+) individuals and is associated with progression to T1DM and increased effector function of T cells [38, 39]. The soluble isoform of RAGE (sRAGE) can competitively bind RAGE ligands and inhibit RAGE signaling. Previous studies have shown that RAGE gene (AGER) polymorphisms result in reduced sRAGE in the circulation which correlates with increased risk of T1DM and seroconversion to islet autoantibodies [9, 40]. Murine studies have demonstrated a role for RAGE in T cell activation, priming and effector function, where RAGE-deficient T cells showed reduced proliferation and production of pro-inflammatory cytokines such as IFN-γ [41]. RAGE also plays a role in DC maturation, migration, and function as well as T cell priming. In children with acute Kawasaki disease and juvenile idiopathic arthritis, RAGE facilitates recruitment and activation of leukocytes and sRAGE is reduced [42].

Another study explored the effects of dietary AGEs in NOD mice. Here, a T cell receptor (TCR) transgenic NOD 8.3 males with $CD8^+$ T cells specific for $IGRP_{206-214}$, one of the main diabetogenic antigens [43], and NOD/ShiLt females and their NOD8.3 female offspring were fed low or high AGEs containing diets from conception to weaning of the offspring. The low AGEs diet resulted in improvements in insulin, proinsulin, and glucagon secretion by the islets as well as reduction in AGEs and RAGE expression in offspring islets. Furthermore, reduced level of immune cell infiltration was seen in the infants whose parents were fed with low AGEs diet in the perinatal period [16]. This is consistent with another previous intergenerational study of low AGE feeding where decreasing rates of T1DM were seen in subsequent generations during feeding with a low AGE diet [44]. In the NOD model RAGE antagonism using sRAGE, significantly decreases progression to overt diabetes onset in NOD mice and preserves β-cell mass and insulin secretory function and that sRAGE therapy did not work following specific depletion of Tregs. This was evidenced through reduced islet infiltration, preservation of islet integrity and numbers as well as insulin expression. Moreover, an increased proportion of Tregs in pancreata, pancreatic lymph nodes and spleens of treated animals was demonstrated. sRAGE-induced improvements in human Tregs proliferative and suppressive ability *ex vivo* [45], whilst exposure to RAGE ligands, AGEs impairs Treg suppressive capacity [45]. These observations suggest that RAGE inhibition may offer protection against future T1DM development [46].

3.2 RAGE and NK cells

Natural Killer (NK) cells are cytotoxic innate lymphocytes that bridge innate and adaptive immune systems. NK cells' importance is firmly cemented in the field of cancer immunology due to their unique ability to recognize and destroy tumors and virus infected cells. Their killing capacity is driven by the activating and inhibitory receptor-ligand interactions as well as cytolytic granules containing perforin and Granzyme B similar to the $CD8^+$ T cells. Some important lectin-like activating receptors include NKG2D and KLRG1 whilst inhibitory include NKG2A and KIRs in humans and Ly49 in mice [47]. Unsurprisingly, NK cells are coming into focus in the context of T1DM as an important effector population for the disease pathogenesis. Their interaction with and ability to suppress other effector cells such as CD8+ T cells is of vital importance, particularly in the setting of autoimmunity [48].

During early human studies it was shown that proportion of NK cells was significantly lower in the peripheral blood of individuals with T1DM compared to controls. This was further linked to reduced lytic and cytotoxic capacity of NK cells and more frequent occurrence of tumors [49–51]. The dysregulation in NKG2D signaling as well as reduction in NK cell proportion was suggested to be a contributing factor to the development of T1DM [52].

HMGB1 a known RAGE ligand plays an important role in NK cell killing ability upon activation. HMGB1 released from NK cells' cytotoxic granules is very effective against oxygen-dependent cancer cells whilst those cells with anaerobic energy metabolism were resistant to HMGB1 mediated killing [53]. These observations are of importance with respect to pancreatic inflammation and associated pathologies. Narumi et al. proposed an NK cell-RAGE dependent suppression mechanism of S100A8/A9 expressing tumors It was proposed that NK cells express RAGE but not TLR4 which is also known to bind S100 family of proteins [54]. The ligation of S100A8/A9 to RAGE led to activation of NK cells, increasing their cytotoxic ability evidenced by elevated IFN-γ production, increased NKG2D activating receptor activity and amelioration of tumor growth. RAGE blockade reversed these effects, highlighting the importance of RAGE-S100 axis for suppression of tumor growth and NK cell cytotoxic ability [55]. Whilst there is as yet no direct evidence linking T1DM, NK cells and RAGE, the clear involvement of RAGE axis and NK cells in T1DM and other autoimmune and proinflammatory disorders warrants future investigation.

3.3 RAGE and neutrophils

Neutrophils are phagocytic leukocytes of innate immune system circulating in the blood in a dormant state. Their activation is initiated in the early stages of inflammation and mechanisms for pathogen clearance include release of cytotoxic granules, cytokines, and reactive oxygen species (ROS). Neutrophils possess a unique ability to form neutrophil extracellular traps (NET) when undergoing altered cell death which have unique antimicrobial properties. Moreover, neutrophils can engage with and modulate activity of other immune cells such as T and B lymphocytes, NK cells and DCs. This can lead to exacerbation of autoimmune disorders such as systemic lupus erythematosus (SLE), multiple sclerosis and autoimmune diabetes [56–58].

In NOD mice activated neutrophils are recruited to the pancreatic islets initiating development of autoimmune diabetes and facilitating recruitment of $CD8^+$ T cells and DCs. Studies in NOD mice shown that migration of neutrophils plays pivotal role in disease progression and preventing it halts or reverses disease development [56, 59]. Similarly, neutrophil infiltrates were found in human pancreata prior to T1DM onset and in individuals with overt disease where there was an evidence of NET formation highlighting pathogenicity of the infiltrating neutrophils. Furthermore, neutrophils from the peripheral blood of autoantibody negative at-risk individuals, displayed a unique molecular signature with overexpression of interferon-related genes [60]. These data reinforce the importance of neutrophils in the initiation and progression of T1DM.

It was previously demonstrated that RAGE expression on human neutrophils and binding to AGEs was associated with impaired neutrophil function, in particular bacterial killing [61]. In the murine streptozotocin induced T1DM model the RAGE ligand S100 calcium-binding proteins A8/A9 (S100A8/A9) are released by neutrophils binding to RAGE on hepatic Kupffer cells leading to increase of IL-6 thrombopoietin production associated with atheroprogression in humans [62]. Albeit limited, these data support the importance of RAGE axis in effector immune populations which may be important for the development of T1DM.

3.4 RAGE and antigen presenting cells

Professional antigen presenting cells (APCs) include dendritic cells (DCs), macrophages and B cells. These cell populations have been extensively studied in T1D due to their tolerogenic and immunogenic properties and importance in therapy development [63].

DCs are categorized into conventional (cDCs), plasmacytoid (pDCs), monocyte-derived (moDCs) and Langerhans cells (LCs). They are important regulators of immune tolerance, can select specific T cell subsets for anergy or deletion and therefore play pivotal roles in the pathogenesis of T1DM. Their immunomodulatory abilities have been widely explored and are targets for various therapeutic strategies in development including antigen specific immunotherapy [64]. Within the pancreata of NOD mice, DCs and macrophages can be detected as early as 3 weeks of age [65, 66]. Interestingly, studies of chronic high AGE feeding of healthy rats also show the appearance of an islet specific infiltrate that is comprised primarily of macrophages [21]. Other studies suggested that plasmacytoid DCs (pDCs) are recruited to the pancreata of NOD mice where they promote diabetogenic T cell activity and initiate T1DM [56]. Many other studies highlighted the importance of DC function in disease initiation and progression (reviewed here [67, 68]). Their maturation status dictates the level and type of response exerted. The immature or tolerogenic DCs usually exhibit low levels of MHC class II and costimulatory molecules expression such as CD80 and CD86, reduced ability to stimulate T cells and produce proinflammatory cytokines, however their phagocytic and antigen processing and presentation capacity is not affected [68]. Several strategies explored immunomodulatory potential of tolerogenic DCs and maintaining them in their immature state for treatment and prevention of autoimmune disorders including T1DM (reviewed in [64, 68, 69]. DCs will continue to be in the T1DM therapy development spotlight due to their proven ability to induce T cell anergy or deletion while promoting and increasing regulatory T and B cell populations.

The exposure of immature DCs from human PBMCs to a high glucose environment and AGEs results in the upregulation of costimulatory markers, increases production of reactive oxygen species (ROS) and proinflammatory cytokines such as IL-12 and IL-6, decrease in regulatory cytokines such IL-10 and enhances expression of AGEs scavenger receptors SR-A and CD36 and RAGE [70, 71]. In another study by Ge et al., AGE-BSA treatment increased DC expression of both SR-A and RAGE but pre-treatment of DCs with RAGE neutralizing antibody halted maturation by impairing upregulation of costimulatory markers and expression of IL-12 [72]. Another study described the effects of AGEs-stimulation in the presence of the antioxidant resveratrol in immature DCs derived from healthy donor PBMCs. Pre-treatment of DCs with resveratrol prior to AGE exposure prevented their maturation, MAPK and NK-κB activation and production of inflammatory cytokines and reduced RAGE expression [73]. This once more highlights that delineating the AGE-RAGE axis in inflammatory or aging processes may have future benefit in understanding T1DM pathogenesis.

Failure of peripheral and central tolerance not only results in autoreactive T cells but also autoreactive B cells and their migration to pancreas and pancreatic lymph nodes. B cells can present autoantigens to islet specific $CD4^+$ and $CD8^+$ effector T cells, which in turn causes destruction of pancreatic β-cells. B cells are necessary for the development of autoimmune diabetes in NOD mice in particular autoantibody production and B cell depletion prevents development of the disease [74–76]. In newly diagnosed individuals with T1DM, B cell depletion using anti-CD20 monoclonal antibody rituximab showed initial preservation of β-cell function and the need for exogenous insulin was reduced for up to 1 year post treatment. However, following a two-year follow up period, initial improvements in C-peptide (a marker of beta cell insulin secretion/function) were diminished and the clinical trial was terminated [77, 78]. Nonetheless, despite disappointing therapeutic results, B cell importance in T1DM progression is well appreciated and several improvements to the B cell depletion therapeutic approaches have since been proposed [79].

In murine models of antibody mediated autoimmune disorders such as systemic lupus erythematosus (SLE) and rheumatoid arthritis (RA) the absence of RAGE tended to cause reduction in germinal center B cells along with decreased anti-dsDNA autoantibody titers and increases in follicular B cells [80]. Germinal centers play important role in B cell maturation, clonal expansion, and class-switching as well an antibody production? [81]. Though these modest changes in B cells in RAGE−/− animals may not be sufficient to prevent autoimmunity, they are indicative that RAGE signaling is an important contributor to these processes [80]. Another study explored the effects of RAGE/HMGB1 interactions on activation of autoreactive B cells. In that particular study, it was concluded that HMGB1 binding promotes activation of autoreactive B cells through TLR9 rather than RAGE [82].

Macrophages act alongside DCs for antigen presentation [83, 84]. Though human pancreatic islets have macrophages present, it is unclear whether there are changes between resident and infiltrating populations in T1DM [85]. The phenotype of macrophages can in general be divided into M1/pro-inflammatory cytotoxic and M2/anti-inflammatory, alternatively activated cells. However, the local microenvironment plays important role in the process of monocyte to macrophage differentiation. Human macrophages represent less than half of the APC population seen in T1DM and form a mixture of both M1 and M2 phenotypes [86]. In NOD mice APCs are represented almost entirely by macrophages and they have an intricate relationship with lymphocytes, although this may be due to limitations in assessing APC phenotypes in mice. Some studied observed that the absence of resident macrophages arrested T1DM development in NOD mice [87]. Depletion of islet-resident APCs caused complete elimination of pancreatic lymphocyte infiltration which was restored upon re-introduction of DCs and macrophages [88, 89]. Following the depletion of macrophages, lymphocytes are also unable to initiate T1DM in the NOD-SCID adoptive transfer mouse model [90].

Monocytes, macrophages as well as RAGE- ligands axis are known players in the diabetic vascular complications. RAGE expression is associated with activation of both monocytes and macrophages which has been well explored in diabetes complications such as atherosclerosis [91, 92] and kidney disease [93–95]. Furthermore hypoxic environments can enhance monocyte adhesion and chemotaxis as well as induction of macrophage proinflammatory phenotype mediated by RAGE activity [96]. Furthermore, HMGB1 signaling through RAGE promotes secretion of IL-10 by M2 macrophages is of particular significance in the hypoxic environments of certain metastatic tumors [97]. In the individuals with T1DM suffering from retinopathy and nephropathy, the mRNA RAGE expression in monocytes was significantly reduced compared to controls. Upon exposure of monocyte cultures to glyceraldehyde-derived AGEs both mRNA and protein levels of RAGE were decreased [98]. This was a surprising result considering that upregulation of RAGE is associated with proinflammatory processes. Another study highlighted increased RAGE expression and activation in the M2 macrophages necessary for tumor vascularization and invasion [99]. Despite significant gaps in our knowledge there is unequivocal evidence that upregulation of RAGE upon binding its ligands leads to activation of proinflammatory cascades which likely impart detrimental effects in autoimmunity.

RAGE is an immunoglobulin type receptor comprised of a ligand binding V-type domain, C1 and C2 domains, transmembrane and cytoplasmic domains. C-truncated soluble RAGE can result from proteolytic cleavage or endogenous splicing of the RAGE gene, *AGER*. RAGE as a pattern recognition receptor can bind a wide range of ligands including AGEs, HMGB1, S100 calgranulins. Commonly, upon ligation downstream signaling via Diaphenous-1 and JAK-STAT pathways ROS production and NF-κB activation occurs stimulating inflammatory processes [11]. In T1DM, RAGE is postulated as important for various mechanisms of central and peripheral tolerance which fail to suppress the escape and activation of autoreactive T cells. This occurs in the presence of already dampened regulatory mechanisms where both function and number of Tregs are reduced This leads to further activation and expansion of pathogenic islet specific T cells aided by antigen presentation by DCs. $CD8^+$ T cells migrate to pancreatic islets facilitating immune destruction and, pancreatic β-cell death and further formation and release of diabetogenic antigens. Pancreatic β-cells may also act as APCs by presenting MHC class I molecules and engaging with cytotoxic $CD8^+$ T cells [100]. Inflamed and apoptotic β-cells can also release molecules that act as RAGE ligands further perpetuating the inflammatory cascade by maturation and activation of DCs and macrophages leading to pancreatic injury. NK cells can directly engage with β-cells through NKG2D-RAE1 interaction known to cause pancreatic β-cells death [101]. Furthermore, NK cells can release large quantities of cytotoxic granules and HMGB1 that may directly interact with RAGE expressed on β-cells [53]. Similar to NK cells, neutrophils can also release RAGE ligands and interact with other RAGE expressing cells including pancreatic β-cells [61].

3.5 RAGE, diabetes and COVID-19

The severe acute respiratory syndrome coronavirus (SARS-CoV)-2 pandemic has affected millions of people globally in recent years [102]. Life threatening severe lung inflammation and infections of cardiovascular and central nervous systems as well as the gastrointestinal tract have been reported during SARS-CoV-2 infection [103].

Emerging evidence suggests that individuals with diabetes have poorer prognosis when infected with SARS-CoV-2. Given that the greatest basal expression of RAGE in the body is within the lungs, it is highly likely that RAGE mediated immune processes contribute to these poorer outcomes. In hyperglycemia priming of neutrophils may result in the uncontrolled formation of NETs and release of HMGB1 further increasing vascular permeability. RAGE levels were elevated in both rodent models and humans with acute lung injury and associated with inflammasome formation and IL-1β release [104–106] Whilst most recent SARS-CoV-2 studies focused on comorbidities associated with type 2 diabetes, a common theme of imbalanced immune responses, upregulation of RAGE ligands such as HMGB1 and S100 proteins, insulin resistance, hyperglycemia and release of pro-inflammatory cytokines is seen [107, 108]. Furthermore, several studies reported a significant increase in diabetic ketoacidosis (DKA) in recent onset T1DM during the pandemic [109–111]. These findings have important implications on future treatment and management of patients with dysglycaemia and severe respiratory conditions.

4. Conclusions

The robust evidence pointing towards involvement of RAGE and its ligands in inflammation and autoimmunity paves a new pathway towards understanding the pathophysiology of T1DM. Valuable lessons can also be learned about approaches to undertake when designing new therapies to target this axis from previous findings. Further understanding of the role of greater RAGE expression on immune cells and pancreatic islets during T1DM pathogenesis is required and is likely to be multifaceted given the myriad of inflammatory diseases which involve RAGE mediated processes. T1DM is incredibly complex and heterogeneous disorder, and it is unlikely for a 'silver bullet' therapy to emerge. This highlights the importance of exploring alternative mechanistic pathways for therapy which have not been previously considered. Indeed, it is likely that the best approach to T1DM may be combination therapies which are targeted towards various aspects of disease and provide greater coverage of the vast immune dysfunction which may be present.

Acknowledgements

JMF is supported by a Leadership Fellowship from the National Health and Medical Research Council of Australia. Her team's work is also supported by an Innovation Grant from the Juvenile Diabetes Research Foundation, the Mater Foundation and the Australian Centre for Accelerating Diabetes Innovations awarded from the Medical Research Future Fund of Australia.

Conflict of interest

The authors declare no conflict of interest.

Author details

Irina Buckle[1,2] and Josephine M. Forbes[1,2,3*]

1 Glycation and Diabetes, Mater Research Institute – The University of Queensland, Translational Research Institute, Brisbane, Australia

2 Faculty of Medicine, The University of Queensland, St. Lucia, Australia

3 Department of Medicine, The University of Melbourne, Austin Health, Heidelberg, Australia

*Address all correspondence to: josephine.forbes@mater.uq.edu.au

References

[1] Atkinson MA, Leiter EH. The NOD mouse model of type 1 diabetes: as good as it gets? Nature Medicine. 1999;**5**(6):601-604

[2] Bonifacio E et al. International workshop on lessons from animal models for human type 1 diabetes: Identification of insulin but not glutamic acid decarboxylase or IA-2 as specific autoantigens of humoral autoimmunity in nonobese diabetic mice. Diabetes. 2001;**50**(11):2451-2458

[3] Yin L et al. Humanized mouse model: A review on preclinical applications for cancer immunotherapy. American Journal of Cancer Research. 2020;**10**(12):4568-4584

[4] Viehmann Milam AA et al. A humanized mouse model of autoimmune insulitis. Diabetes. 2014;**63**(5):1712-1724

[5] Luce S et al. Humanized mouse model to study type 1 diabetes. Diabetes. 2018;**67**(9):1816-1829

[6] Luce S et al. A humanized mouse strain that develops spontaneously immune-mediated diabetes. Frontiers in Immunology. 2021;**12**:748-679

[7] Tripodis N et al. Physical map of human 6p21.2-6p21.3: Region flanking the centromeric end of the major histocompatibility complex. Genome Research. 1998;**8**(6):631-643

[8] Burton PR et al. Genome-wide association study of 14,000 cases of seven common diseases and 3,000 shared controls. Nature. 2007;**447**(7145):661-678

[9] Forbes JM et al. Receptor for advanced glycation end-products (RAGE) provides a link between genetic susceptibility and environmental factors in type 1 diabetes. Diabetologia. 2011;**54**(5):1032-1042

[10] Gao P et al. Genetic and molecular basis of QTL of diabetes in mouse: Genes and polymorphisms. Current Genomics. 2008;**9**(5):324-337

[11] Le Bagge S et al. Targeting the receptor for advanced glycation end products (RAGE) in type 1 diabetes. Medicinal Research Reviews. 2020;**40**(4):1200-1219

[12] Chiappalupi S et al. Hyperactivated RAGE in comorbidities as a risk factor for severe COVID-19-the role of RAGE-RAS crosstalk. Biomolecules. 2021;**11**(6):876

[13] Yamamoto Y et al. Short-chain aldehyde-derived ligands for RAGE and their actions on endothelial cells. Diabetes Research and Clinical Practice. 2007;**77**(Suppl. 1):S30-S40

[14] Forbes JM et al. Role of advanced glycation end products in diabetic nephropathy. Journal of the American Society of Nephrology. 2003;**14**(suppl. 3): S254-S258

[15] de Courten B et al. Diet low in advanced glycation end products increases insulin sensitivity in healthy overweight individuals: A double-blind, randomized, crossover trial. The American Journal of Clinical Nutrition. 2016;**103**(6):1426-1433

[16] Borg DJ et al. Perinatal exposure to high dietary advanced glycation end products in transgenic NOD8.3 mice leads to pancreatic beta cell dysfunction. Islets. 2018;**10**(1):10-24

[17] Ramasamy R, Yan SF, Schmidt AM. Receptor for AGE (RAGE): Signaling

mechanisms in the pathogenesis of diabetes and its complications. Annals of the New York Academy of Sciences. 2011;**1243**:88-102

[18] Forbes JM et al. Advanced glycation end products as predictors of renal function in youth with type 1 diabetes. Scientific Reports. 2021;**11**(1):9422

[19] Diallo AM et al. Association between the tissue and circulating advanced glycation end-products and the micro- and macrovascular complications in type 1 diabetes: The DIABAGE study. Diabetes Therapy. 2022;**13**(8):1531-1546

[20] Beyan H et al. Glycotoxin and autoantibodies are additive environmentally determined predictors of type 1 diabetes: A twin and population study. Diabetes. 2012;**61**(5):1192-1198

[21] Coughlan MT et al. Advanced glycation end products are direct modulators of β-cell function. Diabetes. 2011;**60**(10):2523-2532

[22] Yang H, Wang H, Andersson U. Targeting inflammation driven by HMGB1. Frontiers in Immunology. 2020;**11**:484

[23] Zhang J et al. Extracellular HMGB1 exacerbates autoimmune progression and recurrence of type 1 diabetes by impairing regulatory T cell stability. Diabetologia. 2020;**63**(5):987-1001

[24] Han J et al. Extracellular high-mobility group box 1 acts as an innate immune mediator to enhance autoimmune progression and diabetes onset in NOD mice. Diabetes. 2008;**57**(8):2118-2127

[25] Marjanac I, Lovrić R, Barbić J. Serum levels of the high-mobility group box 1 protein (HMGB1) in children with type 1 diabetes mellitus: Case-control study. Central European Journal of Immunology. 2019;**44**(1):33-37

[26] Yao D, Brownlee M. Hyperglycemia-induced reactive oxygen species increase expression of the receptor for advanced glycation end products (RAGE) and RAGE ligands. Diabetes. 2009;**59**(1):249-255

[27] Donato R et al. Functions of S100 proteins. Current Molecular Medicine. 2013;**13**(1):24-57

[28] Huang M et al. S100A9 regulates MDSCs-mediated immune suppression via the RAGE and TLR4 signaling pathways in colorectal carcinoma. Frontiers in Immunology. 2019;**10**:2243

[29] Kierdorf K, Fritz G. RAGE regulation and signaling in inflammation and beyond. Journal of Leukocyte Biology. 2013;**94**(1):55-68

[30] Yan SF et al. Tempering the wrath of RAGE: An emerging therapeutic strategy against diabetic complications, neurodegeneration, and inflammation. Annals of Medicine. 2009;**41**(6):408-422

[31] Walker LS, von Herrath M. CD4 T cell differentiation in type 1 diabetes. Clinical and Experimental Immunology. 2016;**183**(1):16-29

[32] Phillips JM et al. Type 1 diabetes development requires both CD4+ and CD8+ T cells and can be reversed by non-depleting antibodies targeting both T cell populations. The review of diabetic studies : RDS. 2009;**6**(2):97-103

[33] Willcox A et al. Analysis of islet inflammation in human type 1 diabetes. Clinical and Experimental Immunology. 2009;**155**(2):173-181

[34] James CR et al. Reduced interleukin-2 responsiveness impairs the

ability of T cells to compete for IL-2 in nonobese diabetic mice. Immunology and Cell Biology. 2016;**94**(5):509-519

[35] Marfil-Garza BA et al. Progress in translational regulatory T cell therapies for type 1 diabetes and islet transplantation. Endocrine Reviews. 2020;**42**(2):198-218

[36] Sims EK et al. Teplizumab improves and stabilizes beta cell function in antibody-positive high-risk individuals. Science Translational Medicine. 2021;**13**(583):eabc8980

[37] Volfson-Sedletsky V et al. Emerging therapeutic strategies to restore regulatory T cell control of islet autoimmunity in type 1 diabetes. Frontiers in Immunology. 2021;**12**:635767

[38] Durning SP et al. The receptor for advanced glycation Endproducts drives T cell survival and inflammation in type 1 diabetes mellitus. The Journal of Immunology. 2016;**197**(8):3076-3085

[39] Akirav EM et al. RAGE expression in human T cells: A link between environmental factors and adaptive immune responses. PLoS One. 2012;7(4):e34698

[40] Salonen KM et al. A drop in the circulating concentrations of soluble receptor for advanced glycation end products is associated with seroconversion to autoantibody positivity but not with subsequent progression to clinical disease in children en route to type 1 diabetes. Diabetes/Metabolism Research and Reviews. 2017;**33**(4):e2872

[41] Moser B et al. Receptor for advanced glycation end products expression on T cells contributes to antigen-specific cellular expansion in vivo. Journal of Immunology. 2007;**179**(12):8051-8058

[42] Wittkowski H et al. Acute Kawasaki disease is associated with reverse regulation of soluble receptor for advance glycation end products and its proinflammatory ligand S100A12. Arthritis and Rheumatism. 2007;**56**(12):4174-4181

[43] Krishnamurthy B et al. Autoimmunity to both proinsulin and IGRP is required for diabetes in nonobese diabetic 8.3 TCR transgenic mice. Journal of Immunology. 2008;**180**(7):4458-4464

[44] Peppa M et al. Fetal or neonatal low-Glycotoxin environment prevents autoimmune diabetes in NOD mice. Diabetes. 2003;**52**(6):1441-1448

[45] Leung SS et al. Soluble RAGE prevents type 1 diabetes expanding functional regulatory T cells. Diabetes. 2022;**71**(9):1994-2008

[46] Manfredi AA et al. Maturing dendritic cells depend on RAGE for in vivo homing to lymph nodes. Journal of Immunology. 2008;**180**(4):2270-2275

[47] Buckle I, Guillerey C. Inhibitory receptors and immune checkpoints regulating natural killer cell responses to cancer. Cancers. 2021;**13**(17):4263

[48] Pallmer K et al. NK cells negatively regulate CD8 T cells via natural cytotoxicity receptor (NCR) 1 during LCMV infection. PLoS Pathogens. 2019;**15**(4):e1007725

[49] Wilson RG et al. Natural killer cells in insulin dependent diabetes mellitus. British Medical Journal (Clinical Research Ed.). 1986;**293**(6541):244-244

[50] Negishi K et al. Natural killer cell and islet killer cell activities in type 1 (insulin-dependent) diabetes. Diabetologia. 1986;**29**(6):352-357

[51] Negishi K et al. Natural killer cell and islet killer cell activities in human type 1 diabetes. Experimental and Clinical Endocrinology. 1987;**89**(3):345-353

[52] Qin H et al. Natural killer cells from children with type 1 diabetes have defects in NKG2D-dependent function and signaling. Diabetes. 2011;**60**(3):857-866

[53] Cerwenka A et al. HMGB1: The metabolic weapon in the arsenal of NK cells. Molecular & Cellular Oncology. 2016;**3**(4):e1175538

[54] Leung SS, Forbes JM, Borg DJ. Receptor for advanced glycation end products (RAGE) in type 1 diabetes pathogenesis. Current Diabetes Reports. 2016;**16**(10):100

[55] Narumi K et al. Proinflammatory proteins S100A8/S100A9 activate NK cells via interaction with RAGE. Journal of Immunology. 2015;**194**(11):5539-5548

[56] Diana J et al. Crosstalk between neutrophils, B-1a cells and plasmacytoid dendritic cells initiates autoimmune diabetes. Nature Medicine. 2013;**19**(1):65-73

[57] Naegele M et al. Neutrophils in multiple sclerosis are characterized by a primed phenotype. Journal of Neuroimmunology. 2012;**242**(1-2):60-71

[58] Villanueva E et al. Netting neutrophils induce endothelial damage, infiltrate tissues, and expose immunostimulatory molecules in systemic lupus erythematosus. Journal of Immunology. 2011;**187**(1):538-552

[59] Diana J, Lehuen A. Macrophages and β-cells are responsible for CXCR2-mediated neutrophil infiltration of the pancreas during autoimmune diabetes. EMBO Molecular Medicine. 2014;**6**(8):1090-1104

[60] Vecchio F et al. Abnormal neutrophil signature in the blood and pancreas of presymptomatic and symptomatic type 1 diabetes. JCI. Insight. 2018;**3**(18):e122146

[61] Collison KS et al. RAGE-mediated neutrophil dysfunction is evoked by advanced glycation end products (AGEs). Journal of Leukocyte Biology. 2002;**71**(3):433-444

[62] Kraakman MJ et al. Neutrophil-derived S100 calcium-binding proteins A8/A9 promote reticulated thrombocytosis and atherogenesis in diabetes. The Journal of Clinical Investigation. 2017;**127**(6):2133-2147

[63] Creusot RJ, Postigo-Fernandez J, Teteloshvili N. Altered function of antigen-presenting cells in type 1 diabetes: A challenge for antigen-specific immunotherapy? Diabetes. 2018;**67**(8):1481-1494

[64] Loaiza Naranjo JD et al. A question of tolerance-antigen-specific immunotherapy for type 1 diabetes. Current Diabetes Reports. 2020;**20**(12):70

[65] Unanue ER, Ferris ST, Carrero JA. The role of islet antigen presenting cells and the presentation of insulin in the initiation of autoimmune diabetes in the NOD mouse. Immunological Reviews. 2016;**272**(1):183-201

[66] Lehuen A et al. Immune cell crosstalk in type 1 diabetes. Nature Reviews Immunology. 2010;**10**(7):501-513

[67] Sandor AM, Jacobelli J, Friedman RS. Immune cell trafficking to the islets during type 1 diabetes. Clinical and Experimental Immunology. 2019;**198**(3):314-325

[68] Khan FU et al. Dendritic cells and their immunotherapeutic potential for

treating type 1 diabetes. International Journal of Molecular Sciences. 2022;**23**(9):4885

[69] Ríos-Ríos WJ, Sosa-Luis SA, Torres-Aguilar H. Current advances in using tolerogenic dendritic cells as a therapeutic alternative in the treatment of type 1 diabetes. World Journal of Diabetes. 2021;**12**(5):603-615

[70] Lu H et al. High glucose induces upregulation of scavenger receptors and promotes maturation of dendritic cells. Cardiovascular Diabetology. 2013;**12**(1):80

[71] Buttari B et al. Advanced glycation end products of human β2 glycoprotein I modulate the maturation and function of DCs. Blood. 2011;**117**(23):6152-6161

[72] Ge J et al. Advanced glycosylation end products might promote atherosclerosis through inducing the immune maturation of dendritic cells. Arteriosclerosis, Thrombosis, and Vascular Biology. 2005;**25**(10):2157-2163

[73] Buttari B et al. Resveratrol prevents dendritic cell maturation in response to advanced glycation end products. Oxidative Medicine and Cellular Longevity. 2013;**2013**:574029

[74] Akashi T et al. Direct evidence for the contribution of B cells to the progression of insulitis and the development of diabetes in non-obese diabetic mice. International Immunology. 1997;**9**(8):1159-1164

[75] Xiu Y et al. B lymphocyte depletion by CD20 monoclonal antibody prevents diabetes in nonobese diabetic mice despite isotype-specific differences in fc gamma R effector functions. Journal of Immunology. 2008;**180**(5):2863-2875

[76] Serreze DV et al. B lymphocytes are critical antigen-presenting cells for the initiation of T cell-mediated autoimmune diabetes in nonobese diabetic mice. Journal of Immunology. 1998;**161**(8):3912-3918

[77] Pescovitz MD et al. Rituximab, B-lymphocyte depletion, and preservation of beta-cell function. The New England Journal of Medicine. 2009;**361**(22):2143-2152

[78] Pescovitz MD et al. B-lymphocyte depletion with rituximab and β-cell function: Two-year results. Diabetes Care. 2014;**37**(2):453-459

[79] Hamad AR et al. B cell-targeted immunotherapy for type 1 diabetes: What can make it work? Discovery Medicine. 2016;**21**(115):213-219

[80] Eichhorst A et al. Relevance of receptor for advanced glycation end products (RAGE) in murine antibody-mediated autoimmune diseases. International Journal of Molecular Sciences. 2019;**20**(13):3234

[81] Chevalier N et al. The role of follicular helper T cell molecules and environmental influences in autoantibody production and progression to inflammatory arthritis in mice. Arthritis & Rhematology. 2016;**68**(4):1026-1038

[82] Avalos AM et al. RAGE-independent autoreactive B cell activation in response to chromatin and HMGB1/DNA immune complexes. Autoimmunity. 2010;**43**(1):103-110

[83] Sica A, Mantovani A. Macrophage plasticity and polarization: in vivo veritas. The Journal of Clinical Investigation. 2012;**122**(3):787-795

[84] Mills CD et al. M-1/M-2 macrophages and the Th1/Th2 paradigm. The Journal of Immunology. 2000;**164**(12):6166-6173

[85] Zirpel H, Roep BO. Islet-resident dendritic cells and macrophages in type 1 diabetes: In search of Bigfoot's print. Frontiers in Endocrinology. Lausanne. 2021;**12**:666795

[86] Wang YJ et al. Multiplexed In situ imaging mass cytometry analysis of the human endocrine pancreas and immune system in type 1 diabetes. Cell Metabolism. 2019;**29**(3):769-783.e4

[87] Hutchings P et al. Transfer of diabetes in mice prevented by blockade of adhesion-promoting receptor on macrophages. Nature. 1990;**348**(6302):639-642

[88] Nikolic T, Roep BO. Regulatory multitasking of tolerogenic dendritic cells - lessons taken from vitamin d3-treated tolerogenic dendritic cells. Frontiers in Immunology. 2013;**4**:113

[89] Nikolic T et al. Dendritic cells and macrophages are essential for the retention of lymphocytes in (peri)-insulitis of the nonobese diabetic mouse: A phagocyte depletion study. Laboratory Investigation. 2005;**85**(4):487-501

[90] Jun HS et al. Absolute requirement of macrophages for the development and activation of beta-cell cytotoxic CD8+ T-cells in T-cell receptor transgenic NOD mice. Diabetes. 1999;**48**(1):34-42

[91] Soro-Paavonen A et al. Receptor for advanced glycation end products (RAGE) deficiency attenuates the development of atherosclerosis in diabetes. Diabetes. 2008;**57**(9):2461-2469

[92] Schmidt AM et al. The multiligand receptor RAGE as a progression factor amplifying immune and inflammatory responses. The Journal of Clinical Investigation. 2001;**108**(7):949-955

[93] Kanter JE, Hsu CC, Bornfeldt KE. Monocytes and macrophages as protagonists in vascular complications of diabetes. Frontiers in Cardiovascular Medicine. 2020;**7**:10

[94] Kawakami R et al. S100A9-RAGE Axis accelerates formation of macrophage-mediated extracellular vesicle microcalcification in diabetes mellitus. Arteriosclerosis, Thrombosis, and Vascular Biology. 2020;**40**(8):1838-1853

[95] Coughlan MT et al. RAGE-induced cytosolic ROS promote mitochondrial superoxide generation in diabetes. Journal of the American Society of Nephrology. 2009;**20**(4):742-752

[96] Zhou J et al. Intermittent hypoxia enhances THP-1 monocyte adhesion and chemotaxis and promotes M1 macrophage polarization via RAGE. BioMed Research International. 2018;**2018**:1650456

[97] Huber R et al. Tumour hypoxia promotes melanoma growth and metastasis via high mobility group Box-1 and M2-like macrophages. Scientific Reports. 2016;**6**(1):29914

[98] Miura J et al. AGE down-regulation of monocyte RAGE expression and its association with diabetic complications in type 1 diabetes. Journal of Diabetes and its Complications. 2004;**18**(1):53-59

[99] Rojas A et al. HMGB1 enhances the protumoral activities of M2 macrophages by a RAGE-dependent mechanism. Tumour Biology. 2016;**37**(3):3321-3329

[100] Hamilton-Williams EE et al. Beta cell MHC class I is a late requirement for diabetes. Proceedings of the National Academy of Sciences of the United States of America. 2003;**100**(11):6688-6693

[101] Markiewicz MA et al. RAE1ε ligand expressed on pancreatic islets recruits NKG2D receptor-expressing cytotoxic T cells independent of T cell receptor recognition. Immunity. 2012;**36**(1):132-141

[102] Chen Y, Liu Q, Guo D. Emerging coronaviruses: Genome structure, replication, and pathogenesis. Journal of Medical Virology. 2020;**92**(4):418-423

[103] Rojas A et al. Advanced-glycation end-products axis: A contributor to the risk of severe illness from COVID-19 in diabetes patients. World Journal of Diabetes. 2021;**12**(5):590-602

[104] Kim EJ et al. HMGB1 increases IL-1β production in vascular smooth muscle cells via NLRP3 Inflammasome. Frontiers in Physiology. 2018;**9**:313

[105] De Francesco EM, Vella V, Belfiore A. COVID-19 and diabetes: The importance of controlling RAGE. Frontiers in Endocrinology. 2020;**11**:526

[106] Uchida T et al. Receptor for advanced glycation end-products is a marker of type I cell injury in acute lung injury. American Journal of Respiratory and Critical Care Medicine. 2006;**173**(9):1008-1015

[107] Egana-Gorrono L et al. Receptor for advanced glycation end products (RAGE) and mechanisms and therapeutic opportunities in diabetes and cardiovascular disease: Insights from human subjects and animal models. Frontiers in Cardiovascular Medicine. 2020;**7**:37

[108] Sandooja R, Vura N, Morocco M. Heightened ACE activity and unfavorable consequences in COVID-19 diabetic subjects. International Journal of Endocrinology. 2020;**2020**:7847526

[109] Beliard K et al. Increased DKA at presentation among newly diagnosed type 1 diabetes patients with or without COVID-19: Data from a multi-site surveillance registry. Journal of Diabetes. 2021;**13**(3):270-272

[110] Gottesman BL et al. Incidence of new-onset type 1 diabetes among US children during the COVID-19 global pandemic. JAMA Pediatrics. 2022;**176**(4):414-415

[111] Dżygało K et al. Increased frequency of severe diabetic ketoacidosis at type 1 diabetes onset among children during COVID-19 pandemic lockdown: An observational cohort study. Pediatric Endocrinology Diabetes and Metabolism. 2020;**26**(4):167-175